Listen To What "Dr. Shoe
About *Desperation Medicine*

—Diane Stephenson, 53, Homemaker, Ohio: "I spent 10 years looking for a cure for my Chronic Lyme Disease, and I must have consulted 50 doctors. Nothing helped ...until I found Ritchie Shoemaker, who told me what was wrong with me, and how to fix it. He has restored my world to me!"

—Marie Moore, 51, Financial Administrator, New Jersey: "I feel like Dr. Shoemaker has given my brain back to me. I struggled along for years, while a dozen doctors told me my problem was 'depression.' Wrong. I was suffering from Lyme and Babesia –two chronic illnesses caused by bacterial toxins. Dr. Shoemaker helped defeat both of them!"

—David Jasinski, 51, Salesman, New Jersey: "I spent five years working in a sick building, and it nearly killed me. My hands and feet were numb all day long, and my nerves were shot. Luckily for me, Dr. Shoemaker finally diagnosed my Sick Building Syndrome ...and then treated it. My symptoms have evaporated, and I sleep like a baby at night!"

The stories of the patients in this book are real ...and the science behind them is rock-solid. The research was performed by an award-winning investigator with impeccable credentials and the scientific publications to back them up.

FOR 10 MILLION AMERICANS AND THEIR FAMILIES...

This book will be the ray of hope that leads toward a healthier, more active life, as patients with environmentally acquired illnesses discover that they can get well again, thanks to: *Desperation Medicine!*

Desperation Medicine

The Inside Story of How An American Doctor Discovered A Threatening
New Family of "Environmental Diseases"...And How To Stop Them.

Ritchie C. Shoemaker, M.D.

GATEWAY PRESS, INC.
Baltimore, MD   2001

Front cover photo:
"Hazmat Investigation of Nursery Site Owned by Frank Fuzzell"
Andrew Smith, *Daily Commercial*, Leesburg, Florida, 2/03/00.

Please direct all correspondence and book orders to:
Ritchie C. Shoemaker
1604 Market St.
Pocomoke City, MD 21851

Library of Congress Control Number 00-136080
ISBN 0-9665535-1-9

Cover design by Janet Kratfel

Published for the author by
Gateway Press, Inc.
1001 N. Calvert Street
Baltimore, MD 21202

Printed in the United States of America

Dedication

With thanks to Ken Hudnell, Ph.D., Neurotoxicology
Division, U.S. Environmental Protection Agency, National
Health and Environmental Effects Research Lab

*More than a neurotoxicology research collaborator, he is a
tempering force who firmly but kindly has kept the leaps
of insight anchored in careful scientific thought.*

Also to Donald Anderson, Ph.D., Senior Scientist,
Woods Hole Oceanographic Institution

His keen insights showed Pfiesteria *to be the model
of a disease process that was larger than anyone
could have imagined.*

Also to Frank Fuzzell, Nurseryman, Leesburg, Florida

*Not even Penelope has waited so long for the
truth to emerge.*

And in memory . . . of George Demas, Ph.D., Soil
Scientist, United States Department of Agriculture

*During his life, he gave us a new definition of soils.
After his death from Pfiesteria-related human illness,
he gave us proof of how chronic, neurotoxin-mediated
illnesses can hurt us.*

Table of Contents

ix   Foreword

xv   Preface

xxiii   Special Thanks

xxv   How to Read This Book

Chapter 1   Everything That Lives
Reflection   Is Food for Something Else
page 1

Chapter 2   Showdown.
Event   Confrontation with a Toxic Invader.
page 9

Chapter 3   Clear As Mud.
Reflection   The Public Health Coverup Continues.
page 33

Chapter 4   A Mysterious Illness
Event
page 45

Chapter 5   Brilliant, Just Brilliant.
Reflection   Sometimes the Best Ideas
page 69   Are the Simplest Ones.

Chapter 6   "Contrast Sensitivity."
Reflection   A Key to Diagnosing Chronic,
page 79   Neurotoxin-Medicated Illnesses.

Chapter 7   Ciguatera. Anatomy of
   Event   A Toxic Nightmare.
   page 87

Chapter 8   Even Ph.D.s Get Sick . . .
  Reflection   But Why Wouldn't They?
   page 111

Chapter 9   Chronicles from
   Event   A Poisoned Landscape
   page 121

Chapter 10   The Appearance
  Reflection   Of Good Science
   page 155

Chapter 11   The Monster in the Lake
   Event
   page 167

Chatper 12   "Fad Medicines"
  Reflection   For America's "Fad Diseases"
   page 195

Chapter 13   Healing Chronic Lyme Disease
   Event
   page 203

Chapter 14   Lion Fish . . . or *Lyme* Fish?
  Reflection   An Essay on Comparative Toxicology.
   page 243

Chapter 15   Lessons from Solving
   Event   The Herxheimer
   page 249

Chapter 16   Jill: 100 Weeks in
Reflection   The Medical Wilderness.
page 277

Chapter 17   Update from Diane Stephenson,
Reflection   March 14, 2000
page 285

Chapter 18   Escape from Naushon Island
Reflection
page 293

Chapter 19   Famous Falsehoods
Reflection
page 299

Chapter 20   Getting behind
Event   "Sick Building Syndrome"
page 305

Chapter 21   How Sick Is Your Building . . .
Reflection   And What Can You Do about It?
page 327

Chapter 22   A New FACT for
Reflection   Occupational Medicine
page 337

Chapter 23   Surviving Chronic Fatigue Syndrome
Event
page 343

Chapter 24   Toxins, Chronic Soft Tissue
Reflection   Injury And Fibromyalgia
page 361

Chapter 25   Lenny Wein. A Survivor—Thanks to
Reflection   Daily Cholestyramine—Was He a Victim
page 373   Of Genetic, Endogenous Neurotoxins?

Chapter 26   Getting behind the CDC
Reflection
page 379

Chapter 27   Why Johnny Can't Read
Reflection
page 395

Chapter 28   Even Ph.D.s Die.
Event   Making the Ultimate
page 413   Sacrifice for Research.

Chapter 29   Struggling Towards the Light
Reflection
page 431

Appendix   Cholestyramine Recipes
page 483

485   Index

495   About the Author

Foreword

Was it all a matter of destiny?

As a youthful physician, I never imagined that I might one day become the center of an environmental and public health controversy involving both the "medical establishment" and the elected politicians who rule our part of the world.

Far from it. In the beginning, fresh out of med school at Duke University, I had dreamed only of operating a rural primary care practice. And the National Health Service Corps (NHSC) had helped to make that dream a reality—by providing a medical school scholarship for students like me who agreed to serve in a rural or "under-served" area after graduation. I could hardly believe that the government was going to pay my way through a few years at Duke Medical School, in order to let me do what I already *wanted* to do!

The residency program I attended at Williamsport (Pa.) Hospital provided additional evidence for my long-held belief that the problems of rural health care delivery were the inevitable result of inadequately trained physicians who worked in inadequately staffed and equipped facilities . . . and who often did an inadequate job of outreach and chronic care management.

While fretting over these problems as a young resident, I also began to notice how such systemic flaws as the political manipulation of public health policy and the cynical acceptance of "situational ethics" among medical authorities provided stark evidence for the fact that those in power intended to *stay* in power, regardless of the cost. Creative change in health care delivery was acceptable only when it suited the agenda of those who controlled the levers of power.

Although I found these distortions of the medical ideal somewhat vexing as a young doctor, the truth is they didn't seem to matter much during my first few years at an NHSC clinic in Pocomoke, Md. After settling there in July of 1980, I found myself living in an idyllic setting—with fresh Chesapeake Bay crab meat and seafood always available "just down the street." Accompanied by my new bride JoAnn and later by our daughter Sally, I took immense delight in the wild birds of the Atlantic flyway—along with the great variety of plants that thrived in the marshes, wooded wetlands and swamps of this bucolic region.

I liked the geography of Pocomoke . . . but I liked my patients even better. These were the kind of people who looked you directly in the eye and told you exactly what they meant! And although I've always been careful to avoid "romanticizing" small town life, I loved the fact that a calloused hand and a firm handshake was "better than a contract" in Pocomoke.

As the years slowly passed, my family and I became active in numerous local initiatives, such as preserving and then rehabbing the historic Election House, which had been scheduled for demolition. We also took great pleasure in restoring the old Pennsylvania Railroad Train Station, transforming it into JoAnn's "Learning Station"—a comprehensive early-childhood learning center. Another rewarding civic project saw us helping to return the William Johnson House (circa 1814) to its original splendor as a 5,000-square-foot Federal townhouse in quaint Princess Anne, just north of Pocomoke.

Was the Lower Eastern Shore to be a paradise on earth, then? Of course not. Our little town had its share of flaws, like any other, and one of them became evident when a newly launched clam processing plant began to spoil our fresh air with the stink of putrefying waste water in 1988. The local elected officials did nothing, and the responsible state agencies also failed to act. Responding to their inertia, our quickly organized protest group —Public United, aka "Peeeeee-*uuuuuu!*"—went to war against the nasal offenders . . . only to discover that the "clam plant" was actually a cover for a marijuana-smuggling operation!

Later, when the Governor of Maryland took credit for the discovery and closed the plant, it became clear that the new stench had been caused by something more pungent than backed-up clam washings!

We left Princess Anne soon after a mysterious fire broke out in our wood-storage bin. Fortunately, no one was injured in the blaze . . . but we were happy to move on, closer to my office in Pocomoke, and to begin building a wetland paradise on 15 acres of fertile land that backed up to the Pocomoke River.

Assisted by some other gung-ho volunteers such as Bruce Nichols, Don Malloy, Jack Spurling and Jim Norton (the Nature Trail Committee), we raised funds in Pocomoke and built several wetland restoration ponds, wetland gardens and a mile-long nature trail through a cypress swamp, complete with a uniquely designed floating boardwalk.

Life was good . . . especially when Sally's fifth-grade ecology club planted 1,500 trees and wetland shrubs on a new wetland pond project that we built and then donated to the local YMCA in 1996.

But it wasn't long after that—less than a year, in fact—that the first reports of "sick fish" in the Pocomoke River would begin to make the local newspaper.

Those early reports sounded even more ominous, after we learned that local residents, including some of my patients and friends who handled the fish, were also falling ill. How could I have known that these early reports of "toxin-linked illness" were about to change my life forever?

How could I have known, in short, that I was about to discover a new *family* of illnesses—along with a brand-new disease mechanism in which the pathogen generates neurotoxins that "hide out" in body tissues, making us chronically ill?

And how did this new group of diseases emerge from the contemporary landscape to torment a growing number of "chonic illness" victims?

In large part, these new pathogens were the result of massive changes in our society. Booming populations . . . accelerating urbanization . . . increasing conversion of agricultural land (with it's natural "buffers" along watersheds and wetlands) into parking lots and apartment developments; these are obvious examples of some of the ecological factors at work in the new pathology. And what about all those recent advances in transportation, which have led to mass migrations of people and animals?

Let's face it: concentrated populations of animals means concentrated amounts of animal waste (nutrients)—along with the proliferation of growth-stimulating compounds, including antibiotics, heavy metals (especially copper) and food preservatives. Concentrated agriculture also provides an open invitation for invading pests, all of which are eager to feast on these ready food supplies. To stop them, we rely on increasing amounts of pesticides, which then trigger all sorts of unpredictable effects in the "microenvironment"—a vast and teeming world as unknown to us as the depths of outer space.

The problem is that nothing in nature stands still. Sure, our antibiotics and our pesticides do a good job of protecting us and our food supply from certain kinds of unhealthy microbes. But these threating bugs are not without some weapons of their own. For one thing, they know how to alter their own genetic makeup (even "trading genes" with one another, when required) in order to increasingly evade our high-tech, chemical artillery. Like a troupe of cunning fast-change artists, they can put on and take off their "biochemical costumes" in a few hours, sometimes with disastrous consequences for the humans who try to eradicate them.

The bottom line here is simple enough: instead of hypnotizing ourselves with the wonders of our own technology—even as we degrade our environment—we must learn to think about biology and living beings as part of a larger ecosystem. We need a broader scientific approach to the new illnesses we face . . . the same kind of approach that's required to be a good primary care physician. (Listen carefully to what the patient—or the *environment*—is telling you, then respond appropriately!)

If we hope to control the bizarre new form of algae now choking Florida's Lake Apopka, for example, we need to understand what these microorganisims really are, and how they relate to the predators and prey that inhabit their endlessly changing worlds.

The science behind *Desperation Medicine* may be complicated, but the message is simple: the illnesses described in this book are largely the result of the damage we've done to our ecosystem. As a result, the struggling patients you're about to meet are "markers" for both the diseases they carry *and* the illnesses that increasingly affect their environment.

As you might imagine, it took me several years to gradually assemble these insights, and to begin building the world's first-ever theory of "chronic, neurotoxin-mediated illness." The process of scientific discovery moves at a glacial pace most of the time, and for a few years nothing in my world seemed to change. My patients still surprised me occasionally by bringing their prize tomatoes to the office, and unpaid bills were often left that way until the "chicken check" arrived. Yet there was something new in the air . . . and my role as a "country physician" had already begun to change. I guess it started with the great outrage I felt, when I saw how local and state politicians by their actions and words, essentially had accused my friends of lying—merely because they had reported the dead fish and the growing human health epidemic along the once tranquil Pocomoke River.

In the end, it was the perpetually repeated litany of the politicians—"No one gets sick from the river!"—that awakened the smoldering determination of a former competitive wrestler. Thoroughly incensed by these double-talking politicos, I vowed with growing fervor: "They aren't going to get away with it!"

My motto became the same one that had gotten me through hundreds of high school matches: "Don't ever stop working to find a way to win honestly, and never give up!" Those wrestling matches had lasted only a few minutes, however . . . while the battle to uncover the truth about environmental disasters that trigger human illness seems to be going on forever!

Every single day, I'm reminded that there *is* a dark side to the politics of medicine and the politics of the environment—a side that few people (especially busy physicians) ever see, let alone understand. I learned quickly that the political climate often controls how we deal with medical problems.

During the past five years, I've absorbed many other new lessons (especially about biology) . . . along with some rather painful political lessons. That experience has changed my life-style, and I now spend more time writing and lecturing and less time listening to the birds of the forest call at dusk.

Still, what *hasn't* changed is my passion for medicine and for the life of the physician. Some of the most emotionally rewarding experiences I've ever had are woven into the pages that follow. The miracle of life—as exemplified by the miracle of restoration of health after 20 years of "brain fog, muscle aches and confusion" in a chronic Lyme patient—has remained the driving motivation in everything I do.

I want to share the excitement of healing with every reader who picks up this book. My chronic Lyme patients usually start to recover in 36 hours, and continue to improve rapidly after that, though healing may take several months. But my great hope is that this book will go on helping people to recover from chronic, neurotoxin-mediated illnesses far into the future.

—Ritchie Shoemaker, M.D.
Pocomoke, Md. 2000

Preface

A man cannot step into the same river twice, for it changes
with every step we take.
    —Heraclitus

As those ancient Greek philosophers so often reminded us,
the only constant in life is change.

It's also true, of course, that "adaptation" to change, along
with the survival of offspring, is as much a part of the cycle of
life as is the death that begins yet another revolution of life's
endlessly turning wheel.

No man (or woman) can hope to control the wheel. And yet
we do influence it. Is there any doubt that our human behavior
—including our life cycles and the residues of our chemical-age
society—has a powerful impact as a "force of natural selection"
on those species whose life cycles are influenced by our own?

The long record of human growth and expansion shows that
as we live, we create changes in habitat for other organisms
around us. Take the ordinary red cardinal, for example. As suburban "sprawl" has expanded everywhere in recent years, "backyard birds" like the cardinal have been migrating north in record
numbers in order to take advantage of their new, human-altered
habitat.

Even as the surge in human housing has allowed the cardinals
to flourish around suburban housing tracts, however, the habitat
for summer tanagers and bobolinks (denser woods and large,
open fields) has been noticeably shrinking—triggering a steep
decline in the ranks of those pleasing birds, along with several

other species that require lots of wide open space or heavy forest in order to thrive.

Let's face it: the "decline of natural habitat" is one of the prices we pay for civilization, and it requires that we balance our disappointment at losing many of the bobolinks and tanagers with our unexpected joy at discovering millions of new cardinals thriving in the northeastern United States. (The first nesting pair in Massachusetts was spotted in the early 1960s, by the way, which shows just how quickly the transformation has taken place.)

In similar fashion, the "advance of suburbia" has triggered recent accounts of cougar attacks in northern California and bear encounters along the northern reaches of Pennsylvania. These kinds of shifts in the ecosystem are predictable, and to be expected, of course. But many other changes are not so easy to forecast, including the recent alterations in reef ecosystems that are now being blamed for outbreaks of toxin-mediated "ciguatera" illness. Similar changes in estuaries are clearly associated with the emergence of *Pfiesteria*-related human illness, and there are now so many *Pfiesteria*-like species of toxin-dispersing micro-organisms that many have not even been named.

Another compelling example of the way in which altering our habitat causes public health problems is "Sick Building Syndrome" (SBS), which increasingly attacks our sealed office buildings and our climate-controlled homes, with their horticulturally perfect backyard plantings (a major new habitat, by the way, for rapidly proliferating Lyme disease and Babesiosis).

Who would have guessed that modern advances in building design, along with computer management of indoor environments, would accelerate the growth of fungal toxins responsible for surging SBS?

In the same paradoxical way, we failed to understand that the powerful pesticides which gave us "blemish-free" produce would eventually unleash a microbial monster on land, in lakes and in estuaries, because of the way they so dramatically affect the survival and adaptation genetics of microbial populations.

But the chronic neurotoxins that increasingly affect the industrialized world don't always emerge from organisms living in the external environment. They are being produced within our own bodies—as in Chronic Fatigue Syndrome and Chronic Soft Tissue Injury, both of which now appear to be caused by toxins spontaneously generated in human tissue via processes that we do not yet fully understand.

While some analysts are quick to blame "the stresses of society" for the widespread rampant fatigue, depression, and difficult-to-diagnose chronic pain in joints and nerves, my recent research strongly suggests that these growing health problems are linked to the spread of "endogenous" (inner) toxins generated by human nerve cells somehow gone awry.

Although medical science has by now accepted the reality of Chronic Fatigue Syndrome, the startling fact remains that most physicians today are required to diagnose it without the help of a definitive lab test—and without the hope of a cure.

For their patients, the millions who drag themselves daily through the debilitating exhaustion of this fast-spreading illness, *Desperation Medicine* offers a new source of hope: the promise contained in a brand-new diagnostic tool for pinpointing an ailment that cannot be detected in the bloodstream, along with a simple, inexpensive drug therapy (more on this later) that has already brought renewed health and restored vigor to thousands of patients.

Wouldn't it be wonderful if those suffering from Chronic Fatigue could change their lives, so that they didn't have to rest during four hours out of every waking eight? Can you imagine the creative opportunities for new life and high-intensity living that would follow—to say nothing of the time that would be saved for new productive activities?

And what about the endless pain and reduced physical mobility caused by Chronic Soft Tissue Injury, another increasingly common disorder in our high-tech society?

Our fast-moving civilization emphasizes safety in transportation, and it's good that high-velocity auto accidents aren't as lethal as they once were. And yet they leave behind patients who are permanently impaired. Like the millions who suffer from obscure-sounding complaints linked to other forms of neurotoxin-mediated illness, the victims of "chronic soft tissue injury" are desperately in need of information—and new forms of treatment—that will take the mystery out of their difficult-to-diagnose illnesses.

For ten million or more Americans who now suffer in silence from these supremely modern forms of disease, this book offers a new vision, and a new hope for cure. But there's no "magic" here, and you can be sure that all of the new diseases created by habitat-change in our new society are not catalogued in *Desperation Medicine*.

The diseases presented here *are* new to the medical field, however. And so are many of the techniques for diagnosing them. In this book, for example, you will learn about a helpful test called "Contrast Sensitivity" (CS)—a simple, inexpensive diagnostic tool that can measure the impact of biologically produced neurotoxins on brain function.

You'll also learn about a health-restoring chemical, cholestyramine, or "CSM," that binds biologically produced toxins. When combined with the CS test, CSM provides a powerful new weapon in the battle against Chronic Fatigue and other neurotoxin-mediated illnesses like it.

Like the medical science research described in *Desperation Medicine*, the patient-histories presented here are factually accurate, although some names have been changed to protect confidentiality. In addition, the often harrowing stories you're about to read—stories of grueling battles fought by patients against uncaring physicians, benefit-denying insurance companies and state regulatory agencies—are also completely authentic.

The descriptions of "stonewalling" by some of America's most respected regulatory agencies (including the Centers for Disease Control and Prevention, or CDC, and the National Institutes of Health, or NIH) are reported with careful attention to accuracy, as are the case histories documenting successful treatments of once hopeless patients who chose to follow my new protocols.

For me, *Pfiesteria* provided the first chapter in a story that has now begun to unfold in earnest, after opening a window on the sudden appearance of neurotoxin-mediated illnesses in the developed world.

This fascinating microorganism quickly became a laboratory subject in which it was possible to see how our civilization has created or expanded a "niche" for new, toxin-forming organisms. At the same time, the discovery of this new type of disease mechanism has been the greatest reward of my own 20 years as a Family Physician.

For more than two decades now, I've lived among the hard-working people of my rural community. I've treated their children in my office on Market Street, and I've sat applauding in the auditorium as those same kids played in the high school band. For a dedicated Family Physician who spends 70 hours a week caring for ordinary folks in a general practice, there can be no greater thrill than diagnosing and then treating illnesses that cause intense suffering—especially when the public health authorities continue to deny that they exist!

The themes of government denial, deceptive science, the "appearance of good science" and dissemination of misinformation to the public about environmentally acquired illnesses are repeated again and again in the stories that follow.

Most of these new diseases often have nothing to do with infection. All too often they are caused—"mediated," if you will —by small, low-molecular-weight toxins released by living organisms. These are not the giant molecules manufactured by bacteria that poison meat or cause tetanus or diphtheria. The morphology may be different, but the symptoms caused by the low-molecular-weight toxins are similar, and the effects these toxins have on nerve, muscle, lung, intestinal bile, brain and sinus are also similar to many of those caused by infectious agents.

It should also be pointed out that some of the solutions to the environmental problems that cause these illnesses are unacceptable. We can't cut down all the trees and shrubs, and then exterminate most of the deer population (as we did in the 1880s) in order to turn back the expansion of chronic Lyme disease.

We can't open our fixed and secured windows on snowy days to let in fresh air, and we can't just stamp our feet and expect the cylindrospermopsis blue-green algae and their toxins to disappear from the lakes of central Florida. But we should at least become *aware* of them, before they threaten the last of the region's beloved manatees, in the same way they are now killing the last few remaining alligators in Lake Griffin.

We can't wave a magic wand over the chemically altered soils that contribute to *Pfiesteria* blooms in submerged sediments and colonies of *Fusarium* fungus in Florida ornamental nurserylands.

What we *can* do, however, is to start opening our eyes about where these environmental problems come from. Instead of automatically accepting the pronouncements of those public health experts who blame agricultural "nutrients" (from animal wastes and fertilizer) for habitat degradation, we need to take a broader look at the full range of chemical substances now being manufactured daily by our high-tech society, along with their continuing interactions over time.

We can also begin to demand that our physicians know what questions to ask in an orderly fashion, and how to give a special CS test—known as the "FACT," or Functional Acuity Contrast Test™, which is manufactured by Stereo Optical Company, Inc., a Gerber Coburn Company.

At the same time, we can also insist that toxin-binding therapy be initiated when indicated, according to the Shoemaker Protocols.

How can you know if your FACT is "normal?" All you have to do is take the simple CS test you will find at chronicneurotoxins.com.

Then show the results to your doctor . . . and be sure to ask for a referral, if he or she doesn't have experience yet in the treatment of chronic neurotoxin-mediated illnesses. (Contact us at the website, if no one seems able to help you.)

As you're about to discover in these pages, it's time to recognize the unhappy fact that toxin-mediated illnesses are here to stay. Some may have been here for eons, in fact, but are just now being recognized. Just ask my friend and colleague, Dr. Ken Hudnell, a neurotoxicologist at the U.S. EPA's National Health and Environmental Effects Research Lab. Almost daily, Dr. Hudnell sends me information he's received about new toxin-forming species—such as algae in Australia, or new rickettsia species from Europe, or the new "mahogany tide" (a different species of dinoflagellate) that is now having a major impact on the Chesapeake Bay.

Are the culprits responsible for these newly recognized illnesses really chicken manure and other fertilizer products, as the politically connected "experts" so often insist? Of course not.

The blunt fact is that the emerging epidemic of chronic, neurotoxin-mediated illnesses has been spawned by our rapidly changing ecosystem, and not by any particular set of chemicals, agricultural or otherwise.

As long as we live on this overcrowded and over-polluted planet, Earth, we must adapt to the daily change that our civilization forces on us. Example: think about the impact of all those millions of plastic containers—many made with "plasticizers" containing toxic isocyanates and cyanide-related compounds—floating around out there on the landscape.

Our new diseases may not kill us quickly; they simply leave us feeling tired, irritable, unhappy and full of pain. They dull our senses, so that we end up walking around in a "brain fog," with our energy sapped and our spirits sagging.

All too often, these new diseases masquerade as *old* diseases —even though the symptoms appear to have changed. Say goodbye to "age-related memory loss," and "irritable bowel syndrome," and "fibromyalgia" and "deconditioning" that causes delayed recovery from activity.

And say goodbye, also, to excuses such as "It's just my sinuses!" and "Of course my joints hurt—I'm overweight, you know; it must be all the stress I'm facing!"

As a parent and spouse of an early childhood educator, I believe the greatest tragedy of chronic, neurotoxin-mediated illnesses is the insidious threat to our children. At the same time, we're going to have to say goodbye to some of the reasons frequently cited for why "Johnny can't read" . . . while recognizing that if he's struggling with vision-deficits caused by toxins, his reading and thinking proficiency can be restored by only three weeks of taking a benign, inexpensive medication.

It's time to strip the façade of false science from all the empty phrases, and to throw open a window onto the world of toxin-mediated illness. Take a good look around, my friends, and then take a deep breath of fresh air. With this book as your faithful guide, prepare yourself for the great public health struggle that lies ahead.

Welcome to the world of *Desperation Medicine.*

Special Thanks

A special thanks to all those who helped with the preparation of this book, including:

Dr. Frank McDonald, Biochemist, Emory University. He showed me the commonality of structure of molecular dipoles of ionophore toxins.

Dr. Allan Bickling, CEO, McCready Hospital, Maryland. He supported my research by providing time and staff, and without ever looking back.

Dr. Tom Tosteson, University of Puerto Rico, Mayaguez. He led the way through the complex physiology of ciguatera toxins and provided strong intellectual support.

Steven Nostrom, RN, Mattituck, Long Island. For more than 13 years, he has fought for his Lyme patients.

Robert Taylor, M.D., Pathologist extraordinaire at Peninsula Regional Medical Center, Salisbury, Maryland. He always had a helpful insight.

Russel Kujan, information specialist at the Medical Chirurgical Faculty of Maryland. What a fantastic resource person. None of my research questions were too obscure for him.

Pat Smith, President, Lyme Disease Association. She believed my approach had merit even before the data confirmed the merit.

Bruce Nichols, District Conservationist, Worcester County, USDA. More than a friend, a solid source of information and support regarding all aspects of biology, ecology, agriculture and politics.

Art Raines, M.D., Dallas, Texas. A man of razor-sharp insights balanced by warmth, experience and human compassion.

Mitch Hoggard, Pharm D and Dana Caldwell, Pharmacist, Chico, California. They took my idea—the neurotoxin basis of Lyme disease—and added an exponential leap of clinical application by studying what works and what doesn't with my protocols.

Don Malloy, Pocomoke River Alliance, Pocomoke, Maryland. He has the best-documented case showing the effect of cholestyramine on Contrast Sensitivity in Chronic Lyme Disease. He has never wavered in his support over the past ten years.

Debbie Hudson, Office Manager, Pocomoke, Maryland. Without question or complaint she has taken countless handwritten pages and turned them into the written force that drives *Desperation Medicine*.

Jack and Marian Spurling, Pocomoke River Alliance, Pocomoke, Maryland. Jack nearly gave his life to the *Pfiesteria* research effort. Has anyone told these two beautiful people today how much they are loved?

Wells Shoemaker. Dad went fishing for Bubba and caught Lyme instead.

Sara Shoemaker. Mom would have all the chronic Lyme patients in the country treated by now if she could.

Sally Shoemaker. No father could be more blessed than I to have a daughter like Sally. She has learned to follow her own way and never give up.

JoAnn Shoemaker. The love of my life. She gives her heart daily to her students, yet still has warmth, beauty, insight and elegance. Many thanks for everything.

How to Read This Book

Desperation Medicine contains many dramatic stories of patients who became involved in life-and-death struggles with chronic, neurotoxin-mediated illnesses such as Chronic Lyme Disease, Sick Building Syndrome, Chronic Fatigue Syndrome and *Pfiesteria*-Related Human Illness Syndrome.

But *Desperation Medicine* is also a book about science, and about some of the ways in which modern scientific research has been contaminated by a distorted political process in which money and power all too often win out over the truth.

Rather than interrupt the dramatic stories about struggling patients and the quest to identify a brand-new family of diseases, I decided to divide the book's chapters into two distinct groups.

One group of chapters, contained under the heading EVENTS, describes the treatment of patients and the continuing battle to come to grips with these new toxin-linked illnesses ... while also challenging the "public health bureaucrats" and the "Appearance Of Good Science" tactic which they so frequently employ in order to promote their own hidden agendas.

A second group of chapters, contained under the heading REFLECTIONS, offers the reader some thoughtful observations about the history of science, the biochemistry of biological habitats, the effect of industrial pollution on such habitats, and many other related topics.

For the convenience of readers, the Table of Contents presents a sequence of chapters in which EVENTS and REFLECTIONS alternate to best effect. But the reader is of course free to order the sequence of chapters differently, depending on mood and particular interest.

—Ritchie Shoemaker, M.D.
   Pocomoke, Md. 2000

chapter 1

Everything That Lives
Is Food for Something Else

Pocomoke, MD –April, 2000

Fifteen years ago, and soon after launching my primary medical practice in this little Maryland corner of the world, I planted a dozen Kwanzan cherry saplings around the parking lot that flanks my office in downtown Pocomoke.

The saplings were real beauties, each five-eighths of an inch in diameter and each holding out the promise of one day producing those pink blooms that have made Washington's Tidal Basin such a famous landmark.

I'm no fan of Washington politics, mind you. But I've always thought that the ugliness of what takes place daily on Capitol Hill is nicely tempered by the beauty of all those cherry trees. The original Kwanzans were a gift from Japan to the U.S., and today you'll find them gracing both our nation's capital and our asphalt-threatened wetlands.

Once my office trees were planted, they grew quickly, helped along by the extra water and fertilizer I offered them. But I noticed a troubling fact: Because they bordered a soybean field and its accompanying biological pests, my fast-growing cherry trees were an available "standing crop"—which is the biological name we use for a ready source of available food-energy.

Make no mistake: nature does not usually permit a standing

crop to exist without some nearby organism feeding on it. Varmints, pests, insect plagues, man—call them what you will, but these biological entities are all consumers of standing crop. Example: If you don't protect your field of soybeans (usually with chemicals, these days), you'll soon discover that your standing crop is a lying crop worth nothing.

Simply stated, biological survival requires transfers of energy, usually from eating and reproducing. Isn't that why the fungus in an orange grove will keep spreading until all the oranges are gone? Give them half a chance, and bacterial speck will ruin your tomatoes, even as fungi such as rust and smut transform your wheat field into something other than "amber waves of grain." Whether we're talking about the behavior of corn- and squash-borers, or the nasty blights that attack potatoes and elm trees, the fact remains: everything out there eats something else, while doing its very best not to get eaten in return.

And so it was with the tent caterpillars who showed up one fine morning to begin devouring the vivid green leaves on my Kwanzan cherry trees.

The egg cases of the tent caterpillars had appeared almost overnight. Hard as asphalt, the ugly casings clung to many branches, just beyond the second-year growth line. That insect cement protected the eggs as they waited through winter cold and spring winds for the lush crop of new cherry leaves to emerge.

The trees are a standing crop of energy, remember. And now the standing crop-*eaters* had arrived in force, safely guarded by their seemingly impregnable cases and intent on attacking the tender, nutritious greenery when it emerged in spring.

During the first "Spring of the Caterpillars," our trees ended up as a nearly leafless Cherry Blossom Festival. Luckily, the buds and flowers didn't house much available energy, so they weren't eaten. The trees lived despite the defoliation, however, and a new growth of leaves quickly restored their vitality. Soon the caterpillars turned into moths and the trees were then safe for the summer.

But winter returned soon enough, and once again the second-year growth line fell prey to the concrete egg cases almost overnight. This time I was ready with my loppers and shears, however. My medical office became a surgical suite, as I worked hard to save the trees by pruning the branches that held unremovable eggs and then disposing of the clippings. Imagine my sense of satisfaction, when the trees put out renewed growth from the pruning, and I noticed that virtually all of the egg cases were cleared.

Imagine my disappointment, a few weeks later, when mellow springtime brought the same number of tents sheltering the same number of hungry caterpillars, who ate the same number of leaves they'd eaten the year before, while once again sparing the buds and flowers!

Sure, the robins showed up on schedule and became my pesticide-of-last-resort, as they gobbled up the free-crawling, bad-tasting, stiff-haired tent caterpillars. (At the same time, the starling babies were thoughtfully picking all the tent caterpillars off our plum and peach trees.)

The cherry trees grew despite the pests, with new smaller trees and shrubs soon taking root beneath the canopy of the cherries. A new community was developing.

Happily for us, the caterpillars didn't kill the cherries in the way that many standing crop consumers wipe out their biological meal tickets. But the scene they left behind wasn't much fun to contemplate: *Just look at those threadbare trees!* There were so many caterpillar egg cases . . . could anything on earth shut down this prolific pest?

The tent caterpillars had made a very canny "habitat selection!" There they were, living right next door to a nutritious food source. Equipped with a physical bunker to protect their young, in the form of those durable egg cases, their position seemed unassailable.

Were we doomed to admiring beautiful Kwanzan blooms on bare-limbed trees for the rest of our natural lives?

Hoping to answer that question, I dialed up my friend, the pesticide expert, who quickly explained that he could treat the trees each year for a few years with a new chemical that killed the caterpillars. No, he hadn't heard about any long-range effects of this newly assembled insect poison. But not to worry: EPA had approved the new DNA-disrupting substance on which it was based. This dandy new product prevented insect cells from dividing, and resistance didn't develop.

Hmmmm . . . the whole thing sounded a bit illogical to me. Was it really safe—or downright dangerous—to put DNA-modifiers around my parking lot? How would the chemical stop killing other things, once the caterpillars were gone?

Another friend, this one an integrated pest management specialist, wanted me to use *Bacillus thurigensis* as an insecticide. Too bad he didn't know about the toxins manufactured by other bacillus species, such as *B. anthracis* (the causative agent of anthrax), *B. cereus* (a known poison in rice products) and *B. subtilis* (another toxin-former). I recognize that many organic gardeners are these days employing toxin-forming bacillus species to aid in crop preservation—but adding uncommon or unknown new toxins to the environment in which I live and play just doesn't sound like a great idea. Man-made or not, these chemical and biological agents are still toxic!

Next, my friend Bruce Nichols, the USDA District Conservationist of Worcester County, Maryland, gently reminded me that the caterpillars were food for other species that used the new cover for feeding and breeding. He also pointed out that my cherry trees were healthy . . . and that they could certainly withstand a few weeks of leaf harvest by the caterpillars. I didn't need to do anything, said Bruce, except open a few of the tents in order to make it easier for grackles and starlings to eat the caterpillars. No, the robins weren't a major predator of tent caterpillars.

Conservationist Edgar Hall, curmudgeon that he is, had already taught me a lesson that applied here. I'd interviewed Hall at length for my 1998 book, *Pfiesteria: Crossing Dark Water,* and he'd impressed me greatly by suggesting that the key to trapping muskrats was to "leave no mark" showing that I'd visited their lair.

(A wise maxim—especially when you remember that "do no harm" is the foundation-stone of the entire Hippocratic tradition among physicians!)

In the end, I decided to follow Edgar's advice and Bruce's advice to do nothing at all about those pesky caterpillars and their even peskier egg cases.

We enjoyed an early thaw this past February. After six weeks of ice on our ponds, the warm air from the South soon awakened a few spring peepers. I enjoyed the sun and hoped those bold peepers wouldn't freeze in the cold front due the next day, or be devoured by the nearly starved herons. If everything in biology ends up as food, is devouring impatient peepers an important way in which herons manage to survive ice, frost and snow?

Well, the mellow sun warmed the branches on the cherry trees, too. The egg cases had protected their occupants from snow and sleet, but now the radiant heat was affecting those rock-hard caterpillar motels.

Heat brings excystment of *Pfiesteria*, too, even in frigid temperatures, as the slack water warms up beneath the sun. In the silty loams (deposition-sites of metals and fungicides) of the dark-bottomed Eastern Shore waterways—including the Pocomoke, Manokin, Wicomico, Chicamacomico, St. Martin, Gargatha, Bulbeggar and Choptank Rivers, along with Corkers Creek—the cysts woke up and triggered mid-winter blooms of toxin-forming dinoflagellates. Of course, the smaller ditches and creeks woke up, too.

Surely, some opportunistic creature would be hanging around, waiting to eat our winter *Pfiesteria* in the cold waters of our estuaries? (Unless the caterpillar poisons—or some other ill-advised toxins from the previous year—killed off the *Pfiesteria*-eaters!)

Maybe that scenario had already taken place, in fact. How could I explain the presence of two new *Pfiesteria* patients on my schedule, or the fact that both hailed from the St. Martin River, located directly across the Assawoman Bay from Ocean City, Maryland—not known before to have been located in the heart of "toxic dinoflagellate" country?

Before leaving the parking lot to see my newest *Pfiesteria* patients, I took one last look at the branches of the cherry tree above my car. Nothing was going to eat those iron-hard cases! Oh, well. The caterpillars bloom for a little while and then change life form. It wasn't any different for *Pfiesteria*, really. They also bloom for a while, feed and breed and then change life form.

The tundra swans flying overhead were calling, a magical sound worth hearing if you've missed it so far. I'm looking up, watching the swans and getting ready for the public relations pressure I know I'll face, if I tell the truth about toxin-formers living year-round in the waters that surround the expensive waterfront homes. How will my Cassandra-like warnings affect Maryland's cash cow resort, Ocean City, and Worcester County's real estate tax base? And how much will that real estate be worth, if it also turns out to be "*Pfiesteria*-front" property?

How much would you pay to live in the Hamptons on Long Island, in the middle of West Nile-like virus, malaria, Lyme disease and Babesia? For that matter, who would want to live *any place* on earth where such life-threatening infectious diseases as malaria and tuberculosis have gained a foothold in an altered habitat?

The branch above me is moving unnaturally. Look . . . there's a red-cockaded woodpecker. Hang on . . . I'm wrong. It's actually a downy woodpecker. Makes sense, too, since the old-growth loblolly pines (the feeding and breeding habitat of the red-cockaded) were logged out years ago. The truth is, those crimson-hued birds are now extinct everywhere in Maryland—except for the two pairs of birds living on the high-ground island of loblollies beside our nature trail in the Pocomoke Swamp. . . .

Look! The downy is banging away on a concrete egg case. Bang, bang, eat, eat. Again and again, the downy tap, tap, taps. Over the next several days, he will clean all the egg cases from all the branches.

All at once, the situation becomes clear: these cement-wrapped pests have become "standing crop" for the ravenous woodpecker!

But what will the hungry robins and grackles eat now, and what will happen to the baby starlings?

Don't fret. As long as we don't get a plague of woodpeckers, the other birds will be just fine. And if we *do* get a "bloom" of downies, their arrival will merely signal another shift in the eternal cycle of life.

I need to learn how to watch. And I must be careful—very careful—to leave no mark on these thriving tree lands!

Showdown.
Confrontation with
A Toxic Invader.

Pocomoke City, MD –July, 1997

It began on a steamy summer afternoon back in 1997, when a worried fisherman named Ray Maddox phoned my Family Practice office on Market Street to report that he was in possession of a dead trout.

Although I didn't know it at the time, I was about to get my first look at the grisly damage caused by a biological mutation—a pollution-spawned microorganism armed with a toxic weapon that also makes people very sick.

"I've got one, doc. We pulled him out of the river just two hours ago."

"Nice job, Ray."

"He's in real bad shape. Covered with fresh lesions, and they're still bleeding. Real ugly."

"Okay. Are they the same lesions you've been seeing on the other dead fish?"

"Yup. We netted at least 30 of 'em, and they're all covered with these same sores. What's wrong, doc?"

I shook my head. "I wish I could tell you, Ray. But the truth is, nobody has an explanation. Let's see what the microscope shows us."

"Fair enough, doc. I'm on my way."

• • •

Covered with blood-oozing lesions, the fish floated dead on the water. And no one could tell us why.

Then the people who lived along the tranquil Maryland river began to come down with a mysterious illness.

Soon they were dropping by my solo Family Practice on Market Street in Pocomoke City. They were puzzled, fearful. They were also presenting symptoms that suggested a syndrome produced by a toxin-related illness.

One by one, they listed the complaints making them miserable: nasty headaches, secretory diarrhea, rash, cough, persistent muscle aches and increasing failure of short-term memory.

I asked myself if there might be anything connecting these patients to a shared toxic exposure?

Yes. The link was the river. Each one of them had spent time working or playing in the slow-moving Pocomoke during the summer of 1997.

• • •

I placed the newspaper-wrapped package from Ray Maddox on the stainless steel table in my lab. Then, wearing latex surgical gloves, I uncovered the sick fish that had come from the river earlier that day.

Puh-*yeeeeewww!* Resisting the temptation to hold my nose, I got down to the serious business of conducting an autopsy that might tell me something about the death of this decaying specimen.

At first glance, this 14-inch grey trout might have been any other member of the "Salmonidae" aquatic family. Covered with light brown speckles, he came equipped with a sleek set of fins and a powerful-looking tail. No wonder he could zip through the water at 20 miles an hour!

A normal fish? Almost . . . but not quite. Because there was something missing.

Where was his coat of protective mucous?

Somehow, this diseased trout had lost most of the slime-like substance that ordinarily covers a fish's scales as protection from predatory microorganisms, including water-borne bacteria, viruses and fungi.

And there was more. Looking closely, I noticed a raw, abraded area on the fish's ventral side. It was about an inch in diameter, and it was covered with tiny bubbles of blood. Had the trout been bleeding internally? Had the blood then leaked out through his skin and scales?

I lifted the scalpel.

On the very first cut, I got a surprise: each pass of the blade released several waves of old, unclotted blood. Underneath the blood, I found more trauma—most of the underlying muscle had been dissolved, as if eaten away by a powerful solvent.

I was looking at "liquefaction necrosis," a fatal condition in which death is caused by the dissolving of cells and tissues.

But what kind of illness could cause such profound devastation in living tissue?

I was challenged and stimulated to find the answer.

• • •

How could I have known, on that humid afternoon in the summer of '97, that I was about to confront a new kind of disease threat—a biological predator which had sprung up spontaneously from the witch's brew of pesticides and industrial chemicals that were now transforming the ecosystem of the eastern seaboard?

Nasty headaches, secretory diarrhea, rash, cough, persistent muscle aches and increasing failure of short-term memory . . .

While I struggled to identify the microorganism that was attacking the local fish population, I also noticed a curious increase in these dramatic, flu-like symptoms among my patients. Were they somehow linked to the organism killing our fish?

According to the newspapers and the TV news shows, our tiny community was under assault.

Our picturesque Pocomoke River—a tributary of the 200-mile-long Chesapeake Bay—had been invaded by a toxin-producing, one-celled dinoflagellate: *Pfiesteria*, aka "The Fish Killer."

This rapidly reproducing microorganism had triggered an outbreak of what I would identify as a new disease in late 1997: *Pfiesteria*-related human illness syndrome. A year later, the disorder would be re-named the "estuarine-associated syndrome" by the CDC.

Remarkably enough, the Atlanta-based federal agency would change the name of the disease *again*, two years after the outbreak—this time labeling it: "Possible Estuarine-Associated Syndrome," or "PEAS."

(That new nomenclature appeared in May of 2000 in the CDC's Medical Morbidity Weekly Report, along with the astonishing assertion that no states had reported cases of PEAS in 1998 or 1999, despite all of the contradictory evidence from my numerous, well-publicized cases.)

Although the outbreak of a new disease always deserves careful scrutiny, I saw no reason for panic. After all, don't new diseases show up fairly often on the microbiological landscape, as bacteria and fungi and viruses contend for "survival niches" in the brutal struggle we call "evolution?"

But this disease agent wasn't just another pathogenic loner, cruising up and down the river in search of its next juicy meal.

Although nobody understood it at the time, this toxin-forming dinoflagellate was leading the vanguard of an entirely new kind of disease. *Pfiesteria* was a "toxin-mediated" pathogen—only one of a dozen new disease agents that were about to declare war on millions of Americans.

Although the Maryland *Pfiesteria* outbreak was a regional event, it would soon take on major epidemiological significance. During the next year or so, this voracious one-celled organism would open a window on an entirely new kind of disease threat.

• • •

After autopsying Ray Maddox's bloody trout for more than hour, I had to admit a very unhappy fact.

I was baffled.

My detailed examination of the specimen had turned up nothing conclusive. I'd found some discoloration of the brain-covering meninges, and the fish's spleen felt swollen. But those symptoms told me nothing about the toxic invader that had taken down this trout.

Face it: I was in the dubious situation of looking for clues for a new disease by doing an autopsy on a fish! As a scientist, I was swimming in quicksand. Where was all of this research headed, anyway?

Only one fact seemed certain, at this point. Somehow, the toxic marauder had managed to knife its way through the protective layer of slime. In those areas, liquefaction necrosis had quickly set in. But what was the chemistry? What was the step-by-step physiology? If the toxin molecules were bullets fired from a gun, what make was the weapon? What kind of microscopic predator had pulled the trigger?

A biological mystery!

And then, within a few weeks of that puzzling autopsy in my medical lab in downtown Pocomoke City, the stakes suddenly got much higher.

All at once, many more people were getting sick. The dead fish floated—tens of thousands of them—on the motionless water, while the rapacious seagulls ripped and slashed at them.

HUMAN ILLNESS REPORTED NEAR SITE
OF MASSIVE POCOMOKE FISH KILLS

It was time for the State of Maryland to step in.

Within a matter of days, of course, the state health bureaucrats would be making matters worse.

• • •

Politics and Medicine: The Two Don't Mix

Imagine my consternation in the summer of 1997, when a team of Maryland public officials came to our small town of 4,000 residents and three stoplights to investigate the increasing reports of toxin-based illness along the waterway.

"The river is safe!" said the Maryland State Department of Health, after interviewing five or six citizens, taking a few water samples and examining a few fish.

"The river is safe; no one has gotten sick from the river!" On TV news programs and front pages throughout the region, the public health officials repeated these lines. Apparently, they were convinced that if they said the words often enough, people would finally begin to believe them. The Secretary of the Department of Health said he would let his family "swim in the river."

Those of us who were watching the bio-invader at work along the infested estuary could hardly believe our ears. Why wouldn't the Health Department conduct the kind of in-depth investigation that might confirm the presence of this new illness? "Before we can do that," explained the health bureaucrats, "we'd need to have a cohort of sick patients!"

Mystified by the state's continuing refusal to alert the public to an obvious epidemic, many area residents were asking themselves: Hadn't the health experts examined the fish with the grotesque, bleeding ulcers?

Hadn't they heard about the fish whose tails had been gnawed off by "The Cell from Hell" . . . or the ones that swam in endless, confused circles—many with their intestines trailing along behind them?

And what about all the sick people with pronounced symptoms? Weren't those ailing watermen enough to make up a "cohort?" Didn't they count as people? Increasingly puzzled by the state's unwillingness to act, I couldn't help wondering if the health officials might be engaged in a cover-up designed to protect Maryland's multi-billion-dollar tourist and seafood industries. Were the health bureaucrats part of an ongoing news distortion orchestrated at the upper levels of state government? Was the truth being blacked out?

I didn't want to believe it. But how else could I explain the endless stonewalling by the health bureaucrats? Increasingly troubled as the long hot summer of 1997 advanced and the *Pfiesteria* plague took off in earnest all along the Pocomoke watershed, I vowed that regardless of the consequences, I would not stay silent. . . .

If the health officials wouldn't do their job, I'd take it on, myself. I'd "go public" with my diagnosis of *Pfiesteria*-related human illness, in order to alert the news media to the public health threat swimming around out there in the brackish waters of the Pocomoke.

The whole thing was painful to watch. As the weeks crept by and a growing number of *Pfiesteria* patients trooped into my office, I concluded that the official deception about *Pfiesteria* was probably as threatening to public health as the microorganism, itself.

My practice had always been quite busy. But now I was swamped by the extra work of caring for my *Pfiesteria* patients. I was also spending a great deal of time in the laboratory and the library, as I searched for a scientific explanation for the *Pfiesteria* plague. By August I was working more than 100 hours a week, while doing my best to balance patient needs with the demands of estuarine research.

It was a difficult period. And yet the struggle was only beginning. Although I didn't realize it at the time, I was soon to discover that *Pfiesteria*-related illness was only one of a dozen new toxin-based disease agents now running loose on the American landscape.

Make no mistake: These toxin-illnesses are making life increasingly hellish for more than 10 million Americans, according to the latest health research.

But the dinoflagellate invasion and the illness it caused were only part of the problem.

All too soon, the arrival of the Cell from Hell would begin to teach us some painful lessons about the thin line that separates medicine from politics, and public health from economics.

• • •

"You Gotta Do Something, Doc!"

Some background, first.

A 1977 graduate of the Duke University Medical School, I launched my medical practice in Pocomoke City in 1980, after finishing my family practice residency. I settled there because I had fallen in love with the slow-paced world of Maryland's thinly populated "Eastern Shore," and with the sinuous river that winds among the scattered villages and "black water" swamps of the coastal plain.

No wider than 50 yards in most places, the Pocomoke ("Dark Water," in Algonquin) is an 80-mile-long ribbon of sun-dappled water that flows south from Delaware. Shaded by nodding black gum and giant cypress, this murmuring waterway drains the tidal swamps of Maryland and Virginia en route to the Chesapeake Bay.

During nearly 20 years of practicing medicine in Pocomoke City, I'd spent many volunteer-hours working to raise funds for a "nature trail" that now flanks the river. Completed in 1994, the mile-long, $300,000 project offers visitors a close-up look at the uniquely diverse flora and fauna of the Great Pocomoke Swamp.

As a "rural Family Practice doc" who thoroughly enjoyed his primary care practice, I had many friends among the local men who work the water, as well as their families. Over the years, they'd come to accept me as part of their extended families. They didn't mind the fact that I wore a sports shirt in the office, instead of a lab coat. (The white coat would have made them uneasy: Didn't the inexperienced medical students all wear white coats on TV?)

When the *Pfiesteria* epidemic arrived in Maryland, I was one of the first to be asked about it. What *was* this new illness, my patients wondered, and how did it make people sick? Notebook at the ready, I quickly began to build the profile of this new toxic disease.

The Maryland epidemic had actually begun back in the fall of 1996, when the local watermen who fished the river and nearby Pocomoke Sound started netting hundreds of dead fish.

As it turned out, this one-celled predator had also killed fish by the millions in the coastal waters of North Carolina during the early 1990s. But there had been no proven cases of human illness acquired in the wild associated with the North Carolina invasion, despite an occasional unverified report.

"You gotta do something, doc!" Lori Maddox, the wife of a longtime Pocomoke waterman and one of my patients for many years, seemed frightened when she visited my office in June, 1997. "Something in the river's making people sick.

"Tommy East had pneumonia seven times last winter and he lost 40 pounds! And Fred [her father-in-law] says his memory isn't right.

"Every time it rains hard, or when we have a big tide, the fish start dying and we start getting sick. And the worst attacks seem to come after they spread those chemicals on the tomato farms around here. What's going on, doc?"

"I don't know, Lori. But I'm going to do my best to find out."

It was no accident that "The Cell From Hell" had decimated North Carolina's coastal fishing industry during the past five years. What would happen to our local watermen, I wondered, when the Carolina-sized fish kills began to appear? And what about the tourist trade at nearby Ocean City—where 250,000 people show up every summer weekend intent on spending their money on "Maryland seafood," while also frolicking along the water's edge?

Pfiesteria would threaten all of that, especially if the rumors that it also caused human illness turned out to be true. Only later would we come to understand that this organism lived sometimes as a plant and sometimes as an animal. In fact, the highly protean invader came in more than 25 *different* life forms, and was quite capable of growing from 10 microns in diameter into a slow-moving amoeba form of more than 460 microns.

Within four hours, this incredible organism could activate its DNA and change its morphology from top to bottom, achieving a feat of differential gene activation that no mammalian cell can equal.

A lethal "ambush predator" in the free-swimming flagellate form (the zoospore phase), *Pfiesteria* releases a powerful toxin that acts on fish like a narcotic. At the same time, powerful chemicals in the toxin attract swarms of other *Pfiesteria*, producing the frothing chocolate-hued "bloom" that is one of the creature's biological signatures. Dead fish and sick people are others.

But the rapid growth of the slowly crawling amoeba form depended, I soon discovered, on the plentiful availability of its main food staples: nutrient-rich, chloroplast-bearing microorganisms—including blue-green algae—living at the interface of the river water and sediment.

Shut down the food supply upon which the amoeba form of *Pfiesteria* relied—because of ground water pollution or other assaults on the waterway—and this crafty organism knew how to shift into a zoospore armed with a nasty suite of toxins well-suited to feeding on animals. And what if fish weren't present to feed on? In that case, the camouflaged marauder would simply drop to the bottom of the river as a long-lived cyst.

When fish were abundant, they became a primary food source for the zoospore, which also scatters the toxins as a sexual stimulant similar to a pheromone. In a *Pfiesteria* bloom, both feeding and breeding take place for several days at a stretch before subsiding.

It didn't take me long to be convinced that the pathogenic agent in *Pfiesteria* was a fat-soluble toxin that first dissolved in muscle, then brain, then equilibrated in reservoirs of surfactant in lung, bile and neural tissue.

Once I understood the toxic physiology, the next step was to figure out a way to block it.

Cholestyramine!

If I could bind the toxin in the intestine with this tissue-cleansing agent, I knew I'd be able to drain the toxin from the brain, the lungs and the bile of any infected patient. (See Chapter 4.)

The biochemistry at work here was quite fascinating. Reviewing it, I quickly realized that if the toxin were water-soluble, the resulting illness would not be persistent. But the substance had to dissolve in water, in order to keep killing fish over several days during a bloom. What if the poison actually dissolved in both fat *and* water?

Then the toxin could move from cell to cell without ever entering the bloodstream. Its point of access was by water droplets, immersion in water, or aerosol . . . but it did its ugly damage in fatty tissues scattered throughout the body. The key point: *Pfiesteria* toxin dissolved in water as a means of transport, but then delivered its toxic punch through fat-containing tissue.

Enter cholestyramine (CSM), the perfect weapon with which to shut down this new disease mechanism.

The exciting news about this 40-year-old, FDA-approved medication was that it removed the toxin from bile, which the body uses to dissolve fats. And when the toxin departed the bile, it also left the body's tissues. Imagine three flasks connected at the bottom. Fill them halfway with water. Now drain one flask . . . and you drain them all.

Treating patients with CSM soon became the foundation stone for a healing process that I decided to call "Desperation Medicine." If you're desperate, you'll try anything! And cholestyramine was the one strategy, I decided, that could actually block the toxins being dispersed by this new breed of disease agents.

During the next two years, I successfully treated several hundred patients suffering from chronic toxin-mediated illnesses. Most of them showed dramatic relief from their symptoms, virtually overnight.

At War with the Bureaucrats

While I struggled to first diagnose and then begin curing this frightening new illness, the State of Maryland was finally doing something to counteract the widespread *"Pfiesteria* hysteria."

In the late summer of 1997, the bureaucrats scheduled a highly publicized scientific conference designed to explore all aspects of the dinoflagellate illness. Summoned to a college campus at Salisbury, Md., the panel of scientists had been recruited by the Maryland Department of Natural Resources (DNR).

Their charge was to study the health implications of *Pfiesteria* and its environmental causes. I felt certain that they'd be interested in my research and findings. And I was convinced that they needed to hear about my research into the "pollution-trigger" that made the bug metamorphose into a toxin-producing source of a human illness syndrome.

It seemed quite obvious, as well, that these health researchers would benefit from hearing about my first-ever *Pfiesteria* patients.

The conference was set to begin on July 31, and it seemed like the ideal place to describe the first diagnosis of this new illness. Still, I felt a bit uneasy, as I made the 30-mile drive from Pocomoke to Salisbury that Friday night.

Already, there was disturbing evidence to show that the Maryland authorities intended to downplay the *Pfiesteria* threat. After trawling the river for dead fish in early July, for example, the DNR had announced that it had found only a few fish with the characteristic *Pfiesteria* lesions. "The river is safe!"

A few days later, when I pointed out in a local newspaper interview that the DNR biologists had trawled the deepest, central sections of the river—instead of the still, shallow pools

where most sick fish could be found—state health officials described me as a "kook" and a "fear monger," according to reporters.

Startled by the violence of their attack, I couldn't help wondering if they were intent on "keeping the lid on" the severity
of the *Pfiesteria* invasion and the reports of associated human
illness.

Those suspicions were confirmed during the conference. Although my case reports and my color photos drew lots of attention, it was soon obvious that the Maryland Health Department
would not change its endless refrain: "No one has gotten sick
from the river!"

That realization seemed especially troubling after one of the
nation's pioneering *Pfiesteria* researchers—aquatic botanist Dr.
JoAnn Burkholder of North Carolina State University—told the
conference that she and several other lab workers had developed
the same illness symptoms I was reporting from the Pocomoke,
while handling the dinoflagellate in their lab back in 1995!

Dr. Burkholder's evidence corroborated my diagnoses of several *Pfiesteria* patients. But the Maryland DNR and the Health
Department remained steadfast, and refused to issue a formal
warning to the public about the illness hazards associated with
the toxic invader.

As far as I was concerned, the "conference" was a fiasco.

I had expected to be able to testify about my diagnosis and
my research on the biochemistry of the toxic invasion. Wrong! In
the end, I wasn't even allowed to attend the technical meeting.
Later, at the health session, I was informed that the panel of experts didn't have time to take comments from the "public."

It was crystal-clear to me that both groups of scientists knew
exactly what I would be telling them . . . and wanted no part of
an honest discussion of the facts about *Pfiesteria*.

Looking back on that conference later, it also seemed clear
that the state had used every possible feature of the "Appearance
of Good Science Strategy" which the bureaucrats so often rely on
to whitewash the truth about environmentally acquired illness.

Pfiesteria was a "window," all right—a window that revealed clearly how science and politics often end up in the same bed together.

That insight seemed even more compelling a few days later, when the panel's "conclusions" emerged. The fish lesions had been caused by "scrapes from crab pots and propeller blade cuts!" How else could the state scientists explain the lesions? The state had carefully documented the fact that every water quality measurement in the river was normal, including nutrient levels that had not changed in over 12 years.

Alarmed by the panel's failure to review my findings, I quickly sent the Health Department the *Pfiesteria* case histories I had assembled. Yet the foot-dragging continued. At one point, then-Secretary of the Maryland Department of Health and Hygiene Martin P. Wasserman even called me at home, urging me to be "patient" in my efforts to protect the public from this obvious pathogen!

It was time to go public with my research on the toxic-producing behavior of *Pfiesteria*, and on the illness it causes in humans. I did my best to get the word out, and the ongoing media uproar was soon compounded by growing public fear throughout Maryland about the possible contaminating effects of *Pfiesteria* in the food supply.

This growing public outcry steamrolled the state into recognizing that my case reports were valid. They quickly convened a blue-ribbon panel of university physicians who confirmed that I was right about the illness outbreak. (Nonetheless, the Health Department did its best during the ensuing months to "spin" the findings of the panel, in order to filter the information that reached the public, or not release it at all.)

During the next year or so, I would give dozens of electronic and print interviews in which I would carefully explain the biochemistry that had triggered a new disease. Whether I was appearing on NBC News or the BBC, or being interviewed for the New York Times, I did my best to tell them what I knew to be the truth.

Three days after the conclusion of the Salisbury conference, *Pfiesteria* attacked again, this time causing a series of massive fish kills in the Pocomoke River. During the next few months, similar assaults would take place along 30 other tributaries of the Chesapeake in Maryland and Virginia. As usual, the State of Maryland officials and their public relations machines did their best to minimize the damage, and formally identified only four rivers in which they said kills had occurred.

But thousands of fish were floating to the surface of the estuary now, and "*Pfiesteria* hysteria" was spreading, as the story dominated the front page day after day in Maryland.

My phone was ringing off the hook, and the reporters were all asking the same questions: Was there really a human illness? What were the symptoms? And what was behind the outbreak? "Dr. Shoemaker . . . Can you identify any of the victims so that we can talk to them?"

Most of the reporters had already talked to the state scientists. They'd been told that the culprit was "nutrients" from the manure (often used as fertilizer) produced by the region's huge chicken-farming operations, which included immense facilities owned by such industry giants as Perdue and Tyson Farms.

At first glance, the Health Department's explanation seemed to make good sense. The reporters could see the chicken manure spread everywhere on the land . . . and it was easy to imagine it washing into the estuary and poisoning the fish. And that was precisely the scenario being described by Democratic Governor Parris N. Glendening, who was reportedly intent on establishing his environmental credentials nationally by protecting the Chesapeake Bay, no matter the cost to truth.

According to the scientists employed by the state, the simplest way to eliminate the *Pfiesteria* outbreaks was to eliminate the nutrients (nitrates and phosphates) in the chicken manure that Dr. Burkholder said in part triggered the blooms. And so what if that policy spelled doom for the chicken growers?

No one seemed interested in blaming the millions of pounds

of "nutrients" produced daily by the huge sewage-treatment plants in Washington and Baltimore and Pennsylvania, and then flushed regularly into the Chesapeake. Apparently, *those* nutrients didn't figure into the equation . . . although they obviously dwarfed the daily chicken manure production around Salisbury!

Interestingly enough, the Salisbury State panel had at first concluded that nutrients were not responsible for the outbreak. But only two weeks later, the state scientists completely reversed themselves on that issue. Suddenly, "high levels of nutrients" became the daily mantra among the health bureaucrats, and politics was once again threatening to distort good science.

That same mantra is now being chanted from coast to coast —from the "Dead Zone" in the Gulf of Mexico, to barren waters in Long Island Sound where lobsters once flourished, to Lake Griffin in Florida, where alligators with lesions in their brains swim through neurotoxin-filled lagoons and then die . . . supposedly from "eating shad that live in waters containing too much phosphate and too few other nutrients!"

What caused the sudden switch in the state's approach to *Pfiesteria*? Obviously, the huge fish kills that followed the conference by only a few days had put enormous heat on the health bureaucracy to come up with an explanation that would stick. Pressured relentlessly by the news media, the state had to pinpoint the source of the kills, even if they had to pretend to have an answer.

Seeking instant credibility, the bureaucrats turned to Dr. Burkholder, who had demonstrated an association between nutrient-enrichment of estuarine waters and enhanced growth of *Pfiesteria*. Dr. Burkholder provided the lynch pin for their campaign to blame the infestation on the chicken growers— although her test results were manipulated toward that end by state employees, including scientists who were induced to come up with an unscientific and expedient answer in order to appease the public. They should have known better.

The villain was nutrients, said Dr. Burkholder, and the state said that was that. It's true that the North Carolina scientist probably knows more than anybody else on earth about *Pfiesteria*. But what about the chemical poisons in the water?

I knew they were present, and other scientists finally admitted it as well. What role did they play?

Suddenly, the poultry producers were in trouble. Loosely organized, and with no political action groups to defend themselves against attacks by government, they were an easy target. Besides, if the legislators made life difficult for the major producers, the large ones could always shift their operations elsewhere and still survive. (Tyson Farms did precisely that, and began departing for greener pastures in Oklahoma soon after the plague began.)

Once the major producers had moved on, the land developers would be able to start building $200,000 townhouses, condos, vacation homes and corporate headquarters where the computer operators could enjoy a scenic backdrop. All over America, the same strategy of fleeing "urban sprawl" for the uncrowded hinterland was now gaining the upper hand. How long would it be before the affluent residents from well-heeled, metropolitan areas everywhere began to invest in abandoned farmlands along our estuary?

Signs that said "Waterfront Property For Sale" began blooming like spring daffodils.

Everybody wins! Well, almost everybody. You didn't have to be a math expert to figure out that the only folks who'd would be wiped out in this kind of scenario were the "little guys"—the small-scale poultry producers who would lose everything if the "*Pfiesteria* hysteria" drove the smaller farms out of production, along with the big producers.

Dr. Burkholder knew the subject inside-out, and her data said nutrients. But I believed it was toxins—and several recent ecological findings, in Florida and elsewhere, have since proved that theory to be sound.

After a great deal of research, I was convinced that the water quality data from the Pocomoke and several other regional waterways demonstrated one fact with compelling clarity: The source of the *Pfiesteria* blooms wasn't nitrates at all, but the copper and fungicides used on a long list of crops including tomato, melons, peppers, apples, tobacco and citrus, up and down the East Coast. Extra nutrients were harmful, but worse were chemicals.

My year-long research into the biochemistry, geochemistry, pesticide degradation, phytoplankton physiology and estuarine limnology involved in the outbreaks had demonstrated conclusively that copper (used both for the leafy crops and to prevent spoilage of animal feed and plant seeds) stored in river sediments wipes out the main food sources, including blue-green algae, on which the harmless amoeba stage of *Pfiesteria* relies for food.

Deprived of their food supply, the *Pfiesteria* amoeba then simply morphed into a toxic zoospore form in order to feed on fish and other vulnerable life forms in the estuary.

At this point, however, the combination of copper and the leafy-crop fungicides (mainly dithiocarbamates) that had been washed into the watershed entered the equation by destroying billions of the microorganisms (rotifers and copepods) that kept the toxic *Pfiesteria* phase under control by feeding on it. Predator-prey relationships are a basic principle of biology and evolution. And the model fit the facts: wherever there was a fish kill, there were toxic chemicals.

But the levels of nutrient-enrichment always remained the same, whether fish kills were present or not.

And when the poisons that I had identified were removed from the equation, the fish kills did not occur, even with extra nutrients!

The bottom line now seemed clear, and highly disturbing.

Instead of accurately identifying the cause of the blooms—chemical substances that could easily be replaced, without upsetting farming operations—the Maryland politicians and their state-employed scientists were pinning the blame for the toxic invasion on the big chicken farmers.

It was an ominous precedent. If the state version of events went unchallenged, any agricultural operation in Maryland could become a target for unsubstantiated political attacks, far into the future. Restrictions on nutrient use take land out of production. These two events were clearly at work in the Pfiesteria episode.

There was no avoiding the obvious question: Were the politicians using the *"Pfiesteria* scare" to drive off the big chicken producers, in a scenario that would also bankrupt the small-scale poultry growers, many of whom happened to be my friends?

What resources would these small producers have left? Only their waterfront land . . . which could prove extremely valuable to regional developers eager to build along the sparsely-populated estuary. It had happened before.

It was a painful question to contemplate, but there it was. Was the *"Pfiesteria* plague" being manipulated as part of a massive land development scheme? All at once it seemed clear that the 21st Century was bringing us a lifestyle that would radically change our environment—just as the industrial revolution had changed air and water quality. But the cause of these new illnesses would be widespread alteration of habitats, and not just industrial and chemical pollution.

The "Health Bureaucracy" Strikes Back

I had no answers for these troubling questions. Yet one fact seemed overwhelmingly clear: my medical diagnoses of more than 50 cases (by January of 1998) of a new *Pfiesteria*-linked illness were now inextricably tangled in political and economic complications.

How could medical researchers and physicians provide the best public health response to this threat, when the state's own public health apparatus was part of a public relations "fix" designed to put a spin—or a cover up—on the medical facts?

During the year or so that followed my first diagnosis of *Pfiesteria*-related human illness syndrome, state health and conservation officials did their best to invalidate my findings and confuse the public about their implications. Among the major attacks on my credibility were the following:

- State environmental and conservation officials, including a Maryland Department of the Environment scientist, discussed in a public meeting in March of 1998 a suggestion that I should be charged with "scientific malpractice" for suggesting that the state's "nutrient theory" for *Pfiesteria* blooms was inaccurate.

- The director of the State of Maryland's *Pfiesteria* Research Program, Dr. Donald Boesch, announced to the news media that "Ritchie has done a good job on the health issue, but he is out of his field in the sciences."

- In the spring of 1998, my office received two "surprise visits" from state and federal medical inspectors who examined our labs and x-ray facilities from top to bottom. Other state inspectors soon followed them into my office. Ostensibly, they were fulfilling their state-mandated duties. But these visits occurred several months before they were scheduled, or for the first time in ten years—suggesting that both the federal and state examiners might have been affected by my part in the continuing controversy over *Pfiesteria.*

- State officials constantly told public meetings and news reporters that my "copper idea" was "off the wall," or "uninformed" —even as an increasing number of estuarine experts were confirming its essential accuracy. The State of Florida, for example, has largely implemented my suggestions for ameliorating copper toxicity, but without formally announcing that copper and fungicides, and not nutrients, are the source of the environmental problem in their affected estuaries.

- While making a presentation to 800 angry Eastern Shore farmers, Dr. Boesch and the heads of the Maryland Departments of Environment, Agriculture, Natural Resources and Health each went out of their way to attack the "copper theory." If the theory were merely "off-the-wall," why were they so eager to destroy it?

- All efforts to obtain research funding for further study of the toxic theory of the *Pfiesteria* organism came up empty. Again and again it was made clear to me that the "Shoemaker copper theory" lay outside the "acceptable" range of findings. On several occasions, I was warned that my approach to the problem amounted to "shouting that the Emperor had no clothes" —and that I would never receive a penny of state or federal funding for research.

• The Centers for Disease Control and Prevention continued to describe my treatment ideas for this new illness as "premature," even as chronic sufferers of estuarine-associated syndrome from Delaware to Florida were getting better in two weeks with CSM, although some had been sick for five years before I began treating them.

Within a few months of going public with my findings about *Pfiesteria* illness and treatment methods, I realized that if I were going to have any success in alerting the public to the danger, I'd have to find a national voice. How could I carry my important message beyond Maryland?

As fate would have it, that problem was solved when the news broke that fish kills had taken place in Florida, and that several cases of dinoflagellate-related illness had also been reported along the now-threatened St. Lucie River (near Stuart and Jupiter, on the east coast). And the record showed clearly that levels of nutrients, including nitrates and phosphorus, were actually *down* in some of the hottest attack zones of the St. Lucie.

After a huge public outcry in Florida, local activists demanded that the state fix the river. They also invited me to come and give a series of lectures on toxin-mediated illness and *Pfiesteria*, followed by participating in a clinic with local physicians. There we examined patients who were unwilling to rely on the State Health Department for diagnosis and treatment, after they learned how the health bureaucrats had handled the outbreak in Maryland.

The Florida version of the disease was identical to the one I had treated in Maryland, and the new cholestyramine treatment proved to be just as effective.

In the end, the Florida state authorities took a very different approach from Maryland's. After concluding that they had to intervene in order to protect the river, they earmarked $30 million to build lagoons that filter runoff from copper-laden citrus groves. Florida officials have also begun buying wetland farms in order to restore them to the estuarine system, and to dredge contaminated sections of the St. Lucie River.

Residents of Martin County levied a supplemental one-percent sales tax for three years to raise funds for the River Coalition to protect the watercourse from toxins by buying wetlands and making other improvements. This was an unprecedented response to the reality of pollution of America's watersheds.

Florida became the national lab that verified my ideas, and the testing that I had sought from Maryland was performed in the Sunshine State. The results showed astronomically high levels of copper and dithiocarbamates in the attack zones. These data verified my ideas about the cause of the outbreak. And I was greatly encouraged when the coordinator of the Florida dinoflagellate research team, Ann Forstchen, in April of 1999, explained in several interviews: "Right now, Ritchie's explanation is the strongest one out there."

An Ominous Turn of Events

Although I was pleased to have identified a brand-new disease threat and to have successfully treated the world's first *"Pfiesteria* patients" with cholestyramine, the euphoria soon evaporated in the face of several troubling questions that had been triggered by the outbreak in Maryland.

Q. What was the physiology involved in the storage and circulation of this dinoflagellate toxin throughout the human body?

Q. Why didn't the effects of the toxin—such symptoms as blurred vision, headaches and diarrhea—clear up on their own within a few days of exposure to *Pfiesteria*? Why weren't the toxins quickly eliminated, as the body metabolized them?

As I studied my patient-charts and read the literature on pathology, toxicology and membrane ionophore chemistry, I realized that I was working entirely in the dark. Was there some new disease principle at work here?

I did not imagine, of course, that my work with toxin-mediated illnesses had only just begun . . . or that I was about to stumble upon a whole new family of diseases that leave millions of Americans defenseless against the ravages caused by the buildup of organic poisons within their cells.

Pfiesteria was an eye-opener that pointed the way to a vast new region of undocumented but very real illnesses. And the pain of these mis-diagnosed chronic, neurotoxin-mediated illnesses isn't just an abstract idea about "human suffering in the face of government and corporate indifference."

These patients are real human beings, and millions of them are suffering as you read this line.

Welcome to *Desperation Medicine*, where simple truths topple entrenched scientific dogma, and where "any improvement is a godsend, and any cure a miracle!"

chapter 3

Reflection

Clear As Mud.
The Public Health
Coverup Continues.

Salisbury, MD –August, 1999

Ask the "science bureaucrats" who run such highly vaunted public health establishments as the CDC and the Maryland State Department of Health to describe the toxic microorganism *Pfiesteria piscicida*, and they'll all tell you the same thing.

"Outbreaks of *Pfiesteria* in U.S. coastal waters are caused by 'nutrients' from agricultural runoff."

Example: Take a quick look at one of the federal government's major websites on *Pfiesteria*, and you'll find such statements as:

"Factors that promote the growth of *Pfiesteria* include warm, brackish, poorly flushed waters and high levels of nutrients. Nutrients such as nitrogen and phosphorus are thought to encourage the growth of *Pfiesteria* populations in coastal waters by stimulating the growth of algae that *Pfiesteria* feeds on when in its non-toxic forms. . . ."

This remarkable statement by the reigning U.S. science bureaucrats perfectly illustrates how the Scientific Establishment relies on "conventional wisdom"—as dictated by the prevailing "scientific paradigm" of the moment—in order to make determinations that powerfully affect public health.

Paradigm or not, however, there is convincing evidence to show that the bureaucrats are dead-wrong about the cause of

Pfiesteria outbreaks and related human illness syndromes. As long as it is "politically correct" to attack nutrient use (agriculture), there's little reason to expect a landscape or systems approach to the scientific testing necessary for evaluating the various hypotheses about factors influencing *Pfiesteria* blooms.

As I explained at great length in my 1998 book, *Pfiesteria: Crossing Dark Water* (350 pages, Gateway Press), the more important trigger for blooms of this increasingly active toxic dinoflagellate is more likely to be dissolved copper and other fungicides that are generally safe on land, but promote the toxin-bearing form of *Pfiesteria* by killing off its micro-organic food supply in estuarine waters. Sure, nutrients are important in laboratory growth of *Pfiesteria*. But the systems approach, the larger perspective, demands that we not overlook the role of toxic chemicals such as the ubiquitously present copper, along with some especially powerful fungicides—the dithiocarbamates —which are present at every kill site (but *not* present at sites without kills).

Since the publication of the book two years ago, evidence in support of the "Copper Theory" has continued to emerge. But public opinion cannot be shaped overnight, and certainly not by an unknown author. Nonetheless, the effort to understand the true causes and effects of *Pfiesteria* is beginning to cut through the layers of political denial that have covered up this key health issue in recent years.

The Copper Theory has important implications for agriculture on the east coast of the United States. In Maryland, especially, the agricultural industry has been targeted as the "source of nutrient enrichment" that "continues to poison the Chesapeake Bay." And so what, if that scenario has never actually been proven by rigorous science?

What matters most, when it comes to this issue, is that "nutrient enrichment" has become the magical buzzword that attracts millions of dollars in research grants to institutions and individuals who can demonstrate that their science projects are focused squarely on nutrients. Let me state clearly: nutrient enrichment has a potential environmental cost. But the fact remains that it is far from being the lone culprit in harmful algal blooms, including *Pfiesteria*.

Like any breakthrough in science, my original Copper Theory had its share of rough edges. As a "scientific outsider" in the world of dinoflagellates, I knew that my research into the *Pfiesteria* epidemic would run up against some formidable opposition from the gurus of Big Science and the Big Money that supports Big Science in the development of new products. But I refused to be intimidated by my outsider status. (After more than 20 years as a practicing family physician, here in Pocomoke City, I'm still regarded as the "new doc in town!")

Of course, it's also true that scientific research on the epidemiology of *Pfiesteria* is less than three years old. Given all of these uncertainties, why should I have expected that anyone would listen to my ideas about the impact of toxic chemicals on food-chain relationships among phytoplankton communities along the Atlantic seaboard?

If nothing else, however, the publication of the book began to spark some penetrating questions from the news media. Washington Post reporter Todd Shields posed a typical question, while reporting on the issues discussed in *Crossing Dark Water*, when he bluntly asked:

"Why should we listen to you on the subject of *Pfiesteria*? After all, you're just a family physician!"

I told him: "Todd, the reason your readers should listen to me is that my opinion isn't for sale!" Somehow, that comment didn't make it into his story. Granted, I've never scored many points for tact or "political correctness." But the record shows that several of my early declarations about the "politics of *Pfiesteria*" have proved to be accurate.

After studying the problem for more than a year, I had by 1997 concluded that the biggest blooms of *Pfiesteria* were taking place in waters where downstream flow of dithiocarbamates (DTC) and copper had built up deposits in sediments. The kills at Shelltown in 1996 and 1997 had taken place directly adjacent to a black-plastic tomato culture operation that used both copper and DTC. Although the Pacific Tomato Company operation—a major player in the Shelltown area which also runs large tomato farms on Virginia's Eastern Shore—has now stopped using DTC as a pesticide, the region is still at risk from other DTC users.

Just as the blue mold epidemic caused tobacco growers in North Carolina to switch from non-toxic metalaxyl to the poisonous DTC (one year before the *Pfiesteria* blooms got started), some other grower will sooner or later feel compelled to resort to DTC when a new mutant arrives. That same scenario occurred in Florida, with a brown root-rot fungus threatening the orange groves that surround the St. Lucie River shortly before the massive fish kills there. In fact, this all too predictable scenario takes place frequently, all up and down the east coast.

Another disturbing example of how these toxic mutations occur involves a large fruit tree nursery alongside the Back Creek tributary of Maryland's Manokin River. That facility opened three years ago, and the *Pfiesteria* blooms started one year later. Why did it happen? To answer that question, just analyze the content of the pesticides being sprayed on America's fruit.

In addition, the multiple cases of *Pfiesteria*-related human illness near the tomato-farming operations along the St. Martin's River (within view of Ocean City) point directly to an undeniable association between heavy metal toxicity and fungicides and dinoflagellate blooms.

After *Pfiesteria: Crossing Dark Water* appeared in a spiral-bound edition in January of 1998, the Copper Theory began to make waves in Maryland's estuarine scientific circles. And the idea that copper might be triggering the blooms seemed to infuriate many members of the scientific elite, who became even more irked when the Pocomoke River Alliance began staging public forums to explore the idea that nutrients might not be the cause of the blooms, after all.

(In a delightful twist of irony, the Alliance was able to use some leftover 1996 Chesapeake Bay EPA research funds to question the Bay Program theories that underlie entrenched policy and public information.)

On one occasion, I was told that the director of the University of Maryland Center for Estuarine Sciences at Horn Point, Dr. Donald Boesch, had been instructed by his scientific colleagues to "engage" me in discussion. We met privately for about two hours at the Ward Museum in Salisbury (July, 1998).

While proposing that we attend a series of meetings designed to "build a consensus" in Maryland about toxics and toxins, Dr. Boesch offered to recommend that my ideas be discussed in a "concatenated fashion." But I felt sure that "concatenated" simply meant building on a set of false data based on false assumptions leading to a false conclusion. (On the other hand, Dr. Boesch was equally convinced that my own theory was flawed.)

You can be sure that I had no intention of going up against Dr. Boesch's entire faculty as a lone scientific voice during these "discussions." All I wanted was a fair test.

In the end, we agreed to disagree. And that's precisely what happened . . . until the announcement, a few months later, of an international *Pfiesteria* conference, to be held at Georgetown University in December of 1998.

When I learned about the approaching conference, I became determined to get there somehow. But I wasn't very surprised to discover that in spite of my numerous publications (including the *Pfiesteria* book) on the subject, I hadn't even been invited to the confab.

Unfazed, I phoned the organizers and complained that the scheduled program included not a single physician who had diagnosed and treated actual *Pfiesteria* patients.

In the end, the conference organizers decided on a compromise. I would be allowed to make a "poster presentation" of the data that Dr. Ken Hudnell (See Chapter Five, "Brilliant, Just

Brilliant") and I had accumulated on both CS testing for *Pfiesteria*-related illness and treatment via cholestyramine therapy.

Of course, I made sure that my conference "poster" also contained lots of environmental information detailing the use and frequency of application of toxic agricultural chemicals that had been dispersed near *Pfiesteria* attack zones in Maryland, North Carolina and Florida. I also added some data describing chemical contamination of porewater, by way of illustrating my thesis that these porewater-based toxic chemicals provide the trigger for the killing process, whenever they become re-suspended in the water column by wind, tide or wave action.

Surprisingly, the conference involved much more than just a predictable rehash of *Pfiesteria* information (See Chapter 7, "Ciguatera: Anatomy Of A Toxic Nightmare"). Dr. Boesch even went so far as to welcome "heretics" into the "official" discussion.

Surely that beyond-the-pale group included me . . . along with several other investigators from Virginia and the U.S. Geological Survey who claimed to have found a fungus—*Aphanomyces invadens*—growing on fish with *Pfiesteria* lesions.

Dr. Joan Bernstein of the Department of Environmental Protection in Florida had been the first to sound the *Aphanomyces* alarm, yet she'd never received the credit she deserved. This fungus was undoubtedly a mutant, not a benign saprophyte like its cousins. An organic monster, *Aphanomyces* crept inside the bodies of fish, then slowly digested them from the inside out. The liquefaction necrosis that I described in Chapter Two was probably the result of *Aphanomyces* action.

Before that could happen, however, a dinoflagellate toxin or some other disruption of the integrity of the protective mucus was required to slice an opening through the fish's slime-layer. Aphanomyces grew better in water enriched with copper than competing species of water borne fungi. In fact, fungus researchers working with *Aphanomyces* added a copper-based compound to their aquarium cultures of fungus to keep the more sensitive wild-type fungal organisms under control.

Aphanomyces was also unusual in another way: it enjoyed a far-flung distribution, and had already turned up in Scotland, Australia, Southeast Asia (where it was known as "red spot," or "ulcerative mycosis"), and the good old Sunshine State of Florida.

If the fungus traveled via ship ballast as some epidemiologists had speculated, that sounded like a highly erratic route. But Frank Fuzzell, the Florida nurseryman who had been at the center of a political storm over public health issues related to pesticide poisoning for more than a decade, had another theory (See Chapter 9: "Chronicles From A Poisoned Landscape"). A canny analyst, Fuzzell was certain that the distribution of *Aphanomyces* matched those areas where particular powerful mutagenic fungicides had been used on land.

There were plenty of data to support his observations . . . but unfortunately, there were almost as many variables involved in trying to prove that Chemical A caused Mutation B as in trying to uncover food chain disturbances caused by toxic chemicals!

Of course, I'd been hearing for years that Uncle Sam had dropped spermicidal chemicals on Vietnam as part of the "Agent Orange" campaign, and also that fungal toxins had been dropped on Laos by the Americans in 1981, as part of the "Yellow Rain" initiative. Were these lurid descriptions of conspiratorial links between the Pentagon and Big Business anything more than somebody's overheated imaginings? Or were the reports of bizarre organisms that made toxins actually true? And were those organisms now turning into aggressive pathogens because of secret alterations of their habitat—rather than as the result of natural selection via evolution?

Had we altered our environment in unpredictable ways with chemicals from laboratories, landfills and exhaust pipes? Of course we had. And what about our ever increasing use of chemicals down on the American farm? Even worse, what about the homeowners who didn't have the training or understanding to follow the instructions on labels for proper use of an arsenal of new commercial chemicals, including pesticides? Yes, it *does* matter that someone "threw in" a little extra of the off-the-shelf fungus killer into the fruit tree sprayer for the backyard trees last Saturday. More isn't better!

In order to attack these kinds of questions, it helps to remember that while physics is dominated by equal and opposite reactions, biology is less straightforward. Disturb one part of a food chain or eco-niche, and you won't be able to predict the "cascade" of changes in checks and balances that soon takes place. In biology, "equal and opposite chaos" is usually the result of sudden change. Long-term change will result from sudden change in ways that no one can predict.

Add fertilizer to an ecosystem, for example, and you'll usually get generalized stimulation of growth. Add chemical toxins, however, and you may find yourself watching a specific drop-off in growth, followed by a process in which an existing organism moves in to fill the newly created void.

Add mutagenic chemicals, and you may trigger the arrival of entirely new species. Now throw in some antibiotics—a form of toxic chemicals, after all—and observe the change in symbiosis between swarming colonies of bacteria and the organisms that live among them. Suffice it to say that billions upon billions of atoms make up the compounds that produce life, and each interacts in billions of ways with other living things.

Call me a "heretic," then. But the fact is that I simply can't accept the conclusions offered by one small group of scientists (regardless of their millions of dollars in research funding!) who have studied only a small part of one facet of the ecosystem.

If "family practice" is based on a "systems approach" to human health, why not employ the same approach when studying the immensely complex world of "ecological health?"

While I mulled these kinds of challenging questions in the spring of 1999, the *Pfiesteria* saga took yet another twist. But one thing remained the same: the political coverup. Although there would be 198 different fish kills investigated by the State of Maryland in 1999, only two were reported to the press . . . and those were after the fact.

But human beings were also getting sick from *Pfiesteria* in increasing numbers, all along the estuaries of Maryland's Eastern Shore.

During this period, Dr. Hudnell and I finished our double-blinded and placebo-controlled crossover clinical trial demonstrating that cholestyramine therapy worked—and that the Contrast Sensitivity test was an effective tool for both initial diagnosis and as a test to follow the beneficial effects of CSM treatment.

By August of 1999, growing numbers of patients were checking into my *Pfiesteria* Illness Center in Pocomoke. At the same time, there were reports that new *Pfiesteria*-like organisms were on the move in our local waters. How many other toxic dinoflagellates would be identified as they came out of the tainted mud? Hoping to answer that question, while also discrediting my data, Dr. Boesch organized a Maryland Technical Task Force meeting to review the "copper issue."

He cordially said he was quite willing to invite anyone I recommended, including EPA and USGS scientists, along with researchers from Virginia Tech who had published data confirming the concept of "adequate amount, adequate time, and adequate exposure" as a working basis for the Copper Theory.

The State lacked the resources to bring in Dr. Chien Wai, the dithiocarbamate fungicide expert from Idaho State University, but I had already forwarded his detection protocols to the Maryland Department of the Environment and they would be available. In a curious twist, the Maryland researchers at the conference told me they'd "never received a protocol for testing for the presence of dithiocarbamates."

Meanwhile, Margaret Maizel of the National Center for Resource Innovation (NCRI) had prepared a careful presentation documenting the need for a "landscape approach" that would parallel my "systems approach" to studying inputs of nutrients and toxins into estuaries. Salisbury State University agreed to videotape the conference, in order to preserve an accurate record for later discussion.

The discussion was spirited, to say the least. For starters, I presented the story of the agricultural disaster caused by an invasion of cylindrospermopsis in Florida's Lake Griffin (See Chapter Eleven: "The Monster In The Lake"), along with our new *Pfiesteria*-human health data. The point I wanted to hammer home was that the adverse effect of ag chemicals on microorganisms wasn't limited to *Pfiesteria*; it included numerous changes in habitat at several locations around the country.

My idea was actually quite simple: chemicals that were used safely on land could become toxic in water, after being captured in porewater and then perpetually recycled.

As the conference unfolded, there were numerous attempts by Dr. Boesch and his colleagues to undermine the copper data. But these obvious attempts at "the appearance of good science" (See Chapter 10: "The Appearance Of Good Science") were preserved for posterity on the university videotape.

In the end, the lead scientist at the Maryland Department of the Environment, Dr. Bob Summers, informed Dr. George Demas and Bruce Nichols (also on tape) that the State of Maryland had been testing "the wrong chemicals in the wrong places at the wrong time." The U.S. EPA and USGS scientists also confirmed the fact that they had seen the ham-handed attempts at data-destruction by the State team. And all of these investigators let me know that their efforts to obtain funding for proper testing would be redoubled.

What next, I wondered, as I held up plastic bottles containing sediment and porewater taken that very morning from a fish kill area in Back Creek, near the Manokin River. The State would deny the presence of the toxins there, of course, until the public outcry overwhelmed their attempts at public relations damage control! Several months later, when the human health data became undeniable, even by the State, the confirmatory test results were released.

The State of Maryland had thrown its very best at me and these other researchers during the conference—and they'd clearly lost the battle of dueling words and dueling data. But would it make any difference? The poisons were in the river sediment to stay, and it was now clear that *Pfiesteria* would continue to flourish in warm weather and cold, regardless of the "nutrient issue."

In short, our poorly planned environmental policies had provided a habitat for an organism that would soon threaten a lot more than just a few fish in a few rural streams.

More than ever, I was convinced that the discovery of *Pfiesteria*-related human illness syndrome had opened a new window on the practice of medicine.

It now seemed clear that toxins which cause chronic diseases were being hatched in altered habitats, and that these "sheltered" new species would not be easy to identify in any laboratory.

Convinced that I'd stumbled upon a new kind of illness, I wondered how I could possibly make a difference in the politically distorted world of contemporary Big Science and Big Medicine. How could I make them listen, when their minds were already made up?

The answer to *that* question seemed about as clear as the black, silty loam-mud in the jar before me.

A Mysterious Illness

Shelltown, MD –August, 1997

The discovery of "chronic, neurotoxin-mediated illnesses" began innocently enough, on a drizzly August morning in 1997, when a young woman named Darla Hutchins walked into my office and presented me with a biological mystery.

Darla was sick, but she didn't know why.

She felt sure that she'd "caught something from the river," but she didn't know what it was.

All she knew was: *I better go see Dr. Shoemaker.*

That's because I'm one of the few "family docs" in my little town on the edge of the Chesapeake Bay.

I'm the one they frequently turn to, whenever they sense that something has gone wrong with them. Maybe it's a lump that they just noticed for the first time. Maybe it's dizzy spells, or shortness of breath, or a cough that just keeps hanging around.

They come to see me because I'm the family physician who's closest to home. Why drive 30 miles over to Salisbury, when you can drop by "Dr. Shoe's" right on Market Street?

"Hello, Ms. Hutchins. Good to see you today."

"Hi, Dr. Shoemaker. Thanks so much for working me in so quickly! Just call me Darla."

"No problem. The nurse tells me you've had severe diarrhea for two weeks."

"I sure have, doc, and that's not the worst of it. I've got a bad cough, my muscles ache like that bad flu I had two years ago, and I've got the worst headache of my life. I've tried everything in the medicine cabinet, and it didn't help a bit!"

Nodding empathetically, I take a good hard look at her pleasant face, her mild blue eyes. *Age: 34. Two kids. Single mother, works part-time at the grocery store. Holding her temples with each palm (a posture I later came to recognize as the "Pfiesteria Salute"), which is a sure sign of painful headache.*

As the "family doc" in this small town, I know Darla well enough to say "hi" to on the street, and to pick her aisle when I need to get checked out fast at the grocery store. But no more than that. Let's see . . . she's pale. Breathing too fast, but not wheezing. No fever, but she has beads of sweat on her forehead. Systemic symptoms, dramatic presentation in a non-complainer. What disease is this?

"Doctor Shoemaker, it isn't just the diarrhea. I've been feeling terrible for about a week. Just awful! To tell you the truth, I think I got sick in the river. I took my kids swimming, and I think there might have been something in the water. Some kind of poison, maybe.

"The kids are still fine, but for the past five days, I've had the worst headache of my life—and the worst diarrhea, to go along with it. Day and night it goes. I can't eat but I still end up in the bathroom."

During more than 20 years of family practice in smalltown Maryland, I've learned the importance of listening to my patients. After literally tens of thousands of consultations, I understand what every Family Physician sooner or later discovers: Let the patients talk—but keep them on track. As Sir William Osler, the great Johns Hopkins physician, once pointed out: "The patient will tell you what is wrong."

"We went over to Williams Point," Darla continued slowly,

"you know, where everybody goes to water ski? This was ten days ago. The kids splashed around in the shallows there, right at the bend in the river.

"I went in with them two or three times, and I dangled my legs in the water for about an hour—"

She broke off suddenly and began to cough. They were deep, wracking spasms. I watched her head drop toward the table as her abdominal cramps set in. This wasn't a simple viral illness. *Headache, bronchospasm, abdominal cramps. Meningitis from a virus like ECHO, or Coxsackie? Some unusual infection? Leptospirosis?*

"Everything went fine at the beach," she said when she'd recovered. "We got home before dark, and I fixed supper like I always do. But the next morning I woke up with this headache. A blaster! I had stomach cramps, too, and this really nasty case of diarrhea. Real watery, you know?"

I nodded encouragingly but didn't speak.

"Well, I told myself: 'I've just got a stomach bug, that's all.' I figured it would ease up after a few hours, so I went on into work. I work days over at Chesapeake Bell in Salisbury. I got to my work station okay, but the bug didn't ease up. Instead, it got worse. I thought my head was gonna blow off my shoulders, and the cramps had me nearly doubled over.

"By two o'clock I couldn't stand it anymore, so I checked out of the office and headed on home. I keep on coughing, but I never have a cold.

"Since then I've tried everything. Kaopectate, Pepto Bismol, Imodium—you name it. But the headaches and the diarrhea just won't go away. I couldn't get an appointment to see my doctor, but he called me in some dicyclomine and ordered blood work.

"But all that did was make my mouth dry. I can't work, and I'm scared . . ." her voice broke for a moment, came dangerously close to a sob. "I'm scared that if I get any sicker, I won't be able to take care of my two kids. I have to work!"

"I hear you, Darla, loud and clear." Then I asked my first question. "How long have you had problems sleeping?"

She blinked at me in surprise. "How did you figure *that* out? It's true. I didn't sleep a wink the first night I got sick—went to work totally exhausted. And things haven't gotten much better, since then. I barely sleep at all now. With this diarrhea and cramps, all I can do is steal a few minutes here, a few minutes there. Then I wake up again."

I listened carefully, and tried to think about a diagnosis. But the pace of Darla's illness just didn't fit what I was now seeing. *Sudden onset, multiple symptoms, prolonged duration, no fever, failure to respond to simple medications. A toxin, perhaps?*

Her physical exam was normal, despite her symptoms. All I found were a few wheezes, slightly reddened eyes, minimal abdominal pain—but no meningitis, pneumonia, or terrible surgical abdomen. Her blood count, urine and other screening tests that the primary doctor had ordered were normal.

Based on what I'd seen in other patients with similar symptoms during the past few days, it seemed quite likely that her cough would only go away when her diarrhea stopped. But why then? This wasn't a summer virus, or some strange "legionnaire's disease." I'd already called a few colleagues in infectious disease, gastroenterology and neurology about these strange symptoms, only to discover that they didn't have any answers either.

Mystified, I turned to my collection of "Shoe's Rules"—a group of medical aphorisms that define what I consider to be a parameter of high-quality medicine in action. "When in doubt, be thorough."

Another rule: "Help the patient; don't make them suffer, just because you, the doctor, can't diagnose the illness right away."

"Darla, the symptoms you describe include what we call 'secretory diarrhea.' It's a disorder in the lining of the small intestine." I went on to explain how the human body manufactures bile in the liver, then stores it in the gall bladder. Later, when we eat a meal that includes fatty foods, that same bile is released into the intestine as an aid in digestion, along with cholesterol. After digestion of the fatty foods takes place, however, the bile salts and the cholesterol are supposed to be reabsorbed in the small intestine and recycled. Our body doesn't waste these complicated molecules that cost so much energy to make.

If that doesn't happen—because of a disease, maybe, or perhaps because of the presence of chemistry-altering toxins—the result will often be painful abdominal cramps and repeated attacks of watery diarrhea, with sleep-disturbing diarrhea a common feature.

One of the most effective weapons in the battle against secretory diarrhea, I explained, is a drug called cholestyramine (CSM). It binds both the cholesterol and the bile salts in the bowel, which prevents them from hanging around and causing the diarrhea attacks. Once these noxious substances are safely excreted, the tormenting "runs" and cramps will gradually subside for most patients. CSM is known to bind a few kinds of toxins as well.

"Darla, I'm going to give you a prescription for cholestyramine, and I want you to check in with me daily on your progress, after you start taking it. I don't have enough information yet to make all your symptoms fit the model of the disease I think you have. But first things first: Right now, I just want to stop the diarrhea and cramps and get you some rest.

"And I want you to stop by the lab on your way home, because we need to do some more tests on that diarrhea of yours. This case is not routine, and I want some facts to back up what I'm doing for you—including telling you what you *don't* have.

"Oh, and one other thing. Starting the day after you swam at Williams Point . . . have you noticed any rashes on yourself or on the children?"

She blinked. "Rashes? No . . . I haven't seen anything like that. And like I told you, the kids haven't been sick at all. What does the rash look like?"

"Small red lesions," I answered. "Most of them are about the size of a dime. And they're fiery red . . . I'm sure you'd have noticed them."

Now she smiled for the first time during our consultation. "I guess I should be grateful for small favors, huh? No, thank heavens—none of us have come down with a rash since we went to the beach. But why do you ask? Has some kind of disease gotten into the river . . . something that could cause a rash?"

I shook my head. "I've heard a few scattered reports of people getting sick around the water, Darla, but nothing conclusive. I'm not certain yet what it means."

"Fine. I've got enough to worry about, as it is." She gave a mournful laugh. "So what do you want me to do?"

"I want you to take the medication four times a day on an empty stomach. It's not easy to take, so I want you to call me tomorrow and tell me how you're doing. I expect your diarrhea and cramping to get better quickly."

She nodded, then sent me another brave smile. "Thanks for your help, doc. I'll catch you tomorrow."

• • •

After she'd gone, I returned to my office and stood looking out the window at Market Street, the main drag in Pocomoke City. Puzzled and frowning, I watched one of the town's three stoplights flash red, then green, then red.

Williams Point, again.

Although I hadn't mentioned it to Darla Hutchins (for obvious reasons), I'd been hearing a great deal about the Williams Point section of the Pocomoke River in recent days.

Only the previous afternoon, in fact, I'd received a phone call from an agitated young man named Roland Parsons, an enterprising businessman who ran his own drywall operation out of nearby Crisfield. As it turned out, the 24-year-old Parsons had been water skiing off Williams Point the same day Darla was there.

While Darla and her two kids frolicked in the shallows at the edge of the river as it made its big turn, Parsons had spent about 45 minutes zipping back and forth in the main channel. A novice who fell frequently, he'd roared with laughter each time his water skis had scooted away from him—plunging him bottom-first into the brackish waters of the Chesapeake Bay estuary.

But Roland Parsons hadn't been laughing when he appeared in my office five days later to show me the astonishing "fiery red zits" that dotted his arms and legs.

Along with 30 or 40 of the inflamed lesions, the troubled dry-waller was struggling with "a brutal headache"—as well as severe muscle aches, stomach cramps and other symptoms of what he suspected was a "bad case of the flu."

Even more alarming than those symptoms were the growing mental confusion and memory loss experienced by the youthful water skier. His wife said Roland was badly frightened by the way he seemed to be losing his ability to think clearly. "He didn't get far in school," she said, "but he's always been able to remember his computer passwords, up until now. He just isn't himself."

Within a matter of days, my worst fears about a potential disease epidemic were realized. I knew many of the watermen who worked the Pocomoke and adjoining rivers day in and day out. I'd spent many enjoyable hours listening to them describe the crabbing, oystering, fishing and muskrat-trapping that provided them with a living along the waterways that flanked the mighty Chesapeake.

These people were my friends. Many of them were scared, but too proud to admit that they knew their river was hurting them. Yet they were convinced that the water was making them sick . . . that some kind of alien, toxic substance had crept into the creeks and marshes of this swampy, tidal region, and that it was triggering many of the symptoms I'd just been looking at —including unusual lesions, bad headaches, aching muscles, blurred vision, secretory diarrhea, violent coughing and most alarming of all: loss of memory and disorienting confusion. (What was it Darla had told me? "I go to the store, and I get so confused—I can't remember what I'm supposed to buy!")

Known locally as "The Cell From Hell," *Pfiesteria* was a "dino-flagellate" microorganism that knew how to manufacture a nasty, fish-eating toxin, then deliver it to thousands of hapless fish of various species. Once affected, the fish would then swim about in confused circles, while the poison ate rapidly through the slimy protective coating around their scales.

It was a frightening scenario, and it was happening with increasing frequency in the summer of '97.

"We're seeing more and more dead fish floating on the water," the fishermen had told me, "and when we pick 'em up in our nets, we find all these bloody sores on 'em. What's going on, doc?"

It was one hell of a question.

And there were many like it, as I struggled to find the best way to help patients like Darla Hutchins and Roland Parsons. Among the major mysteries to have been triggered by the "*Pfiesteria* hysteria" that was growing rapidly along the Chesapeake Bay watershed were the following:

- Why did local watermen such as Tommy East and Ray Maddox keep finding dead fish floating on the waters of the Pocomoke and other Chesapeake Bay tributaries?

- Why did the Maryland State Health Department keep insisting that "our rivers are safe," when it seemed perfectly obvious to those of us who lived and worked along the waterways that something was attacking the fish population, and that local residents were getting sick left and right?

- If the humans who were falling ill along the watershed had come down with *Pfiesteria*-related illness, why were their symptoms so varied? Example: If Darla Hutchins' diarrhea and headaches were *Pfiesteria*-related, why hadn't she developed the same lesions that were being displayed by Roland Parsons and several other patients whom I'd examined?

- And finally: If "The Cell From Hell" really did cause a toxin-related illness in humans, how did the disease process work?

What was the specific physiology of the body's response to physical contact with *Pfiesteria*?

Was the toxin delivered through spores or by enzymes, as often happened with illnesses caused by *clostridia* bacteria and fungi? Or were the toxins released when the cell died . . . as in the case of Florida's notorious "red tide," and also in situations where the *cylindrospermospis* blue-green algae was killed by copper-based pesticides in Australia?

Another theoretical possibility also loomed: the idea that the toxin, alone or ascending in the food chain, might be responsible for the symptoms.

Did the organism have to get inside the human body in order to do its dirty work, like the "Traveler's Diarrhea" bug of Mexico and Central America?

• • •

While I wrestled with these medical problems over the next few days, Darla Hutchins was taking her medication and updating me daily on her progress.

Imagine my surprise on Day No. 3 when she called to say that all her symptoms, including her diarrhea and her killer-headaches, had vanished without a trace. I accepted her thanks, but I really didn't understand the basis for her improved headache. The diarrhea, sure. But her cough and memory, too? I'd certainly never cured a headache or a cough with CSM before!

There was no doubt that the substance lowered cholesterol. But few doctors still used it for that purpose, because better cholesterol-lowering drugs had been created in recent years.

Besides, as most practitioners and patients will quickly tell you, CSM often produces unpleasant side effects—including bloating, reflux and constipation.

The truth was, I didn't understand the biochemistry. Why had Darla gotten better? Her improvement was surely connected to the binding accomplished by the CSM. But this binding agent isn't absorbed. If the *Pfiesteria* toxin was causing her headaches—and that made sense—how did binding bile salts shut down that distinctively severe symptom?

Maybe the *Pfiesteria* toxin had been dissolved in her bile. But that would mean that the toxin dissolved in fat. And if that were true, then **other** fatty tissues (such as those found in the brain, and in lung surfactant) could also serve as reservoirs for the toxin.

What if the toxin was equilibrating throughout the body, with the bile providing the only "faucet" to the outside world?

If the toxin was secreted with bile into the duodenum (the upper small intestine) as part of her normal enterohepatic recirculation, would it be reabsorbed farther along in the ileum (the lower portion of the small intestine)—in the same way that bile and cholesterol get reabsorbed? That, after all, was how CSM works . . . by disrupting the circulation of cholesterol into intestine and back to bile.

The implications were fascinating. If the toxins were indeed moving from bile to intestine and back to bile, then the disease they caused would be chronic, and not just some short, self-limited illness. Darla had been sick for two weeks. Was that "chronic" enough to qualify for the disease model I was slowly building?

Still, maybe the cure-all had been nothing more than a happy coincidence? Had Darla's headaches simply been caused by her stress over the violent diarrhea attacks, so that eliminating the latter also took care of the stress factor? Had the rapid disappearance of her cough also been a coincidence?

At this point, I was fairly certain that Darla had been suffering from a *Pfiesteria*-related illness. But how could I prove that, and who would ever believe me, without clinical proof that the disorder even existed? Also, how would I be able to diagnose other patients—let alone treat them—in the absence of an authoritative lab test?

Questions, questions.

At this point, only two things seemed clear. First, a major

biological predator was loose in the river, and it was killing tens of thousands of fish.

Second, there was a great deal of convincing epidemiological evidence to suggest that the same predator was also making human beings who lived along the water very sick.

With a sigh, I ran my eyes along the medical bookshelf that covered one wall of my office on Market Street. No help there. If I were going to make a difference in diagnosing and treating this new disease, I needed a new medical education fast. This toxin-based epidemic was a new disease. It wasn't in any textbook and nobody was an expert.

It was time to begin learning more about the secret life of toxin-related diseases.

• • •

A Frankenstein for the 21st Century

Question: What is "disease," and how does it actually work to sicken or disable or kill people? You'd think a question as basic as this one would have a simple answer, right?

It doesn't. As a matter of fact, entire libraries have been written by biologists and physicians who tried to provide the elusive answer.

Disease is an immensely complicated phenomenon. For example: It can include both microscopic attackers (pathogens) and functional disorders that operate to deprive human cells of the vital ingredients they need in order to maintain the delicate physiological balance required for life.

These days, we can talk in great detail about the molecular biology of cancer and atherosclerosis, and we have some treatments that work. But we don't know the "why" of these common killers any more than the ancient Greeks did.

The truth is that our understanding of disease hasn't really progressed much beyond the ideas of such ancient physicians as

Aristotle and Galen. Those two early geniuses were convinced that the diseases they encountered around them were caused by "imbalances" in the unstable relationships between earth, air, fire and water.

These days we know a lot about DNA, TNF, nitric oxide, PCR, differential gene activation and enzymes with impenetrable names. And yet we are hard-pressed to understand the functioning of such biochemical entities as the "prion" (the culprit in Mad Cow Disease)—which is a protein that takes over genetic machinery, in the same way that the nucleic acids of DNA and RNA routinely perform this feat.

Given these kinds of biological imponderables, maybe there's something to be learned even in the Year 2000 from the ancient idea that life and health depend on maintaining a proper balance among the elements! Even the Ancient Greeks talked about "ecology" and "habitat."

It's important to remember that the early physicians were also philosophers. And the concept of "disease" as "lack of physiological balance" still has much to teach us. Without the required chemicals—food, oxygen, and substances necessary for electrical transmission (including minerals from the earth)—the individual human cell is no longer able to maintain its place in the "watery world" that we call the human body.

And when cells begin to malfunction or die because of lack of these nutrients, illness will not be far behind.

Perhaps the best way to understand disease is to ask ourselves: What goes on when a cell is living a healthy, well-balanced life? The answer is "homeostasis": the condition in which all of the complex energy needs of the cell are being met, and such vital tasks as excretion of waste products and cell reproduction are taking place in orderly fashion.

As long as homeostasis is successfully accomplished, the cell will be able to effectively take in energy and then expend it in order to protect itself against both organic invaders and internal ailments, should they suddenly make themselves known. This continuing "preparedness" on the cell's part is vitally important, because anything that interferes with the orderly transmission of "chemical messages" inside the cell will immediately cause a deterioration in its ability to maintain homeostasis.

If you're among the millions of Americans who followed the news reporting of the recent wars in the Persian Gulf and Kosovo, you probably remember how U.S. Pentagon officials talked repeatedly about their first military priority—which was "destroying the enemy's command and control systems."

The same principle applies to attacks on the cell by outside invaders. If you recall a bit of your high school biology, you'll remember that for most cells, the "command and control" mechanism is found in the "DNA," the complex substance (deoxyribonucleic acid) which makes up most of the "genetic blueprint" that ultimately dictates what goes on in the cell.

Immensely complex in terms of chemistry, the process of "command and control" is nonetheless simple as a concept. What happens is that the "blueprint messages" from DNA are converted into proteins and enzymes which then "manage" the moment-to-moment life of all parts of the cell. All of this activity takes places at the molecular level, however—which means that there are a myriad of ways in which the "messages" can be distorted or interrupted, whether by disease or accident or environment.

Most of the time, of course, the complex operations of the Command and Control Center go forward smoothly, without being interrupted. This happens in spite of the potential hazards that everywhere surround the cell . . . hazards such as excessive heat, radiation, ultraviolet light or harmful chemicals. If these hazards damage the DNA, they pose a huge threat to the regulation of the cell. A change in the DNA—a mutation caused by outside factors—could disrupt the command and control, killing the cell, or it could change the cell's ability to handle harmful threats from the environment. If the newly changed cell survives and reproduces, we call it a "new species."

Darwin didn't know all the reasons for "natural selection,"

only that the phenomenon was real.

Certain enzymes monitor DNA and cell functions, looking for adverse changes. When these are found, the enzymes set off a series of reactions that kill the altered cells. We call this programmed cell death "apoptosis." A key step in the process occurs when enzymes activate a powerful protein called "tumor necrosis factor alpha"(TNF). In biological terms, TNF is a "cytokine," an inflammatory substance released by white blood cells and other tissues.

Apoptosis is a part of the cycle of life and death. And cells that should die but don't are implicated in a series of diseases, such as osteoporosis, cardiomyopathy, lung disease and neurologic disease, along with many others. Defective apoptosis is the end result of TNF and other cytokines doing the wrong thing at the wrong time.

Example: because a toxin known as "fumonisin," made by a fusarium fungus, can short-circuit the process of apoptosis, the mutated or defective cell can sometimes live on. And if that cell reproduces, we could end up with a new organism—one with less bone, perhaps, along with fewer normal neurons and fewer normal cardiac muscle cells.

The key concept to remember is that the cell is constantly adapting to its changing environment. Awash in freshly oxygenated blood, in people (or in water, for a Pfiesteria organism), that environment consists of both nutrients (various forms of glucose from sugars, for the most part) and electro-chemical "messages" from the central nervous system, which are also arriving moment by moment with information designed to help the cell monitor traffic, control motility, digest foods, eliminate waste and guard against potential invaders.

If all of this sounds staggeringly complex, it is. But that complexity is absolutely essential to the life of the cell—because the threats arrayed against it are numerous and powerful. And disease always involves disruption of the cell's dynamic, second-to-second regulation of its own physiology.

Types of Diseases: A Thumbnail Sketch

A simplistic way to understand the functioning of diseases is to group them in terms of their attacking methods. If, for example, we are confronting a disease that interferes with the "messengers" coming to the cell from the bloodstream or nervous system, we know that it will involve the "hormones" (the messengers, in most cases), and thus belongs among the "endocrine" (hormonal) illnesses. Our concept of endocrine-mediated illnesses is evolving as we understand more about the role of cells releasing locally-distributed messengers (the "neighborhood endocrine system").

Another type of toxic chemicals, the "cytokines" mentioned above, are released by white blood cells, especially lymphocytes, monocytes, macrophages and fat cells (yes, the adipocyte has an endocrine function!) that serve as messengers.

On the other hand, if the disease agent attacks sugar digestion or energy production inside the cell, we define it as a "disease of metabolism." This group of ailments would include such common disorders as diabetes and obesity caused by malfunctioning insulin. Not surprisingly, cytokines such as TNF-alpha that serve as hormone messengers can interfere with other hormones, such as insulin. Medicines that help treat diabetes—such as the new wonder drugs, the "glitazones"—in part do their job by defeating the effects of TNF on insulin receptor function.

Vascular diseases are those that involve problems in the delivery of oxygen and nutrients to cells via the bloodstream. "Hardening of the arteries," or atherosclerosis, is the classic example of a vascular disease which destroys cells by gradually shutting down their supply of oxygen and nutrients.

Some toxins cause symptoms by setting off spasm of small blood vessels as the result of muscle contractions in their walls.

Other toxins produce narrowing of the inside passageways of blood vessels. This happens when white blood cells "marginate," or form a thick sludge along inside walls. Our recently identified "bad guy" chemical—TNF—is a major player in this phenomenon, as well.

Of course, there are many other diseases in which foreign invaders attempt to choke off the normal functioning of the cell.

These microscopic marauders can include both bacterial diseases (such as pneumonia), which attempt to enter the cell and "steal" its nutrients, or viral agents (such as influenza), which "trick" the cell's DNA into replicating the invader's own genetic material, in order to take over and consume the latter's store of precious energy.

The parasites are another powerful group of diseases. They often attempt to penetrate cell walls ("membranes"), in order to feed on the nutrients within. Malaria is a good example of a protozoa which debilitates human beings by literally "stealing" the energy from their cells, one cell at a time. Parasites change the cell membranes of the host, making the host's bloodstream supply the parasites ensconced in red blood cells with nutrients and minerals, especially calcium. Newer treatments, not yet released for use by patients, kill the parasite by shutting off the membrane-based feeding tube, which prevents the calcium-dependent invader from obtaining that chemical from the bloodstream. Goodbye, parasite.

Another example of an intracellular parasite that lives "by the kindness of passing strangers" carrying calcium is Babesia, a pathogen commonly found co-infecting patients with Lyme disease. This ailment has been making headlines nationally, as more and more people are bitten by the ticks that carry this chronic disease. Babesia has always depended on red blood cells to aid in feeding the parasite as it gets ready to reproduce.

The idea that illnesses from toxins involve cytokines, including TNF, is closely linked to the models presented by those diseases.

Pathogenic Toxins: The "Gunfire" of Disease?

Some of the most complex (and interesting) diseases are the result of the work of organisms that produce poisonous substances—toxins—that work in one way or another to disrupt or even destroy cell functioning.

As every good zoologist or botanist will quickly tell you, the biological process in which living creatures produce and then deploy toxic weapons against both predators and prey is nearly as old as life itself.

Poisonous snakes are a good example; they manufacture toxins (aka "venom") to help subdue their prey, or as a weapon to fend off potential attackers.

Seemingly harmless walnut trees provide another interesting example of the use of poisons for survival. These forest-edge creatures release a substance from their roots, "juglone," that kills (or at least inhibits the growth of) plants in competition for the water and nutrients that the mother tree needs.

And most predators would never dream of eating a poison-producing tree frog along the Amazon. Why? It's simple. Some of the frog's toxins are among the most lethal toxic substances on earth—to the point that merely touching the substance can bring rapid death to many species.

Almost as frightening, at least for humans, are the toxins manufactured by various types of "*streptococcus*" bacteria. These powerful germs can destroy host DNA, muscle and red blood cells at will. Along with their thoroughly nasty cousins—the "flesh-eating" *staphylococcus* bacteria that can trigger "Toxic Shock Syndrome," along with "Scalded Skin Syndrome" and other dangerous diseases—this group of pathogens has likely been a tormentor of our species since those distant epochs when we first began to walk upright. (On the other hand, the upright walking may have been one of the many biological/enzymatic changes that helped man survive staphylococci, by protecting the hands and arms from cuts that could have allowed bacteria to enter the body.)

But the toxin-producing germs are hardly alone in their quest to take over human cells by first poisoning them. Another huge group of organisms that use poisons as a kind of "cellular gun-fire" are the fungi. These curious organisms have in recent years enjoyed a pretty good reputation among *homo sapiens* . . . since many of the toxins they produce as weapons against bacteria are today used by humans as antibiotics.

What is life-saving penicillin? Seen from the perspective of the fungi, it's nothing more than a means of seeking a "selective advantage" in the struggle for survival, by poisoning any local bacteria which happen to be competing for the same food and space that the fungi need in order to thrive. Toxins are frequently used as antibiotics.

But you can be sure that the bacteria, themselves, are not standing idly by, while their competitors develop increasing ability to manufacture and employ lethal toxins. Take the scourge known as cholera, for example. What causes the massive diarrhea that results in rapid dehydration and kills so many victims of this dreaded disease? The answer is toxins: poisons that are produced by the cholera bacteria after it successfully invades its human host.

Botulinum, gas gangrene and tetanus are other ugly examples of ways in which bacteria have learned to cook up a nasty menu of cell-threatening toxins, in order to stay on an equal footing with their evolutionary competitors.

Short-Term Vs. Long-Term Toxins

The toxin-mediated illnesses described above include some of the most virulent pathogens known to the human species. Yet there is one merciful component in all of these ailments, and its name is "duration." Almost without exception, the bacterial, viral and parasitic organisms I've mentioned all stop producing toxins when they, themselves, die. And if the patient survives the attack, those pathogen-hatched toxins will soon be flushed out of the body, allowing the patient to regain his health and get on with the business of living.

Survive the bloody diarrhea and enervating dehydration caused by cholera, for example, and your exhausted system will gradually cleanse itself of the toxins left behind by the now-vanquished pathogen.

In most humans, this "flushing out" of the "leftover poison" takes certain predictable forms. For starters, the toxins are excreted in urine or stool. But they can also be neutralized and transformed by the metabolic machinery of the liver enzymes. Or the body's immune system can attack and destroy them, molecule by molecule, as the healing and cleansing process unfolds.

So far, so good.

Kill the invading germs, and the bug's leftover toxins become a mere nuisance—garbage left on the street until the sanitation crew comes along to sweep it away and hose down the affected area.

But ask yourself: What would happen if the body were unable to clean out those toxins, and thus restore the cells to their normal, healthy chemistry?

What would happen if a group of diseases underwent genetic change because of a pollution-altered environment . . . *and then produced a chemically altered toxin that the body didn't eliminate, because the body had never encountered this kind of "toxic mutant" before?*

According to the latest research, many of today's toxin-predators have never been observed in such numbers before. In central Florida, for example, certain toxin-producing blue-green algae, *cylindrospermopsis*, were not found in freshwater lakes until 1995. Yet these toxic microorganisms now account for 95 percent of the *total* algal biomass in the lakes of the Ocklawaha watershed! In other words, a life-form that would normally represent no more than one percent of 4,000 botanical species in that habitat now accounts for 95 percent of the biomass.

The bottom line here is simply that the ever-increasing use of chemicals in our contemporary lifestyle—or changes in our landscape—has helped to create new "habitats" for toxin-linked microorganisms. And it's not just chemicals that create new habitats for these pathogens. In many ways, our contemporary lifestyles are equally to blame.

As millions of city dwellers and suburbanites move into rural areas and occupy former farmlands, they alter habitats by providing food and cover as well as by eliminating predators for a growing deer population—and thus help to create a habitat for ticks that transmit *Babesia*, *Ehrlichia* and Lyme disease.

And what happens when these organisms release toxins that end up circulating through the fat-containing tissues of human beings?

In that nightmarish scenario, the body cannot excrete or metabolize or immunologically rid itself of the disabling toxins . . . which gradually pile up, traveling from fatty tissue reservoirs— including nerves, brain, muscle, tissues lining joints, eyes, sinuses, lung and bile and back—without ever having to face the attack of an antigen-primed white blood cell.

In most cases, these stored toxins don't cause cell death, since the attacker that made them has already been wiped out, shutting down poison production.

But these stored toxins do not go away, either.

Housed indefinitely inside the body's various systems, these threatening substances move from fatty tissue to intestine to liver to brain to muscle to lung and back again, triggering endless problems inside cells that cannot be cleansed.

And the result?

Meet "chronic, neurotoxin-mediated illness," which has recently emerged as a new class of painfully debilitating illnesses that are making life difficult for millions of Americans.

These subtle, often misdiagnosed new illnesses, targeted for the first time in *Desperation Medicine*, represent nothing less than an "evolutionary leap" in human pathology. They are frightening if we don't understand them—but facts can cure fear, and the necessary facts are contained in this book.

As often seen in medical history, we cannot diagnose a group of diseases by using a standard blood test or culture. Those vital diagnostic tools can tell us nothing—since the "stealth toxin" does its damage without being alive!

The patients cry out for help . . .
but no one can hear them!

For ten million desperate Americans today, toxin-mediated illness is as real as the agonizing headaches, the aching muscles, the fatigue, the cough, the light-sensitivity, the night blindness, the shortness of breath, the blurred vision and the impaired memory that constitute its major symptoms.

Ask yourself: If physicians can't administer a clinical test to scientifically validate the presence of toxins that make us sick, how can they hope to convince skeptical observers that the poisons are really at work in the bodies of their victims?

Imagine the daily life of a patient suffering from a chronic, toxin-mediated illness. No one can even prove that the disorder exists, because there are no diagnostic tools.

Yet the victim struggles to find the strength to get out of bed in the morning—and why not? With so many parts of his or her body not working properly because of retained toxins, is it any wonder that the patient often can't find the strength to make a cup of coffee? (But they really *aren't* sick, are they? They're merely tired, and suffering from a brain-fog that their hurried physician has named "depression.")

Horrible? You bet. And there's more. Because the victims of toxin-mediated illness—unlike those suffering with such old-fashioned complaints as asthma or diabetes—soon discover that their painful symptoms also change from day to day.

Depending on which organ isn't working right because of the fat-circulation of soluble toxins, the symptoms can shift without warning, and within a few hours. Fatigue, weakness, muscle ache, headache, difficulty with memory or concentration or both, red eyes, blurred vision, hypersensitivity to light, nasal congestion, sinus congestion, cough, abdominal pain that defies anatomic diagnosis, metallic taste, wheeze and shortness of breath that acts like asthma: This is only a partial list of the afflictions caused by toxin-pileup in the human body.

Now add nausea, abdominal cramps, secretory diarrhea and

joint pain that acts like rheumatoid arthritis to the mix, and you can see why some of my toxin-afflicted patients have stayed home from work for weeks and months at a time. Yet they rarely succeed in obtaining disability compensation for these ailments, because no test confirms the diagnosis.

Oh, you'll be given a diagnosis, all right: "Irritable bowel syndrome." Or maybe it will be "stress," or "sinus problems," or "fibromyalgia" or "memory loss due to age"—anything in order to process you through the medical care system.

But as you'll discover in the chapters that follow, these are breathing, struggling, suffering human beings. They are real people with real illnesses . . . with diseases that have been caused by a fast-growing population of predatory organisms.

Who are these hydra-headed toxin-makers now invading the waterways and forests and once-pristine estuaries of the industrialized world?

Think of them as the "New Frankenstein"—as a bio-monster unwittingly hatched by our runaway technology, as the planet increasingly becomes awash in pesticides, acids, plastics, chemical solvents used in manufacturing and a thousand other toxic substances that our new lifestyle requires.

And how does the dark synergy between our lifestyle changes and the ecosystem actually operate?

Let's think about Lyme disease for a moment. In recent years, as the Lyme epidemic had spread through the northeastern United States (300,000 new cases per year, but only a fraction reported), many of us have learned how ticks can harbor certain bacteria, called *Borrelia*, a spirochete distantly related to the syphilis spirochete.

If an infected tick transmits the spirochete to a human, the result will often be continuing, low-grade fever, along with fatigue and listlessness, rashes, Bell's Palsy, arthritis and even damage to the heart. Those of us who treat chronic Lyme patients know that the illness does many other awful things to its victims, as well.

Science has known for a long time that antibiotics can kill the spirochete. So why does this syndrome persist for years—even decades—after the "bug" has been killed in many patients? We know that "Chronic Lyme" can act like rheumatoid arthritis, with disabling, disfiguring joint problems.

And we know that other Chronics begin to develop memory problems and concentration problems as well as continuing pain.

Is there a sanctuary for the Lyme organisms that live on despite antibiotics? Is that the explanation for this chronic disease? Or is the illness due to toxins released by the spirochete while it lives within you—poisons that cannot be cleansed from your body later? Lyme is just one of the illnesses in which toxins play a major role.

Genetically altered by our fast-changing, pollution-soaked environment, this new type of microorganism-produced toxin is rarely eliminated successfully by the human excretory and immune systems. To understand why, we need to understand how industrial and agricultural chemicals can alter the balances of ecosystems in water and soil. Obviously, every new "niche" we create for some new organism by changing the environment will have some unpredictable effect on other parts of the community of organisms that invisibly surrounds us.

This is precisely what happened to Lyme disease. Until April 9th, 1999, there was no proof that the Lyme spirochete actually manufactured a toxin. But then a Boston University microbiology Ph.D. named Mark Cartwright shocked the scientific world with a sudden breakthrough, after he was able to demonstrate the presence of a new kind of neurotoxin made by *Borrelia*.

Dr. Cartwright's findings dove-tailed nicely with my own continuing research on how environmentally acquired toxins actually work on the human body. His great breakthrough was to show that the Lyme spirochete can manufacture a neurotoxin.

Well why not? If Lyme disease included neurotoxins, I could diagnose and treat that kind of problem. I was certain I could show that my treatment protocols worked on antibiotic-treated patients with chronic symptoms.

Yet the immensely gratifying experience of helping my Lyme patients get better paled in the face of the revelation that came upon me, when I realized that Lyme was only one of a dozen new chronic illnesses mediated by biotoxins.

For me, the discovery of a new illness triggered by *Pfiesteria* was the doorway into an entirely new dimension of disease. And like Alice falling down the rabbit hole into Wonderland, I found myself struggling to understand a world full of strange new creatures—the biologically produced neurotoxins—that no one had studied in this way before. The chapters that follow will tell the stories of patients who were healed, usually beginning within a few days, of debilitating, chronic diseases that had been haunting them for years.

Nothing previously used had helped provide relief for these long-suffering victims, some of whom had been carrying their afflictions for as long as 20 years. Some had even contemplated suicide, in order to escape the daily suffering from an illness that the "experts" insisted didn't even exist.

After ten years of chronic pain, what would the victim of a chronic, neurotoxin-mediated illness do to start feeling better in just 36 hours?

Patients with longstanding illnesses will do just about anything to feel better, so desperate are they. "Just make the pain go away, doctor. If that's all I get from your treatment, I will be grateful!"

In order to help these struggling patients, I invented "Desperation Medicine."

"Any relief is a godsend; any cure is a miracle!"

chapter 5

Reflection

Brilliant, Just Brilliant. Sometimes the Best Ideas Are the Simplest Ones.

Research Triangle Park, NC –August, 1998

Do you remember that wonderful old Chinese saying: "Less is more?"

The ancient philosopher who coined that memorable phrase surely understood something important about the nature of elegance.

I suspect that he understood how it depends, above all else, on a quiet and understated simplicity.

Take architecture, for example. While some critics will praise the ornate, complex flourishes of the Baroque or the Rococco and find them exquisitely elegant, my own temperament leads me in a different direction. For me the crisp, uncluttered lines of a Frank Lloyd Wright building speak volumes about the elegance to be found in simple things. At the same time, I've always appreciated Hemingway's famous remark about the craft of writing . . . his wry comment that the "most important part of any story is the part you leave out!"

If you think about it, you soon realize that the best science is also simple and elegant. The most significant discoveries— whether we're talking about Einstein's Theory of Relativity or Heisenberg's Uncertainty Principle—usually take place after a thinker manages to find a clear, direct path to a simplified concept, while ignoring the tangle of complexities on every side.

One way to picture this kind of "scientific elegance" is to remember the medieval symbol of "Occam's Razor." In that famous metaphor, the razor's edge becomes the super-sharp edge of thought that gradually shaves away everything inessential, leaving behind only the brilliance of a perfectly crystallized idea.

But what could be more out of fashion in today's noisy, contentious world of Big Politics and Big Media than philosophical principles from the Middle Ages? Look around you, and what do you see? Endless political posing, and the quest for the "ultimate sound bite." Talk-show "experts" who insist they can solve every human problem—everything from nail-biting and obesity to preventing outbreaks of nuclear war.

Is it any wonder, given this modern cacophony, that our fast-growing epidemic of chronic, neurotoxin-mediated illness has not yet been *recognized*, let alone confronted and addressed by the Medical Establishment? Fortunately for all of us, however, one scientist's voice has remained calm, clear and uncluttered during the recent debate over the pathology of such difficult-to-diagnose illnesses as chronic Lyme Disease and Chronic Fatigue Syndrome.

Dr. Ken Hudnell has made a quiet but magnificent contribution to this area of medicine. Occam's Razor in action! In a brilliant movement of thought, he brought logic and simplicity to the diagnosis of *Pfiesteria*. Then he worked with me to unravel the mysteries of many other human illnesses. His particular gift was to have realized that he could use an obscure neurotoxicological test as a reliable and reproducible method for demonstrating deficits in the brain's ability to discern visual patterns, as a result of damage caused by neurotoxins.

Starting about four years ago, Dr. Hudnell began giving this test—which is especially good at detecting neurotoxicological effects—to patients who had been exposed to North Carolina estuaries where major fish kills had occurred. His tests made one key fact compellingly clear: the same deficits did not occur in other residents ("control patients," in scientific lingo) who had been exposed to waters without fish kills. Dr. Hudnell's work also demonstrated that the deficits were detectable for months after exposure.

The "razor" had done its job!

Almost overnight, the great debate about whether or not it was possible to accurately diagnose *Pfiesteria* evaporated into thin air. The mystification had ended . . . because the diagnosis could now be made in five minutes, using a simple bedside test. At the same time, the politicians found that they could no longer announce: "This disease is self-limited," since the deficits had proved to be persistent. Dr. Hudnell was obviously *right* . . . which meant that the scramble to obscure the importance of his findings would have to begin.

It did. Within a matter of days, the "spin masters" and the double-dealing public health bureaucrats were hard at work, doing their best to weaken the impact of Dr. Hudnell's breakthrough. (For a quick look at how the process works, check out Chapter 10, "The Appearance of Good Science.")

The bureaucrats did their best to knock Ken Hudnell off the playing field, but he wouldn't allow it to happen. And that was right in character. From the day I met him, Dr. Hudnell has demonstrated the kind of personal integrity—along with the unstoppable tenacity—that is required to continue to press on despite lack of recognition and understanding from organizations like the CDC.

When the *Pfiesteria* epidemic exploded in my Eastern Shore neighborhood back in 1996, I spent a lot of hours calling up academic scientists in search of answers about the toxicology and physiology of this noxious invader. In most cases, I received very little help. Who had time to talk with an obscure "Family Practice Doc" about an illness that was supposedly being spread by a one-celled microorganism way out in rural Maryland?

But Dr. Hudnell was different. He hadn't heard much about my research, but so what? Far from regarding me as an annoyance or as a drain on his precious time, he was genuinely interested in my findings. He also kept his promise to send me his published papers on *Pfiesteria*, manganese, learning disability, Contrast Sensitivity and more. And he soon introduced me to CS, while explaining the basics with the patience and eloquence of a born teacher.

Dr. Hudnell knew his stuff. Even better, he understood the "politics of *Pfiesteria*" and the insular, labyrinthine world of government-funded research. He was also familiar with most of the researchers on this toxin-linked illness, but he refused to be drawn into their personality conflicts and squabbles. Dr. Hudnell wasn't interested in personalities or egos; what he wanted was a chance to apply his "razor" to a few potentially useful scientific concepts.

Armed with a Ph.D. in experimental psychology (including a minor in neurobiology) from the University of North Carolina, Dr. Hudnell had earned undergraduate degrees in chemistry and psychology (and most of a degree in philosophy). Always unpredictable, however, he had postponed his scientific career for three years, while operating a scuba-diving enterprise in the Virgin Islands. But it wasn't long before his special gift for understanding the physiology of vision and the nervous system brought him back to academe—and to the study of "neurotoxicology and the environment."

He spent three years associated with the EPA, as a Research Fellowship recipient from the National Research Council, where he would conduct research showing how Contrast Sensitivity testing can provide an excellent measurement of changes in stationary and motion correlates of vision.

Beginning in 1988, Dr. Hudnell became a permanent principal investigator for the Neurotoxicology Division of the U.S. Environmental Protection Agency's National Health and Environmental Effects Research Lab at Research Triangle Park, N.C.

While raising three children (Alex, Caroline and Max) with his wife Marla, he noticed the problems that were confounding North Carolina farmers and agriculture experts alike. One of those problems involved major changes that were occurring along the Neuse River watershed, after the recent development of hog farms on the sandy soils of eastern North Carolina. Ken worried about the changes in the river environment and he had a personal interest in the area where the Neuse flows into the brackish Pamlico Sound near New Bern . . . since this particular patch of ground happened to include his original family home.

The nutrient-enriched waters of the Neuse were now contaminated with blooms of toxic blue-green algae, also known as "cyanobacteria." He was also well aware of the fact that some rivers in eastern North Carolina flow over phosphate-enriched bedrock laid down during the Miocene and Cretaceous geologic eras . . . which meant that they had been the subject of phosphate enrichment long before the arrival of the Carolina hog farms, which were allegedly the source of growing environmental pollution.

When Dr. Hudnell took a closer look, he discovered that the nutrient-enrichment problem had been magnified by the recent failure of retaining walls around some large lagoons, which had permitted millions of gallons of liquid hog manure to surge into waters already full of phosphates. The practice of spraying lagoon sludge onto fields that drain into rivers via local creeks had also contributed to the problem. And the situation was only exacerbated by the fact that the sandy soils of the coastal plain of eastern North Carolina permit rapid influx of contaminants from manure (and pesticides too) in groundwater.

The emergence of metalaxyl-resistant blue mold and the subsequent switch of tobacco farms from using metalaxyl back to the old standby, dithiocarbamate fungicides, didn't attract much attention from the news media. But that key environmental change was significant, because it was one of the first-ever examples of how chemicals could change the biological habitat and thus promote the development of new, toxin-wielding microorganisms. In the case of blue mold, the results were catastrophic—with tobacco growers throughout the region looking on helplessly, as the unstoppable mold destroyed crops worth $5,000 an acre or more.

Soon the *Pfiesteria*-linked fish kills of the early 1990s were also taking off in earnest. What was going on along the Neuse? One of the first breakthroughs in the struggle to understand the physiology of this toxic invader took place at nearby North Carolina State University, where researchers Dr. JoAnn Burkholder and Dr. Howard Glasgow were able to show that this unique predator displayed "multiple life forms"—while also generating toxins that seemed impervious to all antidotes. In 1995, these two investigators reported several cases of laboratory-acquired illness from exposure to the toxins.

While most scientists in the field of toxicology accepted the validity of the Burkholder-Glasgow reports without question, there was far more opposition to early descriptions of *Pfiesteria*-related human illness syndrome that had been acquired in the wild.

Patients who reported such illness were instantly labeled as suffering from "*Pfiesteria* hysteria," and then resoundingly ignored. And this politically inspired refusal to face the epidemiological facts continued until the publication of my scientific paper on human acquisition of *Pfiesteria* illness in the wild. As it turned out, that document was also the first paper of its kind to be published in the world literature.

After a momentary blip of reality in Maryland—during which affected rivers were closed and some of my cases were confirmed by state health workers—the politicians once again took control of the "spin" on the *Pfiesteria* story. Suddenly, the "confirmed" cases became "possible" cases, and the 60 *Pfiesteria* patients whom I'd already identified were being described as a "handful" of cases. In the same way, media descriptions of "the 30 rivers that had experienced fish kills" metamorphosed into "fewer than five rivers."

Later still, when I reported successful treatment of chronic cases of *Pfiesteria* illness, the disease somehow became identified as "self-limited."

Soon after that, the CDC convened a conference designed to explore diagnosis and treatment of *Pfiesteria* . . . and I learned to my chagrin that the confab would be restricted to "academic physicians"—they had never seen or treated any *Pfiesteria* patients as primary physicians—whose assignment was to develop the guidelines for an entity known as "Possible Estuarine Associated Syndrome [PEAS]!"

What we really needed at that point, of course, was an objective test that would allow us to pinpoint the symptoms of *Pfiesteria* by identifying their neurotoxic basis.

Enter Dr. Hudnell, who had already begun using Contrast Sensitivity as a diagnostic tool among a small cohort of North Carolina watermen. Because of his training, this scientist understood that the retina was actually a "microcosm" of the brain; indeed, he had been experimenting with Contrast Sensitivity since his days in grad school. Ken was also well aware of the fact that a new form of the CS test—a "second-generation" version, if you will—had already solved many of the methodological problems that had dogged the test in previous years. Known as the "Functional Acuity Contrast Test," or "FACT," this exciting new diagnostic tool had been designed by Dr. Arthur Ginsburg.

The concept was simple enough. What Ginsburg had figured out was that you could effectively test the limited outputs of neurons in the visual system by presenting them with sinusoidal wave patterns among lines printed on a special card.

As opposed to unlimited outputs from cortical (or "cognitive") impulses, those from vision system neurons are limited to color, pattern, motion, central, peripheral, binocular, contrast and a few other effects, according to Dr. Hudnell. Access one and you access them all!

Ken and his fellow neurotoxicologists had done a great deal of work with laboratory rats, as well as humans, mainly using electrophysiological and neurobehavioral techniques. And when the State of North Carolina asked the EPA for assistance with its *Pfiesteria* investigation, Dr. Hudnell was ready to add a battery of visual tests to the broad-based series of clinical, laboratory, neurologic, neuropsychological and neuro-behavioral assays that were already planned.

In the end, only Ken's test showed a deficit. His diagnostic tool located a persistent sensitivity-impairment that matched persistent symptoms. Excited about his discovery, he agreed to start working with me in August of 1998 on my own fast-growing cohort of *Pfiesteria* patients. And it was at that point that that he began to break new ground in the area of diagnosing neuro-degenerative effects from the environmental acquisition of toxins. By combining his own researches with my deployment of FACT to measure successful treatment of CSM-mediated therapy of chronic illnesses, he joined me in the discovery of a whole new family of diseases characterized by chronic toxin-injury to patients.

During the same period, the amazing Dr. Hudnell was instrumental in obtaining a $200,000 EPA research grant to test my environmental theories. Studies investigating the relationship between copper contamination of porewater by pesticide runoff into the estuaries and *Pfiesteria* blooms would be conducted in Dr. Burkholder's lab and in an EPA research facility.

That research will probably not be able to answer the question: "Why *Pfiesteria*?" But it now seems certain to open some exciting new windows on the complex relationships between "alteration of the habitat" (via widespread use of pesticides and other chemical substances) and the spreading epidemic of chronic, neurotoxin-mediated human illness.

It took another two years before Ken could present the results of our "Residential and Recreational Acquisition" scientific paper at a "Maryland *Pfiesteria* Task Force" meeting. But his message came across loud and clear: FACT had been instrumental in restoring the health of 54 patients from Maryland who'd visited my office for treatment.

Elegant simplicity! Dr. Hudnell's genius in this scientific episode had been his innate ability to recognize a very uncomplicated fact: the idea that vision presents simple "endpoints" which can be used to measure the effect of neurotoxins. And that insight led to a major shift in thinking about *Pfiesteria*. During that same meeting in Annapolis (March, 2000), the renowned biotoxin researcher Dr. John Ramsdell presented data showing for the first time the presence of receptors for toxins (found in water from tanks containing *Pfiesteria*) in the retina and glial cells of the optic nerve and brain, as well as specialized white blood cells. Activation of the receptors causes an inflammatory response which begins to cause chemical changes inside nerve cells.

Dr. Ramsdell's remarkable findings dove-tailed nicely with the elegant insights of Dr. Ken Hudnell. The model of illness, for which FACT remains the best diagnostic test, predicted just such a distribution of receptors.

Ken Hudnell was there first. His decision to use FACT was brilliant, simply brilliant.

"Contrast Sensitivity."
A Key to Diagnosing Chronic,
Neurotoxin-Medicated Illnesses.

Chicago, IL –November, 1999

It's one of the simplest, quickest, least expensive—and most reproducibly accurate—diagnostic tools in all of modern medicine.

Brought to the forefront of the battle against *Pfiesteria*-related human illness by Ph.D. neurotoxicologist Ken Hudnell of the U.S. Environmental Protection Agency (See Chapter 5: "Brilliant, Just Brilliant"), the Contrast Sensitivity Test of a patient's vision requires only five minutes to determine toxic effects on nerve tissue, including the brain. Taking the test involves nothing more strenuous than reading the orientation of wavy lines on a printed card.

Contrast Sensitivity has been around for more than 35 years and is often used by ophthalmologists to diagnose glaucoma and cataracts. This method of measuring the brain's ability to perceive contrasting shades of white, gray and black has been described as "a five-tone hearing test for the eyes." And it's true that the loudness or volume of the hearing test is analogous to the contrast level.

The CS test gives us a powerful weapon, because it is a physiologic test that demonstrates the effect of neurotoxins on neural tissue. It can separate changes in visual functioning caused by neurologic problems from those caused by toxins, and also from those caused by 'post-bulbar' disorders. It's important to remember that organic toxins may cause deficits in all three categories —and the pattern of the CS deficits provide help in differential diagnosis of confounding CS deficits.

There are relatively few kinds of nerves that, working together, create the phenomenon we call "vision." Some of those nerves register light and darkness; others respond to stationary objects, motion, color, and peripheral images. Other sets of nerves work to create near and far vision, along with contrast. By isolating the nerves that transport information about contrast, during the test, we are actually isolating toxicity effects on a single kind of nerve—and thus eliminating confounding variables.

There's no doubt that the human mechanism for achieving sight is extraordinarily complex and delicate. We've got nerves that respond to changes in subtle light, and changes in intense light. And these nervous system structures are not the same. For example: We know that in the human hearing system, there are all kinds of hairs that will 'turn on' with low-frequency sound versus high-frequency, or soft tones versus loud tones.

When we access the low-frequency-contrast neurons, we essentially are assessing the effects of diffuse neurologic processes affecting the brain. Mid-range frequencies assess the retina, optic nerve and optic radiation. The highest frequencies show post-bulbar deficits and also those caused by repeated glare exposure. For the record, the frequencies involved are 1.5, 3.0, 6.0, 12.0 and 18.0 cycles per degree. By progressively reducing the density of coloration of each frequency at a rate of 0.15 log units per step, we can isolate a point where the neuron can no longer distinguish black from gray from white.

That "point of extinction" is converted into a score that we can graph. The individual frequency contrast scores form a distinctive pattern in normal patients, and abnormalities are easily recognized.

Because we carefully identify the point of extinction during the test, the results are reproducibly reliable, without the "stair-step improvement" seen in many other neurophysiologic tests. (Stair-step improvement can make test results difficult to interpret, because it often reflects benefits that were obtained in learning how to take the test.)

Test-variations as slight as perceiving changes in a single box on a single row can become statistically significant, if enough patients are tested. And perceiving changes in two boxes provides a useful yardstick for demonstrating Contrast Sensitivity in a single individual.

It's easy to understand what happens when the brain's ability to register contrast is compromised. To picture the effect, imagine the loss of visual definition that occurs on a TV screen when you turn down the "contrast adjustment." Even better, try to visualize a girl with blonde hair wearing a white blouse and a white skirt, as she steps from a snow-white automobile on a sunny afternoon. For this visualization, imagine that you are driving another car toward the girl, and that she stands poised against a background of dark trees.

How much of the detail in this scene will your brain perceive? If you have average Contrast Sensitivity, you probably won't find it difficult to distinguish the white dress from the dark background. But to the degree that you suffer from impaired Contrast Sensitivity, you will find it difficult—maybe even impossible—to separate the girl from the car.

Non-invasive and remarkably accurate, CS has been employed for many years to measure the effects of nerve and brain disorders on vision. Until about 15 years ago, the eye care industry used this outstanding diagnostic tool to detect the presence of many different kinds of eye disorders. But then the industry began to rely more on "acuity" than contrast as a diagnostic yardstick. The shift took place at the urging of health insurance carriers, many of whom began demanding the kind of "reproducible results" they decided acuity could provide them.

Their decision was an unfortunate development for many patients, in the opinion of experts in contrast testing, because the Contrast Sensitivity test is extremely effective at measuring rapid changes in optic nerve and brain cortex functioning, which makes it ideal for diagnosing disorders that impede neural activity.

But Contrast Sensitivity became much more important to medical practitioners a few years ago, after Dr. Hudnell recognized that this simple tool could also help confirm the persistent effects of *Pfiesteria* toxins on the optic nerve and the visual cortex of the human brain.

Soon after Hudnell began employing the CS test to measure the brain's ability to distinguish black from gray from white (a key indicator of toxin effect in brain tissue), I was fortunate to make a second important discovery while treating several patients with neurotoxin-mediated illnesses in my Family Practice.

By giving the test to these patients at regular intervals, I proved that I could use the changes in Contrast Sensitivity to measure rates of improvement which followed treatment with cholestyramine (CSM). In this way, while correlating physiologic improvement with clinical improvement, I was able to provide the medical profession with the necessary clinical parameter for effective diagnosis and treatment.

After subsequently studying test results from hundreds of patients suffering from various toxin illnesses (including chronic Lyme, chronic fatigue, sick building syndrome and several others), I recognized that the CS test would soon become the standard diagnostic tool for confirming the presence in patients of this new form of chronic illness.

The good news about this discovery for patients everywhere is that the defects caused by organic toxins are not durable. Unlike the damage produced by such heavy metals as lead, cadmium, manganese and mercury, or by solvents such as toluene and xylene, which is permanent, the effects of organic toxins can be reversed, and the patient's health restored—but only if toxin-binding therapy is employed, according to a strict protocol.

The key to helping the chronic Lyme or Chronic Fatigue patient get better is CSM, which flushes the circulating toxins out of human tissues molecule by molecule, until all of them are gone—while at the same time avoiding the pitfalls of side effects from this medication.

In recent years, I've given the test to more than a thousand "chronic" and "control" patients alike. And I've found Contrast Sensitivity to be vitally important, because it offers us the one thing we must have in order to help these patients—a verifiable diagnostic test that provides a necessary "biomarker." Once we have that in hand, successful treatment of toxin-based illnesses via cholestyramine is relatively easy to achieve, although Lyme disease presents some significant complications. The combination of CS and CSM is a powerful medical tool, because it allows us to show improvement of symptoms in patients and also improvement in a physiologic test.

Moreover, since re-exposure to the toxin brings back the same syndrome, we can use these techniques to once again measure —and once again cure—the illness by using Contrast Sensitivity to monitor CSM periodically throughout the treatment. It's important to remember that the immune system doesn't protect us from these neurotoxins, which means that we must re-treat the illness if it recurs (while also doing our best to prevent that from happening).

The Contrast Sensitivity test allows patient and doctor alike to feel completely confident about diagnosing the often vague and confusing symptoms of disorders such as chronic Lyme, sick building syndrome and *Pfiesteria*-related human illness syndrome. For millions of patients with toxin-based illnesses, this test will now make it possible to obtain a clear diagnosis, followed by effective treatment—rather than relying on medical guesswork (which is always vulnerable to political influences).

The point is that the eyes show the greatest susceptibility in the entire human body to the acute and chronic effects of neurotoxins. And now we've got a tool to measure those effects! That's why this test is so powerful as a diagnostic tool for toxin-mediated illnesses.

How important will the CS test become as a way of measuring toxin-effects on brain-functioning, in the years immediately up ahead?

According to marketing executive Tom Judy, whose Stereo Optical Company, Inc., of Chicago, Ill., a Gerber-Coburn company, now ranks as one of the world's largest manufacturers of vision-testing equipment, the new diagnostic tool is already having a major impact in medical circles.

"I talk to ophthalmologists every single day of the week," says Mr. Judy, whose company produces the most popular version of the Contrast Sensitivity exam (known as the "Functional Acuity Contrast Test"), "and they're usually astonished at the assurance offered by this inexpensive, five-minute exam. I've also looked at the epidemiological data that Dr. Shoemaker has gathered by using Contrast Sensitivity in recent years, and I'm just amazed.

"The medical evidence shows that physicians can use Contrast Sensitivity to detect chronic, neurotoxin-mediated illnesses, and that it can also serve as a powerful yardstick with which to chart improvement in patients.

"We feel that our version of Contrast Sensitivity, the FACT, which was initially developed by Dr. Arthur Ginsburg in 1993, is the most modern—and best—of the Contrast Sensitivity tests available. That's why Dr. Shoemaker uses FACT, and one reason why his findings have been so successfully reproduced by other physicians using FACT.

"Dr. Ginsburg and others have performed a great deal of research validating FACT, including correlating it with many electrophysiologic studies (including 'visual evoked potentials'), while also studying thousands of normal patients and measuring the 'normal curve' that defines their visual contrast function.

"The pattern of abnormalities that Dr. Shoemaker has documented in patients with these diseases—along with the resolution of these abnormalities with treatment—is a giant leap forward for both humankind and FACT.

"It's also true that since the rapidity of resolution of the FACT deficits affects *all* frequencies, the only logical explanation for those FACT scores is a reduction of blood flow to the capillaries of the optic nerve head caused by the disease. That reduced flow is corrected by the treatment protocols.

"Glaucoma often exhibits a similar kind of visual distortion, and it is frequently corrected by the use of special eye drops. We also know that glaucoma is usually caused by excessive pressure exerted by the anterior chamber on blood flow to the optic nerve. But what Dr. Shoemaker has shown is not related to glaucoma; his work has simply demonstrated reduced blood flow (hypoperfusion) that is likely matched by reduced blood flow elsewhere in the body.

"The direct effects of neurotoxins, themselves, must also be factored into this analysis. In short, this use of contrast-measurement in the diagnosis and treatment of chronic illnesses that affect many people is a spectacular medical advance, and I'm looking forward to the next step—in which thousands of primary care physicians like Dr. Shoemaker will begin learning how to use FACT in the same way it is employed by our research ophthalmology colleagues.

"Rest assured that I will help in any way I can!

"The Centers for Disease Control and Prevention (CDC) now estimates that there are at least five million Americans struggling with chronic fatigue syndrome, alone, in this country. Add five or ten more million sick building, chronic Lyme and other 'toxin-mediated' patients to the list, and you can see that the pool of patients who stand to benefit from this test is immense.

"I've been traveling the country in recent months, telling doctors and patients alike about the dramatic implications of the new test. I really don't think I'm exaggerating, when I tell you that Contrast Sensitivity is going to change the way medicine gets practiced in this country today!"

chapter 7

Event

Ciguatera.
Anatomy of a
Toxic Nightmare.

Key West, FL –June, 1998

> *Somethin' strange, in the neighborhood . . .*
> *somethin' strange, and it don't look good!*

Barracuda!

Like a runaway torpedo, he zooms through the turquoise shallows of Key West's Six-Mile Reef.

Powerful tail thrashing, he opens his huge jaws to reveal a double row of needle-sharp teeth. *Pow!* the flashing incisors snap shut on your trolling "white tail" . . . and all at once, you're going eyeball to eyeball with one of the most awesome game fish in the tropics.

If you love to fish, there's no thrill on earth that will match the Quest for the Deepwater Barracuda.

With your rod bent double and the sweat flooding into your eyes, you'll spend the next half-hour or so locked in a titanic battle with one of the swiftest predators in the Florida Gulf-stream: the mighty *Sphyraena barracuda*, aka the "Great Tropical Barracuda."

A word to the wise, however.

If you do succeed in landing that sleek-finned beauty, do not make the mistake of filleting him for your patio grill.

Like more than 400 of his tropical game fish cousins (including the grouper, the red snapper and the amberjack), this gorgeous-looking marine specimen, which dominates the Caribbean from Puerto Rico to the British Virgin Islands, is a carrier of some of the world's most potent toxins.

Meet "ciguatera," which is pronounced "SEE-gua-terra" by most citizens of the region, but "CHEE-gua-terra" by some who know the disease. Although few lay people realize it, this tiny microorganism dispenses a suite of neurotoxins—known as "ciguatoxins"—which ascend in the food chain and cause more outbreaks of non-bacterial, fish-borne poisoning than any other organism on earth.

Once restricted to case studies from isolated outposts in far-off Australia and the South Pacific, this reef-dwelling dino-flagellate is reportedly on the move (though no one knows why) throughout many regions of the world where industrial pollut-ants continue to degrade water-quality, and especially among tropical reefs in the Caribbean and Atlantic. According to the latest research, these one-celled creatures live symbiotically with filamentous algae and bacteria (including *Pseudomonas)*, and they are thriving with increasing frequency along reefs from Japan to Hawaii, and near the Mexican resorts of Cozumel and Cancun.

When these reefs are sufficiently disturbed and their ecological balance is disrupted—whether by pollution, temperature changes, storms, or nearby manmade development—the ciguatera-causing organisms respond with the same strategy employed by *Pfies-teria* . . . which is to spawn a virulent toxin. The difference be-tween them is that the ciguatera toxin eventually makes its way into the bodies of fish, doesn't get destroyed, and ascends in the food chain. The *Pfiesteria* toxins (based on our current knowledge) don't do that.

That same poison then triggers violent illness in those who eat the seafood.

All too often these days, restaurant diners in Chicago or Boston or Sushi eaters in New York are falling ill after eating fish shipped from the Caribbean and sometimes even the Pacific. It doesn't matter whether the fish are served hot or cold or drenched in spices, and it doesn't matter if they're "marinated" in lemon, lime or tomato. If you eat fish contaminated with ciguatera toxins, you might get sick—even if you consume the seafood with a glass of wine, a cold beer, or a frothy Caribbean "Bahama Mama." (As a matter of fact, research shows that alcohol often exacerbates attacks of illness in those suffering from Chronic Ciguatera Syndrome.)

At first glance, there would hardly seem to be a link between the kind of toxin produced by a tick bacteria, a fungus living deep inside an air conditioning vent, and a one-celled marine dinoflagellate hiding beneath sea-green algae fronds in the hope of surviving for one more day in the shallows of a tropical reef.

But there *is* a link—and its name is "neurotoxins."

In this chapter, you'll get an up-close look at the hidden connection between the seemingly disparate illnesses caused by these very different organisms.

The key to the puzzle, in a phrase: *Change the habitat (sometimes with pesticides, heavy metals or agricultural and industrial chemicals), and you change the nature and/or the abundance of the organisms that live there.*

The Captain and the Cookout

Sometimes, if you're patient enough, the answer to a scientific puzzle will come looking for *you.*

Sounds absurd, doesn't it?

But it's true. I can't tell you how many times I've spent an entire day—or an entire week—reading, writing and listening in a fruitless effort to come up with a scientific explanation for some difficult-to-understand phenomenon.

Then I finally throw up my hands and decide to shelve the problem for a while, so that I can think about something else.

Guess what happens next?

Here's what: more often than not, the solution to the problem suddenly appears out of the blue!

And that's exactly what happened to me, a few years ago, as I wrestled with a tantalizing thought that had been offered to me by Dr. Donald Anderson of the Woods Hole Oceanographic Institution.

Dr. Anderson's key insight—unveiled during a conversation we shared at the Georgetown *Pfiesteria* Conference in December of 1998—occurred as he speculated about whether or not my theory of *Pfiesteria*-related human illnesses might "generalize" to other forms of "chronic" disease that involved dinoflagellate neurotoxins, such as those produced by ciguatera.

What if the chronic, endlessly painful symptoms of ciguatera-linked illness were, like those caused by *Pfiesteria*, the result of organic toxins that circulated throughout the body, and seemed to linger there indefinitely? Would Contrast Sensitivity detect the toxin, and would CSM treat the disease?

Interesting! But how in the world was I going to check his idea out? Most of my patients lived in rural Maryland—and it was a long, long swim to those regions of the tropical Caribbean where a physician might reasonably expect to treat a few ciguatera cases now and then. Still, the idea had merit. After vowing to myself to give Dr. Anderson's speculation some further thought, I returned to Pocomoke and my busy office-and-research routine.

Less than 48 hours later, I would receive a telephone call that was destined to play a major part in the discovery of an entire family of neurotoxin-mediated diseases.

That call came around 10 o'clock on a bright Wednesday morning, only a few days before Christmas of 1998.

The man on the other end of the line turned out to be one of my Maryland neighbors—I'll call him "Harry"—and he said that he was in urgent need of some medical advice.

"Ritch, I need your help. I've been feeling rotten for six months now, and I'm sick and tired of it."

"Sorry to hear it, Harry. What's the matter?"

There was a long pause on the other end. Then: "I feel a little silly about saying this, but I've had the worst case, and the *longest* case, of diarrhea in my entire life. It's making me absolutely miserable. I've tried every remedy under the sun, and I can't seem to make it go away!"

I nodded. "Sorry to hear that, Harry. You were right to seek advice, because chronic diarrhea can trigger dehydration, and you don't want that. It can also signal the presence of some other major health problems. It needs to be addressed. So tell me: When did these attacks begin?"

Harry talked fast after that, and I could hear the relief in his voice. Just getting the worry off his chest seemed to help.

"It started when I was down in Key West last summer, on maneuvers with the Naval Reserve. Do you remember that trip?"

"Sure. You brought us that big conch shell, bright pink."

"That's right. Well, while I was down there in good old *Cayo Hueso*, I attended a cookout. Our unit threw a party for the CO—you know, we stood around in some guy's backyard grilling a bunch of Florida seafood and drinking a whole lot of Michelob. . . ."

All at once I was sitting up straight in my chair. Unbelievable! Was this the "ciguatera disease connection" that I'd been fantasizing about making . . . being handed to me by my own next door neighbor?

"Did you say 'Florida seafood,' Harry?"

"You bet. We had a bunch of amberjack and grouper, fresh off the boat. I think they bought it right off the waterfront, next door to Captain Tony's."

"Jack and grouper, Harry?"

"You got it, Ritch. Marinated in lime juice . . . really great stuff, you know? Some of the fish was smoked, and some was cooked in a bag. We even ate the leftovers in a stew. If it was on the plate, we ate it!"

There was another pause, and when he spoke again, I could hear the pain in his voice. "The only problem was, that fish made just about all of us sick as hell. Nausea, diarrhea, abdominal cramps, the works. A couple of the guys even wound up in the hospital, and missed the flight home. They gave a few of them mannitol treatment, but that didn't do anything except make the guys pee a lot.

"I was pretty sick, myself, although I did manage to make it back to the plane. But I haven't been right since. I still get hit with this really nasty diarrhea at least once a day, and the stomach cramps aren't much fun, either."

I was on my feet now, mind racing.

"Harry, did the doctors at the hospital run any tests on you?"

"Well . . . not on me personally. But I know they checked some of the other guys. They said they were looking for salmonella . . . vibrio . . . camp . . . camp-something—"

"Campylobacter, Harry."

"That's it. Anyway, they didn't find anything."

"No bacteria?"

"No bacteria of any kind, as I remember. They were really mystified."

Without even knowing it, I had begun to pace back and forth across the living room, trailing the phone cord behind me. This is a frequent habit, when I'm wrestling with a scientific problem; my wife JoAnn often remarks that I will "wear holes in the tile" if I keep it up.

"Harry, will you do me a favor? Will you drop by my office at the clinic, later this afternoon? Three o'clock?"

"Sure, Ritch. Hey, I'll do anything it takes, to get rid of this damn thing. What do you think's going on?"

"I don't know for sure. But I want to give you a vision test . . . what's known as a 'Functional Acuity Contrast Test.' I'll tell you all about it when you get there!"

• • •

Mysteries of the Tropical Reef: A Primer

Buckle up. Before we learn more about Harry's eventual diagnosis and successful treatment, we're going to take a little boat ride.

Settle back on your padded seat, and let's watch the flying fish take to the skies, as our 26-foot outboarder skims across the Gulfstream en route to Key West's fabled Six-Mile Reef.

Look at the sunlight on the rainbow-wings of those flying fish.

It's enough to make you stand up and salute the mystery of life. Look at how the water keeps changing color . . . shifting from that Gaugin-inspired turquoise at the island's edge to a deeper midnight-blue, as we clear the coastal shallows and zip toward the foam-flecked hulk of bone-coral that makes up the distant reef. The Florida Bay is dying, they say, but I sure can't tell it from topside. Too much pollution? Too much sediment? Too much water being vented from Lake Okeechobee? Too much damage to the Everglades?

I don't know what's been killing the reefs, but the folks who live among them say they're changing fast now, and changing in a way that no one can understand.

So how do organic toxins fit into the picture?

In order to understand the chemistry of fish toxin, let's think about the reef as a *habitat* . . . as a "biological neighborhood" in which thousands of different life forms are all out there working the street in order to make a living—even as they raise their young and do their best to keep out of harm's way.

The center of everything that happens on the reef is coral. Tiny marine polyps surround themselves with limestone and keep adding to their fortress as the years go by. The reef looks hard to the eye, iron-hard, but it's actually quite alive and quite fragile—even as it breaks up the currents of the warm-water oceans all around the world.

This backwater in the shallows is home to an astonishing array of plants, invertebrate and vertebrate animals, crustaceans, echinoderms, sea urchins and fish of all species, along with many other forms of marine life.

The Reef Neighborhood changes from day to night, as the tropical water changes from warmer to cooler and as endlessly changing weather patterns make their presence felt. Look more closely, however, and you'll find that the changes are all part of a larger design that can be predicted quite accurately, as the billion different creatures who inhabit the reef pass through their inexorable cycles of life and death.

As an ecosystem, the tropical reef stretches back into ancient biological history, when sponges and sea worms were taking the first steps on the immensely long journey toward *Homo sapiens*. And although they have witnessed their share of cataclysmic events—volcanoes and hurricanes and tidal waves that destroyed everything in their wake—the great tropical reefs have been fundamentally stable as ecological systems based on a balanced sharing of all the resources of life.

But then human beings arrived on the scene in force.

With them they brought their tools . . . their heavy metals and their plasticizer solvents and their pesticides and industrial chemicals, which began to trigger enormous (and enormously rapid) changes throughout the world of the reef.

Like the poltergeist-chasers in that recent smash-hit movie, "Ghostbusters," the polluting humans now find themselves confronting:

> *Something strange, in the neighborhood;*
> *something strange—and it don't look good!*

As you might expect, the effects of these toxic chemicals have been catastrophic. Example: a new plague is now affecting the coral. Called "white-band disease," it has begun wiping out entire sections of the tropical reef system in ways we do not fully understand.

But recent reef-borings show clearly that the problem is of recent origin; there is no evidence of it in coral deposits that extend back 3,800 years. According to marine experts, staghorn and elkhorn coral organisms are now dying in record numbers, to be replaced by "lettuce coral," which creates an entirely new ecosystem wherever it flourishes: new coral, new food sources, new currents.

Something strange . . . and it don't look good!

In order to understand how our industrial and agricultural chemicals have "altered the habitat" in these fragile ecosystems —thus triggering explosive new growths of ciguatera, among other newcomers—it might help to think of the Reef Neighborhood as a thriving local economy in which all sorts of creative business deals take place from morning to night.

The filamentous algae and their one-celled neighbors, the dinoflagellates, provide a revealing example.

Here we are, anchored directly above the coral reef and examining its sandy bottom through four feet of crystal-clear water. Now look closely . . . do you see that greenish hair anchored on the white rock, and waving slowly back and forth each time the gentle current laps against it?

That "hair" is filamentous algae, an underwater plant that makes a living by converting sunlight and carbon dioxide into glucose and then feasting on it.

So far, so good. Mild-mannered and inoffensive, the algae harm no one—and it seems almost unfair that they should be the dietary targets of a group of tiny, rainbow-hued fish (the "marine herbivores") who feed on them relentlessly from morn to night. But that's how it goes, out here at what Shakespeare in *The Tempest* described as "full-fathom-five" (five fathoms of water). In most sections of The Undersea Neighborhood, you'll find that one critter only survives on the basis of eating the next one—and so it's a mad scramble a lot of the time, as the residents do their biological best to make ends meet.

All right, then: As we study the glittering bone and staghorn coral that dominates a healthy reef, we notice how scores of gold-and-amber-splotched herbivores are feeding on the algae. What we *can't* see, however (at least, not without a microscope), are the microorganisms who also make up part of the local census. These little guys are so small and powerless that they might be expected to have no defense against the predators around them.

But looks are often deceiving, and the dinoflagellates are far from defenseless. Over eons of evolution, they have painstakingly developed an arsenal of secret, chemical weapons, a group of formidable "toxins" that can deliver a knockout-blow to many other species.

Armed with the toxins, the dinoflagellates have worked out a complicated series of business relationships in the Neighborhood.

After endless biochemical negotiation, the filamentous algae and the one-celled dinoflagellates (they're actually "protists," if you want to get technical) have come to an agreement. The deal is this: The algae will permit these swarming micro-animals to occupy some space on the block, provided that they perform a necessary service in order to pay their "rent."

As you might expect, these "services" vary from species to species.

In the case of the dinoflagellate we call "ciguatera" ("cigua" means "snail" and sometimes "conch"—remember that gorgeous pink shell Harry brought back to Maryland for us?), the service-on-demand turns out be an extraordinarily interesting one. It also has major implications for other dinoflagellate toxin-forming species, including *Pfiesteria*.

As several researchers have noted, the ciguatera serve as "filters" for the algae, by straining noxious heavy metals from the water and protecting the algae from the "heavy metal death" similar to that suffered by algae in heavy metal-poisoned estuaries and lakes.

Like most living things that depend on complex cell chemistry to get through the day, the filamentous algae cannot abide heavy metals—and especially copper—in the Neighborhood. Why? It's simple enough: Copper is a marvelous disrupter of enzyme systems. Just pour some copper fragments through the cell membrane of most organisms, and watch what happens: no enzymes, no order, and with no order, chaos in the streets!

Interestingly enough, symbiosis also turns out to be the basis for the survival of the coral reefs, themselves. To understand how it works, imagine the plight of the coral polyps, which must find a way to obtain fresh oxygen, even though they spend their lives deep inside the mini-caverns that are their homes. How can they obtain this vital element, when the flow of water through their coral cavities is so minimal? Lacking the ability to pump fresh water through the caverns, the polyps have solved the problem by hosting a specialized form of algae (in the same way that ciguatera often partners with a filamentous algae) to provide oxygen that would otherwise be lacking.

These specialized algae live inside the coral cavities and generate several organic compounds—along with oxygen—that are used by the coral polyps. The algae manufacture these essential items from carbon dioxide and other nutrients released by the polyps. But if you cut off the sunlight (with silt or other forms of pollution), the algae will soon perish. Change the habitat in this way, and the entire ecosystem of the reef will eventually vanish, to be replaced by other forms of life.

Understanding the "Cell Chemistry" of Ciguatera

Do you remember, back in Chapter Four, when we talked about the cell as an "energy-processing plant" fueled by glucose and controlled by an elaborate electrical system that runs around the clock? You may also remember, from that chapter, the descriptions of the "biological cascade"—the complex set of biochemical interactions in which an initial reaction sets off many others.

It doesn't take much intracellular poisoning to shut down the one-celled creatures and the few-celled plants.

So how can the hard-working algae stave off these threatening metals, in order to maintain stable cell-chemistry?

Enter our old pal, the hardy dinoflagellate, "ciguatera."

By ingesting heavy metals as a full-time occupation, these vigilant little animals "protect" the cell chemistry of their algae neighbors from interference.

Everybody's happy, right?

Well . . . most of the time, anyway. But sooner or later, just as in human life, something will happen to disrupt this pleasing state of affairs—and thus to threaten the "arrangement" between the ciguatera and the algae. Let's say that a hurricane comes whirling up the Caribbean and slams hell out of the delicate reef. Or maybe a group of humans from Miami launches dredging operations nearby, intent on deepening a channel so that petroleum barges from the Middle East can more easily make their way to the great ship terminals at Homestead. . . .

By the time the silt settles in the tiny windows and doors of the coral neighboood—which now looks like an underwater version of a small town bombarded by Mt. St. Helen's—the reef has been forever changed.

Something "strange" has taken over the neighborhood.

All at once, the denizens of the Six-Mile Reef are forced to break off the "arrangements" and scramble for new defenses, a new equilibrium, as the entire Neighborhood goes through a top-to-bottom shakeup.

When that happens, the one-celled dinoflagellate appears to respond exactly as *Pfiesteria* responded when denied its food supply . . . by suddenly "turning on" a gene that directs the manufacture of an attacking toxin. Is this the scenario that actually unfolds in this situation? It seems likely, but the truth is that science doesn't know for sure.

Is the weather a key factor in galvanizing these massive changes along the reef? What about levels of silt? The arrival of new pathogens? The sudden appearance of some unknown factor? Regardless of the ultimate explanation, one thing seems clear: the dynamics of the microbial world depend primarily on the interaction of organisms.

From moment to moment, billions and billions of invisible bacteria are living out their anonymous lives, far outside the narrow focus of our human perceptions. Food-webs, predator-prey relationships, toxin production, nutrient processing and the metabolism of toxic chemicals: these processes are all unknowns in this largest biomass (by weight and volume) of faceless and nameless creatures.

Does anyone really know why ciguatoxin species join cooperatively with bacteria—gram negative rods, including Pseudomonas —to begin to produce toxin? No.

But they do.

When ciguatera microbes are forced out of their defensive symbiosis with their algae neighbors, they soon form a new alliance with a group of adaptable gram-negative bacteria.

Because this highly cooperative strain of bacteria will be taken into the cells of the dino, we call it an "endosymbiont." And once it's safely aboard, the new ally starts "helping" its host to make toxin. To what end? Is it to stop the predation of fish on the exposed algae? But these herbivorous piscivores aren't supposed to be killed by ciguatoxin! Maybe they merely vomit and get diarrhea (like their human counterparts)—and are thus more easily devoured by larger fish?

The implication here is that the ciguatoxin doesn't kill the fish that eat the algae. Instead, it simply weakens them so that they become easier prey for the larger predators.

As always, the toxins from the dinoflagellates are stored in fatty tissues—which means that when the tiny herbivores are gobbled up by larger predators, the poison simply takes up residence in the bigger fish. Give this unfolding scenario a few months, and what do you get?

Toxic barracuda.

Now, the good news in all of this is that the ciguatera toxin has probably been studied more than any dinoflagellate toxin, and we know a great deal about it. As a matter of fact, a few researchers have even been able to synthesize the poison in the laboratory through a brilliant, 30-step process of organic chemistry that remains a marvel of scientific engineering to this day.

The bottom line on the biochemistry is clear: ciguatera toxin makes humans sick because it creates powerfully charged particles—know as "ionophores"—that sneak into cells and disrupt the "sodium channels" that form the heart of the intracellular messaging system.

Translated into "jawbreaker-ese" (the language of the medical textbooks) ciguatera toxin operates as follows:

The mechanism of action listed in the textbooks on ciguatoxin appears to be activation of voltage-dependent sodium channels with presentation of symptoms in three major categories: gastrointestinal, neurologic and cardiovascular.

• • •

What I have also found out, however, is that the symptoms of ciguatoxin-poisoned patients, broadly speaking, are identical to those of *Pfiesteria* patients, Lyme patients, Chronic Fungal Syndrome patients and many other victims of neurotoxin-mediated illnesses, as identified for the first time ever in *Desperation Medicine.*

All of which takes us straight back to my neighbor Harry, who showed up promptly at 3 P.M. that day at my clinic on Market Street.

It didn't take me long to explain my theory to him. If my suspicions were on target, it might be possible to demonstrate that toxins from ciguatera can be detected on the Contrast Sensitivity test in the same way that poisions from *Pfiesteria* are pinpointed with it.

Why not? After all, they both were toxin forming dinoflagellates, right? And the neurological symptoms (along with nausea, diarrhea and cramps) were also identical to those generated by

Lyme disease, Sick Building Syndrome and other chronic, neuro-toxin-mediated illnesses.

Now, as we saw with *Pfiesteria* back in Chapter 1, the CS test is unquestionably the best diagnostic tool for uncovering neurological deficits caused by toxins—because it directly measures the effect of neurotoxins on the optic nerve and the neurons that register perception of contrast. In this way, it tells us at a glance whether or not brain functioning is being interfered with by a biological toxin.

My neighbor Harry listened to all of this . . . and then promptly sat down and began the test by examining patterns of light and dark on a specially designed grid, and then doing his best to identify them.

When his FACT results showed the same deficit that I found uniformly in *Pfiesteria* patients, I wanted to jump out of my chair and slap him on the back. Resisting that impulse, which he might have found unnerving, I instead explained:

"Harry, I think we're going to be able to get rid of that diarrhea that's been bugging you, and fast."

His eyes were huge. "How so?"

I pointed at the test-grid on the desk before us. "The FACT surely demonstrates that you're suffering from chronic toxicity. That poison that was in the grouper and the amberjack has been stored in your fatty-cell reservoirs, including nerve tissue, for the past six months. Your body couldn't eliminate them, and that's why your diarrhea never went away."

He was staring hard at me. Suspicious. "Okay, but I don't understand. If I couldn't get rid of the poison before this test, how am I going to get rid of it *now*?"

I sent him my brightest smile. "Simple. Ever heard of cholestyramine?"

He nodded slowly. "It's an anti-cholesterol medication, isn't it? I seem to remember my Aunt Mildred taking it, a few years back. She had hypertension, and the doctors were worried about clogged arteries."

"You got it. Same stuff, exactly. But here's the good news. Although the researchers have known for years that the drug serves as a kind of filter, by leaching cholesterol out of bile in the small intestine, nobody realized that it can do the same thing with other substances that move through the gall bladder and fatty tissues."

"No kidding?" Harry eyes had lit up; he was beginning to feel some brand-new hope.

"Are you telling me that this stuff will flush the fish-poisons out of my body?"

I was reaching for a prescription pad. "Everything I've seen so far tells me this will work for you, Harry. I think the cholestyramine offers us a very promising avenue of treatment in your case."

Now it was Harry who grinned from ear to ear.

"Okay, doc, you've sold me! When do I start?"

Ciguatera: Some Case Studies

Because Harry's CS test had revealed a "distinct defect" in neurocognitive functioning, I felt confident that he would respond favorably to regular doses of cholestyramine. And my hopes were realized, as I later noted in a scientific paper for publication, entitled, "A New Approach To Diagnosis And Treatment of Chronic Ciguatera Syndrome" (presented October 2000 to the American Society of Tropical Medicine and Hygiene):

"Repeat Contrast Sensitivity testing done at one week showed a marked improvement, with mild additional improvement seen at follow-up one week later. His diarrhea symptoms resolved shortly after cholestyramine treatment was initiated. Patient reported that he had noticed an improvement in night-time vision, as well as reading vision, at his two-week visit. He has remained asymptomatic."

Like my friend Harry, several other patients obtained permanent relief from ciguatera symptoms by first taking the FACT

to confirm the presence of neurotoxins and then taking cholestyramine. Some examples:

Case No. 2

A 52-year-old white female presented to the author for
complaints unrelated to ciguatera. She had experienced
mild nausea and post-prandial bloating for seven years, starting soon after completion of a two-week "bareboat cruise"
through the British Virgin Islands. The patient reported that
she had stopped for meals on numerous islands, where she
ate prepared foods and took some back to her boat.

At the time of her office visit, this patient was taking
dicyclomine regularly for "irritable bowel syndrome." Her
symptoms had not responded to anti-reflux medications,
motility agents, low- or high-fiber diets, several classes of
anti-depressants, or various elimination diets. Her EGD
and colonoscopy were normal and she had no other symptoms.

Her physical exam was unremarkable, except for mild
obesity (BMI 30), and no abdominal pain was elicited. Lab
studies were normal. Contrast Sensitivity was mildly reduced
at 6 cycles. Cholestyramine was initiated. At two-week follow-
up, the patient had resolution of abdominal symptoms, improvement in FACT and a three-pound weight loss.

Case No. 3

A 51-year-old white male yachtsman presented for a routine physical, having recently returned from his annual two-
week sailing trip to the Caribbean. He had no symptoms,
except for chronic "acid stomach," for which he used H2
blockers daily. A prior work-up indicated normal EGD and
GB sonogram. Lab studies, including H. pylori, were normal.
His abdominal symptoms were of prolonged duration, following "something I ate in St. Thomas one time."

His physical exam was normal. But his FACT showed a significant deficit at 6 cycles. Treatment with cholestyramine was tolerated well. The H2 blockers were discontinued after one week. His CS improved slowly, with moderate improvement in two weeks. The patient remarked that he no longer needed to wear sunglasses outside on overcast days, since his eyes were less sensitive to sunlight than before.

• • •

Chronic, Neurotoxin-Mediated Illnesses: Making the Link at Last

The case studies were interesting, but I was still lacking complete proof.

While treating the patients described above, I was slowly increasing my roster of people suffering from the long-term effects of chronic ciguatera illness. These early patients included a writer for National Geographic, who could have gotten sick anywhere in the world, and a tourist who made the mistake of eating seafood at a famous New Orleans restaurant. Such sporadic treatments kept my interest up—but they hardly provided the kind of detailed, documented medical evidence that would allow me to reach conclusions about neurotoxin-mediated illnesses such as the one caused by ciguatoxins.

As Dr. Sherwood Hall—the noted foodborne-illness expert for the U.S. Food and Drug Administration—soon reminded me, I did not have convincing medical proof that these cases were actually the result of poisoning by ciguatera. And I knew he was right. For one thing, I had no way to measure cholestyramine-bound toxins in the stools of my treated patients. Nor were the patients linked by a definitive exposure. On that basis, a skeptical scientist would be completely correct in challenging my ciguatera diagnosis.

Without an unequivocally demonstrable "point source exposure," I would not be able to convincingly link the similar CS deficits (along with the similar corrections of symptoms and vision deficit, via CSM) among these different patients. In the end, the evidence for a ciguatera diagnosis would have to be based on mere "statistical probability"—and that simply wasn't good enough to prove the effectiveness of my diagnostic method and treatment program.

On the other hand, it was also true that Dr. Hall's observation about "lack of proof" nicely summarized the key difference between the diagnostic approach of the primary care physician, who works "under the gun" in a clinical setting, and the lab-based scientist, who can afford to wait until all of the evidence is in before making medical judgments.

Understandably enough, Dr. Hall's approach to solving a medical puzzle would call for much more detailed evidence than could be obtained by a primary care doc, whose "out of desperation" decision-making must often proceed on the basis of incomplete and uncertain information.

Understanding the difference between the two approaches is extremely important, when it comes to the business of thinking through public health policy decisions regarding chronic illnesses such as those caused by ciguatera and *Pfiesteria*. For the doctor, decisions about treatment methods are usually based on practical, down-to-earth observations such as "I tried this and it worked."

For the lab researcher, on the other hand, each and every scientific finding—no matter how obvious—must be buttressed with exhaustive and repetitious experiment, until all conclusions have been convincingly demonstrated.

Although the implications of CS testing for the diagnosis of ciguatera-related illness remain open to debate, the accuracy of the measuring device is plainly evident. There's no doubt at all that if the FACT shows a deficit in nerve function, then biologically produced toxins (along with their breakdown-products, or "metabolites") are affecting the optic nerve, the brain and multiple peripheral tissues.

Ciguatoxin has long been known to bind particular receptors on membranes, which then allows them to cause disruptive injury throughout the cell. And the binding appears to be specific and prolonged—meaning that the process leaves very few toxin molecules floating freely in affected tissues.

While struggling to pinpoint the biochemistry involved in ciguatera poisoning, I called as many experts as I could find. Dr. Mark Poli, one of the world's foremost ciguatoxin researchers, explained early on the vital importance of showing that the toxin was actually contained in the fish eaten by patients diagnosed with this illness. He had already published a scientific paper showing how a widely accepted test for such toxins worked. Unfortunately, the seafood industry is acutely sensitive to increases in cost, and so far has rejected the idea of routinely testing its products for safety, before sending them on to consumers.

Faced with the impossible task of testing fish that had been consumed by my patients before they fell ill, I turned to another expert for whom I already had a great deal of admiration. Dr. Tom Tosteson knows as much about ciguatera as anybody in the world. He lives and works in Mayaguez, Puerto Rico, where the microorganism is endemic. Dr. Tosteson frequently studies these toxins in the lab, and in elegant electron microscope studies he has demonstrated the morphology of the endosymbiont bacteria, while also describing the mechanism by which ciguatoxin acts on its victims.

One of Dr. Tosteson's post-doctorate fellows, Dr. Arnaldo Olivieri, called me at one point and urged me to confer with both Dr. Tosteson and Dr. John Ramsdell, who directs the NOAA Marine Biotoxin Molecular Biology Lab in Charleston, S.C. Olivieri had described my case studies to Ramsdell during a recent international conference on harmful algal blooms, conducted in the Philippines, and he wanted to know more.

One of the most difficult problems I've faced while researching the health effects of ciguatera is the dearth of patients here in rural Maryland. How likely is a mass outbreak of this tropical disease (seen frequently in such locales as Puerto Rico and Hawaii), here among the corn and soybean fields of the mid-Atlantic coastal plain?

Not very!

In an effort to help me solve that problem, Dr. Tosteson referred me to several physicians on the island of Puerto Rico. Perhaps they might be willing to investigate an outbreak? Unfortunately, that initiative failed to light any fires, so I called several public health officials in the Caribbean.

As I'd feared, they quickly let me know that "we don't have a problem with ciguatera" . . . even though eating barracuda in August or September was either prohibited or severely frowned upon throughout the region.

One of these physicians, who shall remain nameless, told me bluntly that if he were to report his ciguatera cases (and he had a lot of them), his action would accomplish "nothing positive." Instead, it would undoubtedly "put a few honest fishermen out of work," while also scaring away local tourists and shutting down area hotels that feature "fresh seafood buffets." In short: Warning the public about the dangers of ciguatera would simply create "economic havoc."

Question: Does this scenario sound a bit familiar?

Of course it does. When the *Pfiesteria* epidemic struck Maryland's Chesapeake Bay estuaries in the summer of 1997, the immediate reaction among public health officials was eerily similar.

"All you'll do is frighten people unnecessarily, while destroying the tourist and seafood industries!" warned the nervous health bureaucrats, while insisting that there *was* no *Pfiesteria* epidemic—and hence no need to "warn the public" about the health menace it now faced.

Infuriating? You bet. The bureaucrats were right about one thing, however: the amazing ability of toxic microorganisms like *Pfiesteria* to scare hell out of most people. Like many Marylanders, I'd seen for myself what a "*Pfiesteria* scare" could do to the local economy . . . even though no poisons ever appeared in the local fish. How would the public respond to the presence of a toxin-former—ciguatera—that *did* leave poisons in fish and also made people ill for years at a time?

In spite of these observations, however, I couldn't deny that Dr. Poli's reservations about my "evidence" for ciguatera were deeply troubling. If the "dissociation constant" (the rate at which toxins leave their cell membrane receptors) was as low as Dr. Poli had defined it, then my binding therapy (via CSM) seemed to stand little chance of working effectively.

Arnaldo remained encouraging, however. He kept telling me: "Just because the dissociation is low doesn't mean it's zero! Perhaps that's why your patients take longer to get better. It just takes more time—when treating ciguatera—to send the toxins down the toilet."

This idea had also been powerfully supported, I soon discovered, by several important journal articles. I studied them carefully, even as the number of my referral cases of ciguatera slowly grew. Several patients had been referred to me by Dr. Ramsdell; others wound up in my office through word-of-mouth. Soon my caseload included several dozen patients from all around the country.

But I still had no point source on which to base a clearcut diagnosis—and I could feel Dr. Hall's cautionary words hanging around my neck like Coleridge's legendary albatross.

But then I got a lucky break.

It happened when Audio-Digest released one of my "continuing education" lectures in June of 1999.

In that talk, which went out to physicians from coast to coast, I had reviewed toxin-binding therapy, CSM, Contrast Sensitivity, *Pfiesteria* and ciguatera. Within a matter of a few weeks, a physician in Florida had contacted me with some very interesting news.

He was treating 11 patients with ciguatera—all of whom had fallen ill after eating fish in a Miami restaurant. The doctor immediately placed all 11 on a CSM regimen. He saw some early improvement . . . but there was no CS testing, no follow-up, and no reporting of symptoms before or after treament.

After months of struggle on my part, fate brought me another significant group of patients. As it turned out, five tourists from Delaware had been vacationing in the Bahamas. All had eaten freshly grilled grouper purchased from a local fish market. All five became seriously ill.

Then one of the patients saw a TV interview I'd done about *Pfiesteria* in fish. During that Q&A, I had compared the impact of *Pfiesteria* and ciguatera toxins on the human body, while describing symptoms in detail. Bingo! The entire Delaware contigent trooped down to my office in Maryland. I soon determined that all of them shared the same CS deficit. Then I placed all of them on the same research protocol. They all improved quickly as a result.

Look out, toxin-mediated illness: here comes an answer to the ciguatera puzzle, based on science.

Along with helping sick patients, the "answer" provided a powerful boost for the idea that scientific discoveries need not be restricted to the university academic research centers or the government-funded labs.

In many cases, those key discoveries should emerge from primary patient care, when creative physicians find the courage to make "the leap" from treating individual patients to coming up with new, inductively based explanations for disease phenomena.

Perhaps the most exciting aspect of the Quest for Ciguatera was the "leap" it required—the willingness on my part to entertain another scientist's speculations, and then to do the detailed, meticulous research required to put that theory to the test.

In the end, the link between *Pfiesteria* and ciguatera would become the foundation stone for a whole new theory—the Shoemaker and Hudnell Theory of neurotoxin-mediated illness.

After treating many ciguatera patients watching all of them improve by taking regular doses of the common and inexpensive substance—cholestyramine—I was delighted to know that I'd discovered an effective treatment for an illness that strikes up to one million people worldwide each year.

But the big news on the ciguatera front wasn't about a new form of disease therapy, however promising that might be.

It was actually about a brand-new "family" of chronic diseases —toxin-mediated diseases such as chronic Lyme, *Pfiesteria*, sick building syndrome and cylindrospermopsis—that had been spawned by alterations in habitat.

Suddenly, it was easy to see how rapid over-development of suburban woodlands had brought people into closer contact with deer ticks, thus triggering the rapid increase in Lyme disease. In the same way, pesticide pollution from new, high-tech agricultural methods had altered the habitat of *Pfiesteria*, and had "switched on" their toxin-making ability almost overnight.

Even as accelerating land development and changes in populations along the world's tropical reefs possibly stimulating the growth of toxic ciguatera, our penchant for building new "climate-controlled" office highrises had helped to create entire new species of toxic fungi that were now making millions of office workers and factory hands sick each day.

With the help of Dr. Anderson's insightful suggestion at the Georgetown Conference, I had managed to make the inductive "leap" from ciguatera back to *Pfiesteria* . . . and then on to a whole new family of toxin-mediated disorders that almost invariably resulted in a group of familiar symptoms: fatigue, headache, shortness of breath, sensitivity to bright light, blurred vision, nausea, diarrhea, aching joints and muscles and short-term memory loss.

With growing excitement and no small measure of alarm, I began to understand the full implications of my ciguatera-*Pfiesteria* breakthrough.

There was a new kind of disease at work in the world . . . and the Medical Establishment didn't even know it!

Even Ph.D.s Get Sick . . .
But Why Wouldn't They?

RTC –June, 2000

The first few times it happened, I was totally surprised. But not any more.

"Dr. Shoemaker, I thought you were describing *me*!"

There I am, gathering up my notes and preparing to depart the lecture hall, after giving yet another presentation on chronic, neurotoxin-mediated illness to yet another audience made up of physicians, academicians and scientific researchers . . . when all at once, a member of the audience stops by the podium to describe some of the same symptoms I've just been talking about.

When that happens—more and more frequently, these days—I usually wind up spending another 45 minutes talking about chronic Lyme disease or sick building syndrome . . . and realizing all over again that academicians and scientists are just as vulnerable as the rest of the population, when it comes to getting wiped out by this new family of diseases.

Let me tell you about a recent lecture I gave at the American Society of Bariatric Physicians annual meeting in Portland, Oregon, by way of example.

That meeting took place back in May of 2000. After spending several days preparing for my presentation on "Environmental

Acquisition of Diabetes and Obesity," I was pleased when the talk appeared to be well received.

No sooner had I answered the last question from the audience, however, than three physicians made their way down to the front of the hall in order to take the Contrast Sensitivity test. All three registered deficits, and all three said they were struggling with symptoms identical to the ones I'd just been describing.

Less than a month later, the same scenario repeated itself at both the Maryland Academy of Family Practice and the Maryland Academy of Osteopathic Physicians yearly meetings, where several more physicians came forward to announce that they had also been struggling with the symptoms of neurotoxin-mediated illness.

Once again, I did my best to help these troubled doctors deal with worrisome physical complaints that they could not readily explain.

My next confrontation with neurotoxic illness among medical professionals came only a few days later, at the U.S. Environmental Protection Agency's National Health Environmental Research Lab meetings on "Human Health and Environmental Indicators." This high-powered confab brought together a distinguished group of environmental researchers with impeccable scientific credentials.

One of the highlights of the conference occurred when EPA neurotoxicologist Ken Hudnell, Ph.D., unveiled a poster that nicely summarized both his environmental research in North Carolina and our collaborative work on the Contrast Sensitivity test and cholestyramine (CSM) as diagnostic/treatment tools for *Pfiesteria*, ciguatera and chronic Lyme disease. That poster drew a great deal of attention at the gathering—and it wasn't just because of Ken's eye-catching graphics.

As I watched the researchers gather around Ken's presentation, I could see how impressed they were with the content. Among the curious onlookers was a U.S. Army virologist who had worked in S.E. Asia studying changing patterns of infectious diseases, including malaria, that were of interest to the Department of Defense.

No longer was malaria confined to steamy, sea-level jungles and crowded cities in S.E. Asia. By the late 1990s, residents of the uplands and mountains were contracting this debilitating illness . . . even though disease-carrying mosquitoes had never before invaded the cooler, higher altitudes in many regions.

For the virologist, this alarming new trend raised some difficult questions. Was the change in S.E. Asia and Pacific areas part of the same worldwide climate shift that seemed to be increasing the range of mosquitoes as vectors for illnesses such as dengue fever, which has been moving north from the Caribbean to the northeastern U.S. in recent years? Probably not. And what about the attacks of West Nile-like virus (a form of encephalitis) that had been making headlines in the American press of late, after cases were reported near Plum Island on Long Island Sound, and also in New York's Westchester County? Had the virus really come from the Bronx Zoo?

Although a virologist would not usually wind up studying parasitic diseases such as malaria, the Army researcher was an exception. Her background included bacterial, parasitic and fungal diseases, including ways to rapidly diagnose infectious diseases.

She knew some of these diseases all too well, in part because of her own past bout with an unusual illness called "Q Fever" (caused by a rickettsial agent, *Coxiella burnetti*), but also because of her academic drive to learn more about infectious disease worldwide.

A bit of background will help explain what happened to her during her last overseas assignment. The Army researcher seemed fit for duty with a regimen of strenuous exercise, a minimum of running 25 miles a week, and also working long hours. In all reviews, she was considered fit for duty and ready to take on her assignment.

One of the areas she would travel to was located in Indonesia, an archipelago of volcanic islands supporting nearly 200 million people on only 800,000 square miles islands. Historically, this tropical environment is teeming with insects. One of the customs in the cities is to spray areas where the public congregates with carbamate insecticide to reduce the insect-swarms, so that tourists and visitors can enjoy dining, movies and shopping with relatively little annoyance from biting mosquitoes. (This practice helped to keep the level of mosquito-borne illnesses at a minimum in the larger cities.)

As you might imagine, mosquitoes are a terrific problem in this crowded, tropical realm. To combat them, local merchants and business people have adopted a complicated set of strategies. The owners of movie theaters routinely "fog the house" with insecticides between showings, for example, in an effort to drive off the pests. (This approach leaves the moviegoers with a difficult health-choice: Should they take the risk of catching a mosquito-borne disease, or the risk of inhaling huge quantities of pesticide every time they attend a matinee?)

Soon after arriving in Jakarta, the Army researcher fell prey to a series of mysterious illnesses. She had of course received every vaccine in the federal arsenal (including a "Q Fever booster" that nearly sloughed her arm), but the vaccines did not prevent her from quickly developing a host of respiratory complaints or suffering from a dental ailment.

On a warm, tropical evening in October during the late 1990s, a dinner took place that the Army scientist would never forget. After a day of viewing several volcanoes on the island of Java with friends, they all decided on dinner at a small, clean restaurant they had frequented before. The menu was the usual choice of a chicken dish or a fresh fish. The others ordered the chicken, but the Army scientist had found the red snapper to be fresh and well prepared.

When the meal was served, everyone noted how large the pieces were, since the red snapper served in the U.S. is typically a small filet. She knew that grouper, amberjack, barracuda and even Mahi Mahi were predator fish and should not be eaten because of the risk of acquiring ciguatera.

But red snapper had always been one of her favorites in the U.S. What she failed to realize, however, was that the smaller U.S. version of that species usually did not prey on and eat enough other fish to allow for a hazardous concentration of ciguatera toxins.

The story was different in this part of the world, however: In these Indo-Pacific waters, the red snapper grew quite large—and they were fully capable of ingesting enough toxins to occasionally cause severe illness in humans. The "large pieces" of snapper she ate that night were from a large . . . and highly poisonous snapper.

It was a mistake she would bitterly regret, and the changes that one meal created—both professionally and personally—would devastate her life. Within 30 minutes, on the walk back to their lodgings, the Army scientist noted an unusual taste in her mouth . . . metallic. She also did not feel well, and began to notice strange, vague symptoms. About an hour later, she began burping massive amounts of what smelled like a sulfur gas. Waves of nausea washed over her.

She knew she was in the first throes of food poisoning. What ensued was a night of cholera-like diarrhea and incredible cramping. The night was spent on the cold tile floor of a small bathroom. What little she remembers of that night most notably are the numb lips, the tingling fingers and toes, and the way her arms and legs kept falling asleep.

She knew it was food poisoning, but the other symptoms didn't fit. Within a few days, the symptoms had eased, except for the continual metallic taste and some strange tingling in her hands and feet. As her menses began, she noted the increasing intensity and severity of the neurological symptoms. On the third day after her illness began, when she started reviewing the entire episode, the logical conclusion was a ciguatoxin-like exposure. After reading and investigating the matter, she realized that in the Indo-Pacific area, red snapper can be quite large in size—and in areas near coral reefs. Suddenly, the source of the toxin seemed clear.

One of the strangest symptoms was the occasional jolt she got when touching something cold, such as a water fountain or faucet. The first time it happened, she was sure that a water cooler had not been grounded properly and checked around to find out if the device needed to be repaired. Another time she was sure that a dishwasher had not been properly grounded, since the "shock" was really severe. Finally, she noted that touching anything cold and metallic would trigger the sensation, and that she was not in danger of being electrocuted. Describing the "shocks" later, the researcher said the sensation felt like "a lightning-bolt" that "bored" into her large muscle-groups and then "exploded." (Lyme patients often report this highly unusual symptom, as well.)

It was not long before the Army researcher's symptoms seemed to improve. But then, after a weekend where she and her friends went to two movies, there was an acute reoccurrence with even more severe neurological symptoms. This time the pain and neurological effects left her only able to shuffle around slowly.

The pain was nearly unbearable and also terrifying. She was not sure where her feet were and every step was an effort. She no longer had any energy and was only able to go to work, come back home and then collapse.

One of the doctors she saw was sure she had injured her back. But that didn't make sense to her . . . since everything had begun with the food poisoning in October. She had not been able to resume her running or any other exercise. Finally she was sent to Tripler Army Medical Center to be evaluated. By the time all the paperwork and phone calls were made, nearly two weeks had passed and her symptoms were easing. Still, there was a decision to curtail her assignment and send her home to the U.S.

Once stateside, the Army researcher began to read more about ciguatera. Most of what she read was reassuring, and she assumed she would be like most of the people who get ciguatera poisoning—that is, she expected to gradually get better. As the weeks passed, things were looking pretty good. Her episodes seemed to be limited to the time of menses, and so she just tried to rest and not do too much on those occasions.

But then another disquieting episode took place. About two months after returning to the U.S., she entered the building where she worked and found workmen running hoses and tubes into walls. The facility was being treated for termites. After raising some questions about the wisdom of treating a densely occupied building with a carbamate-like termiticide, she was reassured that this was done all the time.

Within 48 hours, however, the researcher started experiencing the same episode of being unable to walk and being unable to feel or find her feet. She was also concerned about her growing inability to read or watch television, due to blurred vision.

From then on, her health deteriorated steadily. She had experienced occasional night sweats since the food poisoning, but now they were constant and severe, with strange blasts of pain in the middle of the night that would yank her from sleep.

As the weeks passed, she spent all her energy just trying to get through work. When she kept a medical appointment and was met with the old-fashioned, medical standby of "depression," she knew it was not true. She felt more angry and resentful than depressed. Her symptoms were being brushed off with cursory examinations and no laboratory tests.

One physician tried to prescribe antidepressants to help her sleep and even attempted to explain the recurrent fevers and night sweats as perimenopausal "hot flashes." Her respect for and confidence in the military medical system was thoroughly shaken by now. She had found one neurologist who seemed to be very interested, but he was headed for reassignment overseas. After nearly two months of worsening symptoms, the Army researcher knew she was sliding into a serious medical condition.

After great effort, she finally succeeded in obtaining some lab tests, even though she was told that she'd have to wait another month for a doctor's appointment. She waited and heard nothing back from the doctor who had ordered the tests. She really *was* beginning to feel depressed by now, and had begun to assume that it was "all in her head." But fortunately the neurologist was busy reviewing her case, including all of the computer-based information from the hospital, in order to prepare a case review for the neurologist who would replace him when he left for duty overseas.

One day the Army researcher received an urgent call that interrupted an important task. Exasperated with the medical community by now and in no mood for questions, she demanded to know what the neurologist wanted from her this time. Then she got a surprise. It turned out that even though no one had called to inform her about her blood tests, the results were in. She had raging hepatitis and no white cells! Her immune system was shot, and whether she had contracted hepatitis as a result (or vice versa) would never be determined. Her only satisfaction that day came from knowing that her illness was *not* in her head . . . at least not yet!

Within 48 hours of that discovery, however, the Army researcher broke out with pneumonia, bronchitis, fever and gastroenteritis. She was extremely ill, and this time she wound up in the Emergency Room. Her recovery was slow, and the elevated liver enzymes and low white count remained a problem for many months. After ultra-sound showed fatty infiltration in the liver and all the usual viral hepatitis tests were negative, she knew that her illness was much more complicated than anything caused by an infectious disease.

Fortunately, she had some good friends who were virologists; they worked in both the civilian and military worlds. She sent her blood around to be tested, and most of the more exotic viruses/rickettsias and bacteria were ruled out: Leptospirosis, Brucellosis, Q Fever, Erlichia, Rocky Mountain Spotted Fever, Hepatitis C, Hepatitis B, Hepatitis A and even HIV. At this point, the best assessment seemed to suggest the presence of a toxic hepatitis, such as those caused by Hepatitis C, and multiple tests for Hepatitis C were performed at several institutes. She was never tested for Parvo virus, Chlamydia or Adeno virus. No answer was found.

After talking with several other researchers, including an immunologist, the Army researcher begain to take maximum doses of vitamins, including Silmarin, or "Milk Thistle," to help her liver repair the damage. She put pressure on an Army allergist-immunologist and literally begged for Immunoglobulin shots (IgG) to stimulate her immune system.

Gradually her symptoms began to improve and her liver enzymes began to stabilize. But it would be nearly a year before they returned to normal. Her white count remains low to this day, in spite of her improved health—an outcome that I have sometimes observed in Lyme patients. But her energy levels have never returned and she has never been able to run since the day of the food poisoning. She has optimistically adjusted her lifestyle, after receiving a "Medical Board" and being removed from military duty, due to medical disability.

These days, she guardedly watches for any exposures that might trigger the neurotoxin in her body . . . including alcohol (even topical applications are a risk), sugar, insecticides, pesticides and nearly every drug on the market that has to "clear" through the liver. She also has infrequent bouts with fever and night sweats, along with indigestion and unusual flashes of pain. Indeed, she has never been completely free of any of the health problems that first took place after the poisoning.

Was there a pattern here? Obviously, this struggling scientist was displaying the signs of a multi-system illness, and the kind of unremitting symptoms that suggested a neurotoxic origin. She had also witnessed the failure of standard diagnostic tests to provide an explanation for her condition. The lymphocytotoxicity was an interesting finding, of course . . . but how could I expect it to "generalize" to other neurotoxin-mediated illnesses?

So much for the background.

As the EPA conference unfolded around us, Ken Hudnell administered my Contrast Sensitivity test to the Army scientist (I never attend scientific meetings without one!). While noted molecular biologist and biotoxin expert Dr. John Ramsdell looked on with interest, the Indonesian disease-hunter came up a clear "positive" on the exam. Her brain's ability to register visual contrast was being affected by ciguatera toxins!

She had the deficit—and she'd already had the other symptoms to go along with it.

After treating hundreds of neurotoxic patients like this world-renowned virologist, I felt confident that the Army specialist would find her health restored in about seven weeks.

What will she do with her renewed energy, I wondered, and where will her remarkable new insights about chronic, neurotoxin-mediated illness take her?

And does she now realize—as I certainly do—that Ph.D. researchers are just as vulnerable as the rest of us to diseases caused by toxin-forming microbes?

Chronicles from a Poisoned Landscape

Leesburg, FL –October, 1998

Frank Fuzzell and the Story of Agricultural Fungicides

He spent ten years in Hell.

Ask him.

"I had no memory left," says Frank Fuzzell. "Nothing. My short-term memory was wiped out, and it was pure torture.

"Do you know what it's like when you can't find your car at the airport? Your head is throbbing . . . your vision is blurred. Your joints ache, and you feel so weak that you just want to sit down and cry. But you can't do that, so you just stumble around the airport garage, unable to locate your car because you have no short-term memory left."

Like millions of other Americans in recent years, 49-year-old Frank Fuzzell suffers from a chronic illness caused by toxins. In Frank's case, the medical evidence is suggestive that he was poisoned by a sequence of "biological cascade effects" that took place at his nursery, after it was sprayed with some of the life-killing chemicals (aka "pesticides") that are now routinely applied to agricultural farmlands all across the United States.

A Florida tree-grower who raised hundreds of thousands of

ornamental plants each year until his toxin-mediated illness drove him out of the business in the early to mid-1990s, Fuzzell believes he fell victim to toxic chemicals and microbial mutations that occurred when his nursery land was sprayed with a widely used chemical fungicide.

Fuzzell will never be able to prove that he was poisoned by the pesticide in a "standard-dose response" clinical experiment—because no researcher would ever be allowed to expose healthy patients to the "life of living hell" that can result from contact with such powerful toxins. Without verifiable experiments to draw upon for evidence, all Frank has going for him is a meticulously detailed and utterly convincing story about the sufferings he and his family endured following the use of fungicides.

Chemically engineered to kill plant-attacking fungi, the pesticide that wiped out Frank's operation was widely used in the 1980s. The product was voluntarily recalled by the manufacturer on two occasions. The first, which occurred in 1989, came after the company reported the discovery of a herbicide contaminating the product. Plant-growers who used that version of the fungus-killer began to notice severe crop damage where the chemical had been applied . . . and stunted plants with yellow leaves don't sell well. Although the source of the damage remained unproven, some growers remained convinced that unidentified chemicals in the pesticide were the culprit.

The product was eventually released again—only to be recalled voluntarily in March of 1991. During this recall, growers were informed of an EPA order stating that the action was necessary, requiring that it be withdrawn from the marketplace, since once again it was found to contain the unauthorized herbicide. Meanwhile, the product liability lawsuits targeting the product were piling up.

Initially, no plaintiff proved prospectively that the fungicide was causing the crop damage, but the manufacturer nonetheless began to pay off claim after claim. Investigations confirmed that crop damage was confined to those crops to which the pesticide had been applied. Fuzzell had done his own "case-control" study in which he treated 30,000 plants with the substance and compared them to an exact matched group of plants. Only the treated plants were damaged.

Claims of human illness resulting from exposure to the fungicide also were never proven. By the early 1990s, thousands of American nursery-workers and migrant farm laborers were developing non-specific illnesses that they believed were associated with exposure to a wide array of agricultural products. The manufacturers of these products weren't required to report health effects because the toxic aspects were never scrutinized or proven by the U.S. public health bureaucracy.

Instead, the bureaucrats engaged in a half-hearted attempt at studying the problem, by looking at just about everything else besides the real problem while employing the classic strategy known as "The Appearance of Good Science" (See Chapter 10: "The Appearance of Good Science"). In this way, the government investigators were able to pretend to be fully committed to solving the problem, even as they stood by and did nothing.

Although the poisons that the workers believe are unleashed by the effects of pesticides surely differ in overall structure from the kinds of toxins produced by Lyme bacteria, sick building syndrome-causing fungi and other toxin-mediated illnesses, the nightmarish symptoms they leave behind are exactly the same. Those symptoms include blurred vision, memory loss, muscle and joint aches, pounding headaches and chronic, debilitating fatigue.

In many ways, the story of Frank Fuzzell's ten-year odyssey through ravaging toxin-mediated illness, medical ignorance and total bureaucratic indifference reads like the typical saga of a Lyme (Chapter 13) or *Pfiesteria* patient. Like those other patients, Fuzzell was overwhelmed by a buildup of toxins in fatty tissues scattered throughout his vital organs, his joints, his lungs and even his brain.

But the good news for Frank Fuzzell was named "cholestyramine."

Because this common substance leaches harmful toxins from body tissue and then expels them harmlessly through the small intestine, it worked to begin cleansing Fuzzell's exhausted body of the pesticide-linked poisons that were slowly destroying his ability to function.

But the disturbing question remained: If the poisons continued to affect his residential neighborhood far into the future, would he ever be free of their effects? Or would he relapse each time he came into fresh contact with these toxic residues?

Ask him how he feels today, and he'll laugh out loud: "I started on the cholestyramine a year ago, and I've made tremendous progress. I wonder how I even survived . . . but now my memory is coming back. I can remember where I parked the car! I don't get lost at the airport! No, I'm not cured, and I probably never *will* be. But this improvement has been a godsend to me.

"It's just been unbelievable. For me, small tasks that once felt like they weighed tons are now being reduced to ounces! But whenever I return to the nursery—or open boxes of documents from the operation we ran there—I get sick all over again. Fortunately, however, the treatment protocol Dr. Shoemaker developed for me works to maintain my health. I'm not 'normal' yet, but compared to the 'life of waking death' that I once led, I'm doing so much better!"

• • •

Chronicles from a
Poisoned Landscape: Frank Fuzzell

Ask Frank Fuzzell to describe his ten years as the victim of a pesticide-linked, toxin-mediated illness, and this normally hard-charging and high-energy entrepreneur won't hesitate.

"It was just horrible," Frank told me during a recent conversation in Leesburg, the central Florida town where he lost his huge tree-farming operation and his health after using a suspect fungicide in the late 1980s and early 1990s. "As you know, I went through a serious automobile accident, back in the early 1980s. But when I compare that accident to this chemical thing . . . the truth is, I'd rather have you break every bone in my body.

"But don't poison me with a bio-toxin. Never again! I'd absolutely prefer a car wreck. I'd take that any day. The thought of regressing back to toxic illness is so frightening, I can't describe it. I spent six months in a body cast, after the auto accident, and I was hospitalized for three months. I went through a stormy hospital course complicated by a fat embolism. I had multiple surgeries, and I needed transfusions of 41 units of blood.

"I'm telling you that I'd go through all of that again, any time, before I'd go through toxin disease again! Thank God that with cholestyramine, I've got something that will help start the process of protecting me from the horror that has plagued me for the past ten years."

A successful nurseryman who supplied ornamental trees and shrubs to customers around the nation each year, Fuzzell had launched his 20-acre Leesburg operation back in the fall of 1986. By the late eighties, when his troubles began, he employed 20 full-time workers at Fuzzell Wholesale Nursery, Inc.

"We grew hundreds of thousands of trees at our place," he says with a nostalgic sigh, remembering the happy days before the arrival of his devastating illness. "I loved that business, I really did. I loved having the nursery absolutely immaculate, and having the crops consistent, where each specimen of any given crop—oak trees, let's say—was the same size. I just enjoyed producing beautiful plant material, and striving for quality.

"I also enjoyed our workforce. Things went great for a number of years, and then one by one, all of us started getting sick. Me, my wife, my daughter Alicia . . . then a few of our workers. Pretty soon, everybody seemed to be struggling to get out of bed in the morning. We lost one litter of pups after another. And when the animals began to die of strange diseases, I knew something had gone terribly wrong.

"We didn't even know that we'd been poisoned. But pretty soon, everything started to go downhill. And we ended up . . . I guess it happened first in 1990 and then in 1992—we ended up throwing all these dead trees into huge piles to be hauled off.

"The trees and plants had been poisoned, too. And you'd think it wouldn't be that bad, right? I mean, some people have to go out and shoot their herds of cattle, right? Well, when we went to pile this stuff up in these huge dump-piles to be hauled away, every one of them might just as well have been a living being, not just a plant.

"They were living things. When the hundred-year-old live oaks began to die, it broke my heart. They might as well have been cattle or horses. I think trees have a life force, a spirit. Not just the majestic oaks which have survived drought, fires and hurricane force winds. The commercial product, too, was part of that concept. I felt a spiritual bond to the trees that I grew and nurtured.

"Now, don't get me wrong: I'm not a tree-hugger, or a Druid. But I do feel like we broke that spirit when we had to pick the trees up and throw them on a dump-pile and send them to the incinerator.

"It was a killer."

● ● ●

By the late 1980s, Frank Fuzzell's world was falling apart. Increasingly weak and muddled, himself, he was stunned to see most of the people he cared about in the world falling sick all around him. His daughter Alicia, for example, was complaining more and more of violent headaches that prevented her first from doing her homework, and then even from attending school.

While Frank's wife Lois struggled daily against agonizing muscle aches and debilitating nausea and diarrhea, the once-easygoing and affable nurseryman found himself grappling with "deep-in-the-bone" fatigue that often left him dizzy and disoriented and gasping for breath. He also endured the misery of watching several of his 20 employees—including veteran nurseryman and friend Ishmael Obregon—become grievously ill with ailments that defied diagnosis and didn't respond to any standard medical therapies.

Fuzzell hired private contractors to sample soil and well water at his site. He spent thousands of his own dollars in this effort. When the specialists found chemicals—fungicides and herbicides—that weren't supposed to be in the pesticide product, Frank became worried. He had meticulously documented each of his own chemical applications, including his use of fungicides.

Where had these contaminants come from?

Frank's anxiety about the unknown chemicals escalated rapidly, after he found pesticide residues in his well water. His concern was understandable, because the well was encased to a depth of 165 feet . . . which meant that the contamination had gone at least 165 feet down into the water table.

Increasingly alarmed, Fuzzell turned to a group of high-tech analysts who specialized in chromatography studies, and these quickly confirmed the presence of the unusual chemicals.

Something was obviously amiss. Badly frightened by the human illness he saw around him—and by the mysterious blight that was also killing hundreds of his trees each day—Fuzzell finally turned to the State of Florida for assistance in assessing the toxicity of the compounds detected in their drinking water. But when he phoned the Florida Department of Agriculture to report that something was "terribly wrong" on his tree farm, he received what he would later describe as "one of the worst shocks of my life."

After officials from the Florida Department of Agriculture visited his operation and collected soil and plant samples on several occasions in 1991 and 1992, Frank was stunned when an investigator from the Department of Agriculture told him to keep quiet about the dubious fungicide. Then, while completely ignoring his environmental concerns, they began to investigate *him*.

They suggested that the poisonings of trees and people had actually occurred as the result of two minor violations—on his part —of state regulations controlling how and where the powerful chemical must be used. (Those state citations against Fuzzell were later retracted.)

"I could hardly believe what they were telling me," recalls Fuzzell. "From day one, we had applied only a few chemicals to our plants, and very carefully. Those products had been placed on our fields precisely as directed by the same Florida Department of Agriculture that was now accusing us of misuse!"

Hoping to obtain some help from the state health bureaucrats regarding environmental contaminants found in water, Frank asked: "Is the water safe? What about the neighbors? What effect will contaminants have on human health?"

But they ignored his concern. Fuzzell was staggered to discover that *he* was now the subject of their investigation . . . even though the honchos at agriculture were fully aware of the fact that the hazardous pesticide had already been yanked off the market by the federal EPA—and that the manufacturer had already paid hundreds of millions of dollars in liability settlements to plant-growers (now more than $1 billion) who had lost their crops due to toxic attacks at sites around the country.

Within a year, in fact, the State of Florida would conclude that Fuzzell had violated no rules at all in his application of chemicals. "They tried very hard to come up with something," says the angry tree-grower today, "and they couldn't do it. So they simply fabricated it.

"They wasted all that time . . . and meanwhile, there were thousands of sites all across Florida that were experiencing this same problem with the fungicide. To this day, they still haven't answered the questions about the impact of this substance . . . to the point that Dr. Shoemaker is now petitioning the CDC for some of those answers.

"We gave them all our data, including all the interactions we'd had with the manufacturer, and they could have been making great strides forward in figuring out the problem. They didn't do it.

"The agency knew that the product contained an unregistered chemical in question, and that it was highly toxic to both humans and plants. And you can't apply any concentration of any unregistered compound to an agricultural crop.

"They knew what was happening, right from the beginning, but they never told anyone about the situation. Nobody was warned about the potential for contaminated food crops. Why? My feeling is, it was so huge that they didn't dare touch it.

"I mean, this product was widely used, *everywhere*. We were looking at one heck of a human health and food crop contamination issue, and the agencies wanted no part of it.

"The Florida Department of Agriculture certainly didn't want to send out a letter to every grower of every crop, telling them: 'You are going to have to destroy your plants, if you've applied this pesticide to them.'

"If they'd done that, people would have started asking the question: 'Well, how long has this been going on? And how long has the public been eating this food?'

"Those kinds of questions could get pretty big!"

• • •

To understand why farmers continue to use potentially hazardous chemicals on their crops, take a few moments to inspect a tray of plants, the next time you're visiting a commercial greenhouse. Which group of plants are *you* going to buy: the fungus-scarred specimens with the discolored leaves, or the perfect specimens with the full, lush leaves?

Now think about the plight of the typical grower, who must find a way to control plant/crop damage from fungal species. Remember, also, that there are hundreds of thousands of different species of fungi floating around out there, and many of them can hardly wait to sink their microscopic teeth into a cantaloupe that's been sitting out on a counter for two days, an orange growing in

Alexander Fleming's chemistry laboratory, or a patch of tender new strawberries. The threat from these fungal marauders is so great, in fact, that virtually every commercial farming operation in the United States now sprays fungicides in order to produce the "perfect" fruits and vegetables that consumers expect to find in the produce department.

The chemical battle against the fungi has been particularly ferocious in the warm, moist soils of central Florida, where plants grow in rows of "black plastic" containers that stretch to the horizon. For these tropical operations, the best defense against silent, invisible (until it's too late) fungi is to spray every plant heavily . . . and then spray it again. Central Florida is America's "ornamental plant breadbasket," after all, so it's no wonder that the growers here always use their chemical weapons "to the max" in order to keep fungi at bay.

As a result, you can be sure that the beautiful *dracena* in the lobby of the elegant Chicago restaurant was treated with fungicides during its early life in some Central Florida nursery.

For those who attempt to make a living by growing plants or food, the fungi loom as a relentless enemy. And these hardy microorganisms can digest just about anything. If some black molds can thrive happily on the surface of a metal heating duct, imagine how many fungal species can be nourished on a Florida cucumber crop?

Fungi export antibiotics (penicillin and cephalosporins, for example), enzymes and unusual molecules called "beta glucans" (known collectively as "mycotoxins") outside the cell. Typically, the fungus fights from behind its own impregnable walls, while sending armies of attackers, including low-molecular-weight toxins, outside to perform their silent destruction.

Given this harsh biological reality, it should come as no surprise that fungicides have become an essential element of today's agricultural system, in which "mega-farms" supply "super-stores" with an endless array of perfect fruits and vegetables. Any marks on that head of lettuce? Throw it away. And what about those massive grain elevators in Kansas, most of them crammed to the roof with corn, wheat and soybeans? With all that sugar stored in the grain, you'd expect these multi-story silos to quickly become fungus factories—especially when you remember that these crops are kept in warm, dark, moist surroundings for weeks at a time. (On a smaller scale, the same scenario threatens our stored supply of "sweet feed" for horses, as well as grain stored for cattle, chickens, turkeys, you name it.)

The USDA monitors cereal grains carefully for fungal contamination and for the presence of mycotoxins (but no testing is done in soils or ground water). Some of these toxins have been identified, then studied and classified for safety in food crops. The USDA is aware of the problem, and there's no reason to suspect that they aren't aware of *additional* problems caused by mycotoxins outside of cereal grains.

In most cases, however, the farmers manage to keep the fungi at bay. How can we ship millions of pounds of wheat to Russia and China and feel confident that it will arrive fungus-free, perfectly preserved? The answer, of course, is that we routinely store (and ship) powerful fungicides—such as copper—in our grain. But what happens when that grain is eaten by people, rather than fungi? Copper has little impact on human physiology, but the other toxic chemicals in these grains are not so easily filtered out of the body's self-cleansing system.

The demand for long-lasting fungus killers will always be with us, primarily because of the way most fungi reproduce themselves. As a matter of fact, the method of fungal reproduction —which results in two daughter cells—resembles mammalian cell reproduction more closely than that of any of the other "lower forms" of life.

Like the developing cells in a human fetus, fungal chromosomes—the structures that contain all of the cell's DNA—double themselves through a process called "mitosis." When this happens, the doubles line up in the middle of the cell. Then, during the "anaphase," they are pulled apart by thin threads, called "microtubules." These separate the doubles into singles.

In this process, a single copy of the dividing chromosome is pulled to each side of the dividing cell, which then splits into two new cells of equal size, with each containing identical chromosomes.

But what if the "microtubule tether" that pulls the chromosome to the side of the dividing cell doesn't work correctly? If that happens, some of the new cells won't end up with the right amounts of DNA in the right chromosomes at the right time. And this is precisely how the fungicide that made life hell for Frank Fuzzell works—by interfering directly with normal microtubular insertion into a specialized protein ("kinetochore") on the central site ("centromere") of a chromosome.

If a fungus is exposed to even a tiny bit of the toxin, it will quickly develop both mis-segregation and dis-segregation of chromosomes. And without the perfect structure of DNA in the chromosomes, the new daughter cells cannot be the same as the parent. On a percentage basis, obviously, these new cells will not be viable. As a result, this type of pesticide works very well to control growth of fungi in most cases.

Researchers also rely on this property in clinical fungal labs, in order to create new species and also evaluate the DNA of established species. At a dose of only five to ten parts per billion, the "mutation effect" is evident. As I reviewed the elegant mutation studies, I couldn't stop thinking about a foreboding 1984 study from Holland. There, the concentration of the Fuzzell fungicide in bulb-growers (who dipped the bulbs into a liquid form of the fungicide) was five parts per billion and easily discernible in urine samples taken from the greenhouse workers.

The Dutch survey raised a disturbing question: What effect does five parts per billion of a mutagenic-level chemical have in populations of people over time?

Recent studies describe scattered reports of genetic defects possibly associated with exposure to the substance, but no definitive proof has yet been demonstrated.

Meanwhile, the hazardous fungal-poison remains a bestselling agricultural product—despite the emergence of these "resistant species" of fungus—due not only to its effectiveness but also to its status as a "systemic fungicide." And yet the fact that this poison circulates throughout the plants it protects means that it can easily enter the human food supply, possibly causing widespread threats to human health.

Starting in 1969, the concept of employing a systemic fungicide—as opposed to a "surface contact" fungicide—against these stubborn microbes led to a brand-new approach to the fungus problem. Since then, many other systemics have emerged (see the discussion of metalaxyl and *Pfiesteria* in Chapter Three, "Clear As Mud"). For the growers, the good news was that once this pesticide had been absorbed, it wouldn't break down or degrade.

Unlike contact fungicides, it would not be neutralized by exposure to sunlight, UV light, rain, soil microbes or other chemicals. Instead, the parent compound could linger on in the plant for the rest of its natural life, unless the poisoned organism could somehow manage to detoxify itself.

But there was a price to be paid for this longevity, and it could be found in the idea that the new pesticide possibly made its way into the human food supply as we ate the rice or squash or lima beans with which it had been sprayed. Reflecting on this unhappy concern, I wondered if those Dutch bulb-growers had absorbed the high amounts of toxins found in their tissues from the pesticide-treated flowers they handled daily. Or had they actually ingested most of the fungicide via their diets?

What were the toxin levels in non-exposed workers who ate a similar diet? We don't know.

Up until now, I don't think those questions have been answered in print. As I struggled with them, I managed to collect several clinical histories in which acute illness had followed confirmed ingestion of such pesticides. Yet these cases remained isolated and sporadic; there was no way to link them together in order to prove an association.

Pick up any modern toxicology textbook or other reference work on poisoning, and you'll find long sections dedicated to organophosphates and organochlorines in contact pesticides— but almost nothing about the chronic health and reproductive problems caused by systemic fungicides. Confronting this lack of resources, I soon saw that any effort at single-handedly solving the puzzle would be an impossible task. Talk about confounding variables!

After thinking it over, I turned my attention back to the chemical toxin that *didn't* make it into the plant. Of course, I knew that the parent compound wasn't stable; it broke down quickly into "degradation daughters" that included MBC (carbendazim) and butyl isocyanate. Remembering that last toxic compound, I did a double-take: how many innocents had died at Bhopal, India, after that incident a few years ago in which deadly methyl isocyanate leaked from a Union Carbide plant? (As a group, the isocyanates are known to be toxic to lung tissue.)

At first glance, using this substance as a pesticide looked like the script for an agricultural disaster. Why introduce a mutagenic compound into a habitat where newly resistant fungi could evolve—and quickly—into some deadly new life form armed with toxins we had never seen before? Perhaps the degradation products would simply evaporate . . . or drift away harmlessly on one of those tropical breezes from the Gulf of Mexico.

No such luck. For starters, what would happen to greenhouse workers—and greenhouse visitors—who breathed in vapors containing isocyanates and who knows what else?

In order to understand the chemistry at work here, we need to understand that the cyanide linkage of carbon, triple-bonded to nitrogen, is one of the most reactive kinds of linkages in all of chemistry. If you want to change the structure of an organic compound, one sure strategy is to react it first with cyanide. The cyanide will break down at the same time it alters the parent compound. But you can be sure that no unaided reaction can ever eliminate all of the parent compounds involved in the process, including the cyanide.

For example, I always remember with sadness the deaths of several college students who attempted to synthesize the hallucinogenic drug, mescaline. Their approach was to react a special kind of organic phenol with cyanide. Unfortunately, a small amount of the latter substance contaminated the bootleg mescaline—and the "trip" they took with it was their last.

As I reviewed the literature that described these cyanide compounds, I wondered about the chemical reactions that might be taking place in the soil around Fuzzell's plants. Whatever fungus had survived that onslaught would have to be a mutant, and a mutant now resistant to the pesticide. It also seemed likely that any surviving bacteria, nematodes or algae in the area would also have to be resistant to the chemical agent in the fungicide, isocyanates and also to carbendazim—which chelates copper, much like the dithiocarbamates (see Chapter 2, "Showdown").

I can assure you that these chemicals are not what I'd choose to spray on *my* potted ferns, while growing them in a south-facing window! Yet this same deadly chemical stew might now be found in the soils of ferneries, ornamental plant nurseries, and muck farms throughout central Florida.

How toxic were these soil-borne chemicals to plants in the region? Hoping to find out, University of Florida plant experts surveyed the patterns of crop losses and stunted growth at more than 400 sites throughout the State of Florida where the fungicide had been used. The results were upsetting, to say the least; microbial testing of affected soils repeatedly identified three bizarre types of organisms: *fusarium oxysporum, fusarium solami* (fungus) and *pseudomonas fluorescens* (bacteria).

The fusarium was a fungus with teeth, just like the aphanomyces mutant strain (see Chapter 3, "Clear As Mud"). As it turned out, this powerful fungus was resistant to the Fuzzell fungicide, copper *and* dithiocarbamates. It also manufactured a toxin, similar to the fumonisins, that was known to cause defects in other cells and learning disabilities, along with several other adverse effects. In addition, this Cell From Hell knew how to make and export a cyanide compound.

The pseudomonas fluorescens species was equally alien. These hardy microbes actually required cyanide (a highly lethal carbon and nitrogen compound) for food! But their penchant for ingesting the deadly substance wasn't really that difficult to understand—not when you remembered that both carbon and nitrogen are raw elements required for life.

The *Pseudomonas* bacteria actually lived in the most important part of the plant: the rhizosphere, where the tiniest root hairs meet the soil and porewater. In this sensitive region, bacteria reign supreme. Install some poison-producing organisms around the roots ("DRB," or deleterious rhizosphere bacteria), and you can be sure that you'll soon be watching the plant die.

Sooner or later, it was only logical to expect the evolution of a biological critter that could withstand the reactivity of cyanide, simply breaking it down to use for fertilizer. This was survival of the fittest, indeed!

Since its unholy discovery a few years ago, *fusarium oxysporum* has itself been recruited as a hard-hitting pesticide. Because it's both persistent and resistant to every known fungicide, it has been enjoying a new life as biological herbicide. Why risk a dangerous invasion of the rugged jungles controlled by the drug lords of Colombia, when you can simply spray their coca plantations with fusarium from the air? No *problema*! And while we're at it, why not aim that spray-gun at Burma's Golden Triangle, where the poppies that form the basis of the international heroin trade can be found nodding and dozing beneath the mellow sun?

This "easy solution" to the drug problem seems to deprive politicians of their wits at times. In one recent, temporary episode of mindlessness, representatives from the office of Florida Republican Governor Jeb Bush went so far as to suggest that *fusarium oxysporum* be applied to the lush marijuana fields of Florida. (As if it weren't a big enough problem in the existing contaminated farmland.)

Madness! Fortunately in this case, the governor learned in time that lethal fungi don't just attack the plants we *want* them to attack . . . and that applying fusarium on a large scale would take out all kinds of other perfectly legal crops, along with the offending pot.

At this point, I'm still not sure how safe—or how dangerous —the new fusarium species may prove to be. Based on what has happened to Frank Fuzzell and his family and friends, however, it seems clear that this scary mutant belongs on the "Top Ten" list of mutant pathogens.

Finding the Link Back to *Pfiesteria*

After interviewing Frank Fuzzell at length in late 1998 and then putting him through our standard Contrast Sensitivity test, I felt certain that he was suffering from a neurotoxin-linked syndrome and that his debilitating symptoms had been caused by it.

During the next year or so, I would interview dozens of other residents of the Leesburg area. Again and again, their Contrast Sensitivity test scores made one fact overwhelmingly obvious: many of these neighbors of the nursery lands in this region of central Florida had been badly poisoned, leaving them with major vision and short-term memory problems, among other disorders.

Although their symptoms varied somewhat in intensity, they were remarkably similar in most other ways, as patient after patient reported suffering from:

- headaches;
- swollen joints and aching muscles;
- excessive fatigue;
- respiratory blockages, wheezing and nosebleeds;
- loss of short-term memory;
- severe diarrhea.

The question was: what if some chemicals that weren't supposed to have *been* in the fungicide drenched on Frank Fuzzell's trees—such as chlorothalonil and flusilazole—had actually caused these persistent and debilitating symptoms?

Or was there perhaps a *better* question . . . as in: What if the active agent making all these people sick wasn't one or more chemicals in the pesticide—*but a genetically altered fungus armed with a new kind of toxin that just happened to attack human beings? An organism, that possibly had been brought to life by the pesticide!*

In other words: What if the culprit in the Leesburg breakout was a microbe, rather than a chemical substance?

Why not? Hadn't *Pfiesteria* been hatched out of an estuarine environment—a coastal "habitat" that had been dramatically altered by the infusion of copper-based fungicides and dithiocarbamates?

And how had the *Pfiesteria* mutation responded to its sudden diet of porewater copper? Answer: By developing a whole new suite of toxins aimed at preserving itself in this changed ecosystem.

Francis Bacon again! There was certainly nothing "deductive" about my leap from pesticide toxins to the possible presence of a genetically altered fungus that thrived in the presence of fungicides and other microbial poisons. But the more I thought about this approach to the human illness syndrome that was at work in the Leesburg area, the more sense it seemed to make.

Why would we ever expect *no* effect on resident populations of microorganisms, after we had dumped untold numbers of pounds of biological poisons on the soil? Clearly, changes we could never predict were now quite possible—and might even persist. (See Chapter 11.)

With growing excitement, I reviewed the "inductive" chain of reasoning that had led me to the discovery of the human illness syndrome caused by the genetically altered and toxin-armed dinoflagellate, *Pfiesteria.* In many different ways, the parallels between that situation and the events at the Casteen Roads nursery in Leesburg were now becoming apparent.

First Step: After treating patients afflicted with symptoms that clearly indicated the presence of neurotoxins, I had looked for a common "exposure." And that exposure was the estuarine waters of the Chesapeake Bay, in which all of the infected patients had been swimming only a few days before. At Casteen Roads, the nursery lands had provided the exposure.

Second Step: After searching fruitlessly for a "measuring stick" that would allow me to establish parameters of illness in these newly diagnosed patients, I had hit upon the idea of using Dr. Hudnell's Contrast Sensitivity test in order to accurately gauge nerve-functioning. And that same test would also serve as a powerfully effective screening and diagnostic tool in Florida.

Third Step: Once I had a diagnostic tool in hand, I could quickly and clearly identify patients who were actually suffering from *Pfiesteria*-related human illness syndrome. At that point, I could begin to collect their medical histories and pass them on to the appropriate public health officials in Maryland (and later in Florida) . . . even if that dramatic step ultimately resulted in a great deal of paper-shuffling and very little action.

The bottom line was clear and compelling: In the case of *Pfiesteria*, I had gone against the Medical Establishment's time-honored tradition of deductive logical reasoning and rigorous "controlled" studies as the best way to attack a scientific mystery. Instead, I'd gone back to an earlier paradigm—*Bacon's* paradigm —and I'd employed inductive logic in order to leap to a key insight about the problem at hand.

Why not do the same thing with the mystery of Frank Fuzzell's toxin-riddled nursery in Leesburg? Why not try to determine how many other sites had been affected, and how many of the 120,000 people who worked at nursery operations in central Florida's fields might have been poisoned? How many neighbors of those sites had *also* been infected in recent years?

Could I find any links between the symptoms and treatment methods for *Pfiesteria*-related human illness syndrome and the neurotoxic disorders that were now taking place around farmlands which had been heavily sprayed with fungicides?

Increasingly fascinated by the problem, I quickly dug out a

report on *Pfiesteria* that I'd published in the Maryland Medical Journal only two years earlier . . . and well before the emergence of any other studies on chronic, environmentally acquired, neurotoxin-mediated illnesses.

TREATMENT OF PERSISTENT PFIESTERIA HUMAN ILLNESS SYNDROME

Patients with exposure to *Pfiesteria* toxins have developed an illness syndrome (PHIS) characterized by skin lesions, headache, myalgias, conjunctival irritation, bronchospasm, abdominal pain, secretory diarrhea, recent memory loss and difficulties with number sequencing. *Not all patients demonstrate all features of the syndrome. . . .*

Until the pfiesteria toxins are isolated, characterized and laboratory diagnostic tests are available, physicians must be able to recognize PHIS and intervene when symptoms, particularly memory loss and diarrhea, cause significant impairment in daily activities.

Let us not forget that recent bit of medical history!

•   •   •

**From "Notes for
Dr. Shoemaker," by Frank Fuzzell:**

It's December, 1998. We have been sick now for roughly 10 years. If our health were plotted out, it would show that we have reached the point where the cyclical lows are lower than ever. The peaks are diminishing, a steady decline.

Days, weeks, months at a time pass during which I do not have the energy to do anything. Can not think. Can not recall. Can't even use a calculator. Pushing the buttons, the numbers don't come out right. It seems like every thing sets me off, putting me out of commission.

A neighbor burning leaves next door, any kind of smoke

is devastating. Fumes from the newspaper, the computer, the exhaust from the car, gasoline fumes from the service station, the new asphalt on the highway. We hate to have to leave the house. At least when at home, we can lay down, wait for the nausea to let up, or drift in and out of a sleep that never really restores our energy.

The pain. It had reached the point where I required pain medication every day, so I could walk. Amazingly, certain medications helped me to breathe better. I had become so short of breath that I would run out of air while conversing, or walking from one room to another.

The feeling that I do not yet have a term for. Call it anxiety. It seemed to hit me mostly in the evenings. If asleep it would wake me up. It was intolerable. Many times it reached the point where I rushed to the emergency room. But what was the problem, how do you treat it?

There was an almost endless list of things that if they were not happening to me, I would never have recognized or understood in someone else. Had I met, or worse, ignored others in my life that had a similar problem? If so, please help me find a way to resolve this.

Did I push or criticize my daughter for not working hard enough, or falling asleep in the nursery/farm for hours after school? Why did it not occur to me sooner that my wife, daughter and I all shared the same symptoms? How many people are similarly affected? And what about the other people who work here with me?

The doctors that treated/tried to help, were dedicated. I was fortunate in this respect, but I was not getting anywhere. I really do not know how they handled it so well for so long.

We had reached the conclusion that an exposure to an agricultural chemical was at the base of our problems. I had heard about a medical doctor from Maryland that

came to Florida. He was a guest on a TV show down south
in Martin County. He had a theory that chemicals/toxins
from agricultural problems were responsible for Florida's
contaminated lakes and rivers, as opposed to the old worn
out "nutrient and outdated chemical" explanation that
virtually every responsible state and federal agency was
promoting.

I personally never bought into the classic government/
industry explanation. According to Dr. Shoemaker, chemi-
cals/toxins currently registered for use were the problem,
and not nutrients. I was interested in the environment,
had believed that agriculture and the environment could
co-exist. The disaster on our site now made me question
this.

I ordered a tape of Dr. Shoemaker's presentation. He
spoke words that we weren't hearing down here in Florida.
There were some key players in what I have come to call
"damage control" sitting on the panel to question Dr. Shoemaker. I had seen this style of questioning before with
Ph.D.s, but had never known a medical doctor to cross
over into environmental contamination issues, at least not
with this group.

The panel seemed a little shy, compared to their per-
formances in the past. One of the panel members, with
whom I am well acquainted, was a dead give-a-way. He
asked of Dr. Shoemaker something along the lines of,
"But you don't actually have a product name, right?" This
was a reference to the family of chemicals responsible.
This was damage control. Keep the product name out, and
limit liability for the chemical manufacturing industry.

When I first contacted Dr. Shoemaker in December of
1998, I did not know that he had been treating patients
in Maryland for environmental illnesses, most notably for
exposure to biological toxins. These toxins were produced
by an organism that lived in water. The toxins were causing fish kills, and human illness. He had a method for

screening patients for toxic exposures. He had a treatment for these patients.

By the end of December, 1998, we had been screened for toxic exposure and were taking the treatment recommended by Dr. Shoemaker and prescribed by my family doctor. The trips to the emergency room stopped. We began to breathe, think, to live. The pain went away. All of this began to happen in a period of several weeks, after years of suffering. Ishmael improved, too.

• • •

Showdown at the CDC: Here's What Happened

After talking to Frank Fuzzell and many other Leesburg residents, I knew it was time to act. I had a working theory about the source of the health problems at his site.

If my theory of an altered microbial population were correct, I also understood that there would be a "cohort" of Frank's neighbors who were suffering with an illness similar to his. After all, there are no artificial boundary lines for a biological organism like a fungus. All you need are a few spores on a windy day—or maybe a dog running through the mud on an infested property —and the fungus or bacteria or algae will begin to travel. If I got lucky, I told myself, I might even be able to work out a "dose response relationship" showing a correlation between the distance from the nursery and illness acquisition.

Coincidentally, one of Frank's neighbors, Marla Story, heard about my work. She lived due east of the Fuzzell site, right in the force of the prevailing winds. She knew all about sick people and sick animals, and her own health was deteriorating fast, she needed a medical doctor to help out—on the double! But I soon ran up against a stumbling block: the fact that no practicing physician near Frank wanted to get involved with Contrast Sensitivity testing and treatment with CSM. Some of the reasons they refused to participate were highly enlightening:

- I don't want get involved.
- I don't want to get sued.
- I don't know anything about this.
- I don't have time.
- This isn't FDA-approved for CSM.
- Things are just fine down here, but those folks are just whiners.
- Let the Public Health Department do it. I don't get paid enough.

One courageous physician agreed to try a few patients. He was starting a new practice, but was fearful of being overwhelmed with too many cases. Still, it only takes one willing physician to begin helping people get better. This bold volunteer didn't end up swamped by chronic, neurotoxin-mediated illness patients . . . but he *did* manage to determine that of the 120 people who lived near the nursery, about 80 were carrying the Contrast Sensitivity deficit. Still, it soon became evident that this illness did not exhibit a dose-response relationship. People got sick, or they didn't; there was simply no in-between.

The Florida physician followed the CSM treatment protocol, then tracked the results with CS testing. He also documented the resolution of symptoms. Soon he observed that both the symptoms and the CS deficit would return to those members of the "neighbor cohort" who continued to sit in backyards located near the abandoned nursery land. Although Fuzzell's former operation had remained idle for many years, with its soils undisturbed, the toxic residue still had the power to make people sick.

Even if these patients could be helped with re-treatment, it was easy to feel empathy for the recurrence of their painful symptoms. Who wanted to live with the memory impairment, severe headaches, abdominal pain, coughing and shortness of breath that are the hallmarks of chronic, neurotoxin-linked illness?

The growing pile of medical reports on the "neighbor cohort" also confirmed what Frank had seen—unusual tumors in horses, fetal wastage in the local dog population and pet birds that died inside the house. Meanwhile, the case histories of area residents continued to reflect their struggle with the poisons that had taken over their bodies.

Marla Story's situation seemed especially poignant. She and her husband had both been felled by the microbial mutants emerging from Frank Fuzzell's tainted acreage. Articulate and angry, Marla called every politician she knew to complain about the foot-dragging by local public health officials. She wrote dozens of letters and phoned the news media repeatedly.

In the end, she was told by Carl Blair—an administrator at the investigative arm of the CDC, the Agency for Toxic Substances and Disease Registry (ATSDR), who was quite aware of the on-going crop and human health problems at the Fuzzell site and many others—that the only workable approach was to find a physician who would agree to submit a formal petition asking for an investigation into the problem.

I was happy to oblige. I filed the petition to the Director of the CDC, Jeffrey Koplan, M.D., and he initiated the process that led to both an ATSDR investigation and a November 23, 1999, "conference call." Here's a copy of the petition that triggered the telephone conference:

October 5, 1999

Jeffrey Koplan, M.D.
Administrator
Center for Disease Control
1600 Clifton Road
Atlanta, Georgia 30303

Dear Dr. Koplan,

I am writing to you at the suggestion of Carl Blair, toxicologist at ATSDR, who called me regarding my work with an enlarging cohort of patients who have a chronic, neurotoxic-like syndrome resulting from exposure and re-exposure to nursery lands near Leesburg, Florida. Mr. Blair informed me that I am permitted to petition the CDC to investigate the site owned by Frank Fuzzell and adjacent areas where similar cases of illness have been identified. Given the clearly documented history of land use and pesticide application, it is reasonable to question whether or not chemicals used on the land are associated directly or indirectly with the development of a suspected chronic, toxin-mediated illness.

The clinical syndrome includes the following symptoms, although not all patients have all symptoms. Following exposure patients may note:

1) fatigue, weakness

2) memory problems, difficulties in executive functioning, difficulty with concentration (including task completion)

3) disorientation, confusion

4) headache

5) muscle ache, cramping, joint pain without inflammatory arthritis

6) hypersensitivity to bright light, blurred vision, burning or red eyes, tearing

7) cough, asthma-like illness, shortness of breath, chronic sinus congestion

8) chronic abdominal problems including nausea, cramping, secretory diarrhea

Our case definition is exposure to the lands in question, presence of at least four of the eight categories of neurotoxic symptoms, a deficit in visual contrast sensitivity (CS) greatest at 6 cycles per degree of visual arc, and lack of confounding medical conditions that produce abnormal CS results.

These patients are screened to exclude those with a history of Lyme disease, estuary associated syndrome

(*Pfiesteria* or morphologically related dinoflagellates), chronic ciguatera syndrome and chronic fatigue syndrome.

Many of these patients have been diagnosed variously as having depression, sinus problems, asthma, irritable bowel syndrome and fibromyalgia, among others. Treatment of patients with cholestyramine at the current approved dosage for treatment of hypercholesterolemia gives prompt improvement in CS as symptom severity abates. The improvement is durable, though re-exposure causes recrudescent illness. Repeat illness is also documented by reappearance of the CS deficits that abate, as does the illness, following re-treatment with cholestyramine. For those with residential exposure to affected land, continuous treatment with cholestyramine is recommended.

A thorough investigation is requested to include expanded exposure and health assessments. Exposure assessment should include a thorough sampling of the soils, surface water and ground (subsurface) waters for the pesticides applied, their degradation daughters and possible contaminants in the pesticide formulations. Since application of pesticides may lead to selective advantage for one or more species of resistant organisms, investigation should be broad spectrum, including all microbial species and toxins they produce. Mycotoxins (especially fumonisins and toxins made by Fusarium oxysporum), bacterial species, especially Pseudomonas species, and blue green algae species that make toxins including microcystin, cylindrospermopsin and anatoxin a-s are obvious analytes that must be included on these sites.

Because the human health syndromes are still being defined, the investigation cannot be limited to a restricted group of organisms or a restricted group of known toxins. In this rapidly evolving field of unusual organisms and unusual toxins, the reasonable scientist must be excruciatingly thorough.

Standard health screening of an enlarged cohort of

individuals exposed on Fuzzell's land and adjacent land needs to include the additional screening instruments that I used to document the presence of a chronic, toxin-mediated illness. By adding a complete neurotoxin symptom questionnaire and CS, some of the confusion and lack of documentation of a distinctive clinical syndrome noted by previous investigations of these sites and others will be avoided. Data on exposure duration should be collected since several patients in my cohort have reported recurrent symptoms even after brief re-exposures. Of course, data should also be collected to disarm potentially confounding factors. For comparison purposes, the screening battery should be administered to a matched-control population exposed to similar locations where pesticides were not used and would not be contaminated by ground water spread or vapor phase spread of pesticides.

If the human illness results from a direct effect of pesticides, the chemical data will be significant. If, however, the human illness is a result of changes in composition and toxicity of the surviving flora, then the specific assays for pesticides becomes less important. For this reason, data must be collected to show the diversity of microorganisms in the affected sites, the adjacent sites and control sites.

Although some environmental sampling has been done at these sites by Florida state agencies and at nearby sites by ATSDR previously, a thorough investigation has not been done. For example, mass spectroscopy data suggesting the presence of anatoxin a-s, various mycotoxins, as well as chemicals that were never intentionally used on the sites were not explained. There was never any consideration given to the possibility that chemicals used on the land (including degradation daughters) either directly caused human illness or disrupted balances of microbial populations, leading to the bloom of certain toxin forming species or caused mutation of resident species, especially fungi, bacteria and blue green algae. The illness seen in our various cohorts must be defined pathogenically, toxicologically and definitively.

A previous health survey in nursery workers (Stabile, Florida State University, 1993, unpublished), did not use CS or a neurotoxic illness questionnaire, but reported the presence of a similar illness syndrome. Symptoms included headaches (63%), stiff and achy joints (49%), shortness of breath (39%), fatigue (33%), rashes (30%), swollen joints (27%), sore and irritated throat (27%), nausea (27%), dizziness (25%), numbness and tingling in the extremities (23%), short term memory loss (20%) and nose bleeds (20%). No follow up was completed.

The chemical-microbial link to human illness is an emerging field of medicine. CS screening for neurotoxic illness was first used by Dr. Ken Hudnell of the US Environmental Protection Agency, National Health and Environmental Effects Research Laboratory/Neurotoxicology Division. His paper on use of CS in Pfiesteria patients (US EPA #600-R-98-132) was cleared for public release following extensive peer-review by EPA and the North Carolina Task Force on Fish Kill Waters (Chair: William Roper, Chairman of the School of Public Health, University of North Carolina at Chapel Hill). My use of cholestyramine as a therapeutic agent in chronic neurotoxic syndromes was first published in 1998. We have four papers nearing completion using CS and cholestyramine. We have been accumulating a data base on cases and controls using CS for the past 12 months.

Dr. Hudnell and I are currently collaborating on several additional studies, including cohorts of sick patients who live or work adjacent to pelican kill sites near Lake Apopka, patients from alligator kill sites in Lake Griffin and the patients in the Leesburg study.

The need for a Federal investigation of the Leesburg site is evidenced by the facts that these once productive farm lands are now fallow, those who worked on the land have been chronically ill, and some state inspectors who visited the land have developed chronic illness. My identified patients, many of whom have been chronically ill for over 10 years, are likely a small percentage of those exposed and suffering from a chronic neurotoxic syndrome. Treatment with cholestyramine fortunately has corrected the illness in a number of patients.

I am ready to assist you in any way possible in your investigation, as is Dr. Hudnell. Our work will continue, as the use of CS and cholestyramine has potential application in many areas of chronic toxicity. Dr. Hudnell and I will be conducting two large clinical trials soon to present to the FDA for consideration of an additional label for cholestyramine.

Our goal is straightforward: we want to identify cases of environmentally acquired neurotoxic illness and successfully treat the illness. An investigation by your agency could document the extent of the undiagnosed neurotoxic illness, identify the environmental factors responsible for the illness and hopefully, begin the process to mitigate the culpable environmental factors.

Sincerely,
Ritchie C. Shoemaker, M.D.

What happened next, however, was a sad commentary on the deterioration that has overtaken our Defenders of Public Health in recent years. Frank will tell you that the state and federal authorities knew that there was a microbial problem involving toxin-forming fungi on lands where the fungicide was used. But nothing was done.

I did my best, however. After receiving a call from John Saunders, who was charged by the CDC with responding to my petition, I quickly signed on for the Nov. 23 conference call. Trust me: that session was a real eye-opener. Public health officials and scientists from up and down the East Coast logged into the telephonic conference. I felt upbeat and enthusiastic about the call, because I knew that the CDC had the resources and the funding to make a difference in the situation, if the agency executives chose to.

I also knew, of course, that ATSDR had investigated this site and others like it during the 1990s, as indirectly related to the numerous lawsuits filed against the manufacturer of the allegedly offending pesticide.

The manufacturer eventually settled many of these cases, but more than 150 other lawsuits remain in litigation. It seemed logical to assume that since my patients were involved in a site of this kind at the Fuzzell nursery, the CDC experts on the conference call would be familiar with the history of crop damages and litigation in the region.

I was wrong.

The call included several officials from the State of Florida Health Department. Another individual identified himself as a "Fellow" of a professional toxicology group, and as an "expert" in the field. Yet he soon pointed out that he'd never even heard of CS-testing for neurotoxins, and could not understand how such a diagnostic tool could have any merit.

I quickly told the "Fellow" that his lack of knowledge didn't matter, then went on to explain how the test had been used for 35 years, and that it was reproducibly reliable, portable, cost-effective and specific.

In addition, EPA neurotoxicologist Dr. Ken Hudnell did his best to help the "Fellow" understand more about the effects of toxins on the optic nerve, along with optic radiation. Betty Phifer, a health officer at ATSDR, also noted that her agency had been using the test for several years.

We didn't hear much more from the "Fellow" that day. After reviewing the facts, the ATSDR decided that the data were authentic, and forwarded them on to the CDC—while announcing that another conference call would be scheduled after the new year began.

The last act in this comedy of errors finally took place in February of 2000—when the CDC brass came on line for our long-awaited conference call . . . more than four months after the filing of the original petition. Once again, the Official In Charge expressed deep reservations about the efficacy of the CS Test, even though he had little experience (and less knowledge) of its decisive importance in helping to diagnose neurotoxin-mediated illness.

As we talked, it became quite evident that the CDC decision on this issue had been predetermined . . . and that the agency had no intention of getting tangled up in a case of this kind.

Somewhere in the middle of this rambling discussion, the epidemiologist asked an unusual question. He wanted to know why a "private physician" had become involved in this matter. Although it was clear that he and his fellow-bureaucrats had already made up their minds, I went ahead and wasted several minutes in a futile attempt to explain the reality.

"It's because these patients have gotten nothing from the Florida Health Department," I told him angrily. "They're still sick, and their animals are dying of strange tumors that no one has ever seen before. And their children can't pay attention, and can't learn, and are being diagnosed as having depression and attention deficit disorder—even though their performance was fine before they moved here! And all of that happened because of exposure to toxins in their environment.

"I've shown these people a new approach to diagnosing and treating their illness, one that works. The public health people here have done nothing to help. All they do is hide behind one bureaucratic smokescreen after another . . . and you wonder why more and more of them are coming to me for help?"

But the CDC spokesman remained unconvinced. "I think we'll need a review of the old records of all these patients, along with an assessment of their emergency room visits, in order to validate your findings, Dr. Shoemaker."

I could hardly believe my ears.

"Excuse me, doctor. Do you really practice medicine? Do you operate in the real world—where patients must be seen and charts completed before the start of each new day? How many patients have you treated for aching muscles and exhaustion? Did you ask them about sensitivity to bright light?

"Why are you so unaware of the realities of front-line medicine? Did you miss something in your training? These toxin-mediated illnesses are *here*, sir!"

"Only *we* can make a decision in matters of this kind, Dr. Shoemaker. I will review those findings and this conversation with my colleagues and then *we* will determine if there is a public health emergency here."

I paused to take a deep, calming breath, while remembering some good advice from my wife, JoAnn: "Speak slowly, and don't make it personal!"

"Not everyone who's tired, short of breath or chronically coughing will be diagnosed as suffering from a fungus, algae or spirochete toxin, that's true. But if we don't know enough to ask the right questions—*how will we identify the ones who are?*"

Before my question could be answered, however, the CDC's John Saunders jumped in to remind everyone that we were "running out of time," with only two minutes left for our discussion. "Do you have any final comments, Dr. Shoemaker?"

I paused for a moment to gather my thoughts. Then: "Dr. CDC, you have argued with my case definition. You raised trivial objections, and made them seem like insurmountable obstacles. You have shown you know nothing about Contrast Sensitivity. You have shown little empathy for these long-suffering patients. You have cast aspersions on my credibility and my honesty. And you are wrong. But regardless, there will be more cases, and not just from this nursery. And even if you don't investigate them now, for whatever reason, the fact remains that the contaminated plant material was put in the landfills—and the workers in those landfills are now beginning to exhibit the same health problems that nearly destroyed Mr. Fuzzell and his employees.

"Other nurseries throughout the state have called me with similar complaints. The contaminated materials have been placed beside estuaries, and who knows what we now have in the water as a result. These contaminated materials are located at 1,200 different sites around Florida. You have a logical and reasonable basis to investigate the biggest agricultural disaster in the history of Florida, and you choose deliberately to do nothing.

"This will not be our final conversation!"

chapter 10

Reflection

The Appearance
Of Good Science

Pocomoke, MD –May, 2000

Rob Sullivan, M.D., a professor of epidemiology at Duke Medical School, years ago taught me how to save a great deal of time when trying to evaluate the usefulness of medical literature.

Dr. Sullivan's approach struck me as wonderfully down to earth and simple.

"Before you do anything else, take a look at the 'Methods' section of the study you're reading," the professor told us on Day One of his course. "Don't start with the 'Abstract'—because most of the time, it amounts to little more than a distilled sales pitch for the argument the investigator is trying to prove.

"I'd avoid the 'Summary' section, as well," said the outspoken Dr. S, "because in most cases, you'll find authors using this part of the presentation to speculate about the meaning of their results. Nor will the 'Introduction' help you—since it's usually designed to convey the 'spin' of the article that follows.

"No, ladies and gentlemen, the secret to quickly getting a useful handle on a piece of scientific writing is to look first at the 'Methods' section. If these seem illogical, or epidemiologically unsound, you can be virtually certain that the article, itself, will be deeply flawed. Don't read it! Use your precious time wisely—by moving on to some other scientific publication in

which the Methods being used by the investigator seem logical
and coherent."

Unfortunately, Dr. Sullivan's tutorial was sparsely attended.
As a result, far too few of my colleagues learned how to take
advantage of his wisdom, when it came to the important business of evaluating scientific theories and scientific literature.

I was reminded of the power of that wisdom only a few years
after leaving Duke, while engaged in my Family Practice residency. As we made our way through rounds one morning, we
found ourselves confronting the case of a Baltimore pipefitter
and shipyard worker who was being studied for a possible lung
cancer.

I've never forgotten the unctuous certitude with which the
intern-in-charge described some recent research on possible
links between asbestos and lung cancer.

"A landmark study on shipyard workers showed that exposure
to asbestos was associated with the development of mesothe-
lioma," intoned the youthful doctor, while assuring us that this
unusual form of lung cancer was undoubtedly at work in the
Baltimore patient.

It didn't take me long to respond.

"I notice that the study didn't control for cigarette smoking,"
I politely suggested to the intern. "You can see that just by reading the 'Methods' section. It seems to me that you can't draw
any conclusions about such an association without controlling
for confounding variables."

The intern waved my objection away, then breezily concluded:
"I would say that this patient is quite likely to have mesothe-
lioma."

He was wrong, however. Within a matter of days, the pipefitter
was diagnosed as having the most common form of lung cancer.

A recent headline from Florida provides another compelling
example of how bad science can result from a failure to design
logically appropriate "methods" for studying a public health
phenomenon.

ALL TESTS FOR TOXIC CHEMICALS ARE NEGATIVE

The headline appeared above an article that reviewed a cluster of cases involving neuroblastoma—a rare form of childhood cancer—in Port St. Lucie, a town of about 30,000 on the east coast of the Sunshine State. This community had already experienced nearly 40 cases of neuroblastoma . . . even though the normal incidence is only one in about 100,000.

Hoping to gain a clear understanding of how the public health authorities had investigated the outbreak, I examined their epidemiological methods. I soon learned that they had sampled well water from several homes in this small "bedroom suburb," and that they had tested the water for several compounds that are known carcinogens.

As the Florida newspaper accurately reported, all of the test results had been negative.

Fair enough. But even a quick look at the Department of Health's methodology was enough to expose serious flaws. Had the public health officials tested for the presence of toxic pesticides that had been used on the land, or the breakdown products of those chemicals? No, they had not. Yet it was common knowledge that the town of Port St. Lucie had been built on abandoned orange groves, and that their sandy soils quickly allow applied agricultural chemicals to filter into ground water —including water contained in the shallow wells that supply nearly every home in the area.

Question: Would a carefully controlled, logically sound study have included tests aimed at pinpointing residues from agricultural chemicals? The answer is "yes," of course. Unfortunately, the editors at the local newspaper didn't know enough about environmental science to provide their readers with a truly *accurate* story, which might have begun:

"A recent study of well water in Port St. Lucie offered the public the 'False Appearance of Good Science'—by purporting to be thorough and definitive, while at the same time failing to address crucially important aspects of the scientific issues involved."

If only those befuddled editors had spent some time reading the "Methods" section of the public health studies on which they were so glibly reporting!

After many years of watching such bad science pretend to be sweepingly authoritative, I've identified the series of steps that are almost inevitably involved in creating "The Appearance of Good Science" (AGS)—and then palming it off on an unsuspecting public as "The Real McCoy."

Experience shows that AGS—a tactic frequently employed by public health policy bureaucrats—usually contains four basic elements, all of which were carefully designed long ago to help the bureaucrats control situations in which the political system must respond to health events.

The most common weapon in the AGS arsenal is the "Consensus Statement," which has a success-rate of nearly 100 percent, when it comes to quashing controversy. Typically, the Consensus Statement will be surrounded by such authoritative, reassuring phrases as "a panel of experts," "a blue-ribbon committee," or even better, "an international consortium of scientific experts." Of course, such terminology usually works to obscure the fact that the recommendations or decisions involved were actually crafted by a few politically connected insiders who cooked them up behind closed doors.

Another sure sign that the Consensus Statement tactic has been put into play can be observed by watching the demeanor of the politicians involved. After praising the "impartiality and objectivity" of the "blue-ribbon panel," they will tell the news media over and over again: "I want the answers, too! This is certainly an issue for our expert scientists to review in detail, and I will follow the advice of the panel carefully. Let the chips fall where they may." (When you hear that phrase, you can rest assured that the chips will soon be falling exactly where the politicians *want* them to fall!)

It goes almost without saying, of course, that the "panel" has already been stacked with political appointees and other "officials" who, on closer inspection, turn out to have a large personal stake (Financial? Political? Bureacratic?) in the panel's findings.

When the panel convenes to "explore" the issue at hand, you can also be sure that anyone who opposes its preordained conclusions will either be limited to a few brief remarks, or barred from the proceedings on some last-minute technicality. Of course, the chair of the panel will lavish praise on any individual who opposes the rigged findings for his or her "open-mindedness and candor" . . . and then completely ignore every suggestion issued from the lips of the doomed outsider.

Once the panel's "conclusions" have been announced, both its members and their allied politicians will quote it endlessly, in the hope of converting their speculations to "accepted fact" among the citizenry. "Our expert panel carefully reviewed the science involved—and there's simply no remaining doubt that the world is flat. That assertion has now been documented by our experts."

In this book you'll find several examples of "expert conclusions" that turned out to be completely false, including such endlessly repeated maxims as, "The river is safe," and, "The lake is safe," and, "The building is safe."

One of the most disastrous and wasteful "panel conclusions" in all of public health emerged recently from the National Cholesterol Education Project (NCEP), an NIH panel which reviewed findings from five large clinical trials. All five studies focused on white males aged 40–65. When lumped together, the findings clearly showed that cholesterol levels above 240 are associated with an increased risk of heart attack.

Responding to this dramatic disclosure, the panel recommended that people of all races and ages (male and female alike) strive to keep their cholesterol level below 200.

Absurd? You bet. Can you imagine the scene in which the gynecologist warns the 24-year-old, five-foot-four and 115-pound woman that she has *got* to get that cholesterol of 220 down?

What data might justify such a recommendation? There are none! Although I have no wish to unfairly attack the NCEP, the fact remains that their analysis of the "problem" of cholesterol in over-65 people who haven't had heart attacks simply will not bear scrutiny. (Don't forget: one of the major reasons for lowering cholesterol is to prevent *premature* heart attacks. Premature means occurring before age 65.) Yet the panel described such cholesterol as a "special problem" for senior citizens. And because "one study showed that reducing systolic blood pressure in the elderly helped to reduce stroke rates," the scientists in this blue-ribbon assemblage decided that cholesterol should be reduced, too. Since when does one study on blood pressure have anything to do with cholesterol?

The next time your father-in-law winds up spending $150 of his $600 monthly Social Security check for cholesterol pills to prevent the heart attack he's already out-lived, you can tell him that he's just fallen prey to the awesome power of the AGS Consensus strategy!

You can be sure that the AGS is designed to instill doubt— and fear—in those who believe that the "panels are impartial." How many patients beyond the age of 65 (patients who have never experienced a heart attack, that is) are faithfully taking their anti-cholesterol medication each day, even though it has no impact on their health at all?

Lots! And yet there has never been a single study (that wasn't paid for by a drug company, mind you) which found a reduced risk for heart attack among this group of patients, merely because they took a cholesterol-lowering drug!

The second AGS tactic seems especially cruel and unfair, yet it happens every day of the week in every profession. This strategy comes into play whenever a "heretic" parts company with the "conventional wisdom" of the hyena pack. No sooner does this lone hyena make it clear that he or she can't support the Consensus, than the other members turn on the outcast with bared fangs.

Unlike the U.S. Supreme Court, which carefully notes "dissenting minority opinions" for the record, the pack cannot bear to be contradicted in its group wisdom.

And the result? You guessed it. In situations where AGS rules, the dissenter will be treated like a zebra by the hyenas. Nipped at from every side, the loner will be driven to the earth and then slashed to pieces by the AGS hyenas, whose bellies are by now bloated with the suppression of dissent.

Silencing the dissenter doesn't always have to be complete and permanent, however; in many instances, a few successful attacks of "character assassination" will often be enough to eliminate the opposition. And so what, if good science is actually *supposed* to be based on healthy skepticism and criticism—both of which, hopefully, serve to refine and perfect scientific concepts?

A couple of years ago, I was able to record a classic demonstration of such a hyena attack on videotape—during a series of "Copper and *Pfiesteria*" meetings that took place in Salisbury, Md. During one of these "blue-ribbon panel" investigations into illness caused by the *Pfiesteria* microorganism, the gentle Dr. Gian Gupta had just finished discussing his findings regarding the enrichment of copper in porewater, and had found it necessary to leave the meeting. As soon as the door closed behind him, several members of the state-run "panel" immediately began to attack the credibility of his work. Hyena attack! It's one thing to question a scientist's findings . . . but what was the point of attacking the integrity of his work while he was out of the room, as if the attack, itself, proved that the attackers were correct?

So much for the second strategy of the AGS-crowd. But what happens when a "loner" is obviously telling the truth, and seems capable of convincing others of that fact? When this happens, the insiders will often resort to Strategy No. 3, "Damage Control," aka "The Smokescreen." It's a simple strategy, and easy to implement; all you have to do is make the public look the other way.

Example: After our presentation to the Centers for Disease Control and Prevention (See Chapter 9), Dr. Roger Inman—then Chief Toxicologist for the Florida Department of Health

—came up with several novel explanations for why people who lived near Frank Fuzzell's contaminated nursery land kept on getting sick. Was Dr. Inman whitewashing the truth? He retired three days later.

Readers will have to decide for themselves. But here's a direct quote from a 1996 lawsuit deposition in which one of Dr. Inman's former employees—Dr. Ted McDowell of the Florida Department of Agriculture (and later at the Florida Department of Environmental Protection)—describes the Inman approach to fact-gathering:

Q. What do you mean by "damage control?"

McDowell: "When I was hired, Dr. Inman said, 'Ted, what we do here is damage control.' And sitting in there with him was Steve Rutz and Richard Budell of Agriculture. . . ."

Q. When you say . . . "damage control," are you telling us that you were asked at some point to make statements that you believed to be false?

McDowell: "Yes."

Next case!

Several different theories (but not the obvious one) were brought forward to account for the illness. Despite Dr. Inman's creative efforts, however, the truth managed to survive this exercise, and bio-testing continues in Florida in an effort to identify the microbial population (see Chapter 29, "Struggling to the Light") that are manufacturing toxins on Fuzzell's land.

Of course, damage control usually involves blaming an environmental problem on nutrients if not some chemical or other substance that is no longer used—after which no corporate liability can be ascribed in order to remedy the problem.

The "nutrient issue" as related to environmental degradations today provides a powerful example of AGS Damage Control at work. During the past 20 years, the Chesapeake Bay has suffered dramatic loss of underwater grasses (Submerged Aquatic Vegetation, or SAV).

The late Dr. George Demas showed that many of the submerged soils have become so inhospitable that replanting of any new kinds of vegetation simply wouldn't work. Dr. Demas did not perform an assay for deleterious rhizosphere bacteria (DRB) —although he was preparing to conduct that very procedure at the time of his tragic death (Chapter 28).

The Chesapeake Bay/EPA Program finally acknowledged the huge problem of heavy metals and toxic chemicals in the bay, although their report somehow asserted that only nine pounds of dithiocarbamates had been used on land in 1998 . . . even though public records make it clear that more than **1.5 million** pounds were actually applied to drainage-area lands during that period in Maryland alone. Of course, no one knows exactly how many additional pounds or where they were used by other states in the Chesapeake Bay drainage area (Pennsylvania, Delaware, Virginia, West Virginia).

According to the feds, the die-off of SAV was due to "nutrient enrichment that stimulates growth of algae which shade the grasses and also consume all the available oxygen." Unfortunately, the EPA gurus seemed to have forgotten a basic principle of biology. . . . which is that you can't grow grass in unsuitable soil! Do we have DRB in the barren, submerged lands of the Chesapeake? If the nutrient apologists have thought about DRB, they sure haven't talked publicly about their critical interface of roots, soil and bacteria.

The Chesapeake Bay program could learn from our small acreage. We have planted over 10,000 trees and shrubs that make our home a wildlife sanctuary. In one section of our local reforestation area however, no trees will live. The grass grows fairly well, but any vegetation with roots longer than six inches soon expires. The former owner of that parcel of land told me that this same area "was where the herbicide spray had been loaded for use on the fields." But, according to the feds, the pesticide and the herbicide he used broke down "in just a short time," and there was "no chance of prolonged toxicity to plants!" Why is the soil so toxic years after the herbicide was gone?

In spite of the obvious evidence of the importance of DRB, or other water column deleterious bacteria, however, the AGS hyenas continue to blame nutrients for the *Pfiesteria* blooms of the Eastern Seaboard, along with the degradation of Florida Bay and the persistence of the Rhode Island-sized "Dead Zone" of the Gulf of Mexico.

Maybe there *are* extra nutrients as the result of runoff. But what else is in that runoff? What other chemicals are poisoning our ecosystem, and working hand in hand with nutrients to accomplish this? If we should discover that toxic chemicals are even partially responsible, would there be a corporate liability? You bet. But who is responsible for the "nutrient" scourge? Why . . . everyone! (And thus . . . *no* one.) No one has even begun to test for DRB. Don't ask, don't tell!

So much for Damage Control. The fourth and final increment in the AGS strategy for preventing dissent is "Burial." If the truth manages to survive Consensus, Hyena Attack and Smokescreen, its final reward will be the oblivion of "We need more study on this important issue!"

"Yes . . . we have gathered here today to honor Dr. Truth. At first, we felt sure he was mistaken. But we have studied his ideas and his evidence carefully . . . and now we feel the need to thank him for his tireless, courageous work. This medal is our highest award, and carries the official *H. pylori* Bacterial Seal of Heroism—in honor of the forgotten scientist who showed us that many stomach ulcers are actually caused by bacteria!

"We are today launching a ten-year series of studies in honor of Dr. Truth, and we are confident that his ideas will continue to enrich our lives deeply, even as we study them forever."

One of the most frequently employed forms of AGS Burial is the "My Idea First" approach. In this remarkably cruel application of the strategy, Dr. Truth eventually discovers that one of his harshest critics has actually *stolen* his discovery and is now peddling it, himself, for considerable personal gain. This final step is the surest evidence that Dr. Truth's Burial is now complete.

"Farewell, Dr. Truth! Have a wonderful life. You did a fabulous job of re-educating the scientific/political establishment about Controversy X . . . but you forgot that bureaucracies *never* grow smaller. They will fight for their lives at all costs. You also forgot that politics usually controls science, and that the truth will usually be sacrificed for ends that have very little to do with public health or the common good."

Question: how can we defend ourselves, as a society, against the destructive impact of The Appearance of Good Science?

Answer: The first step—the absolutely essential step—is to recognize it when you see it. And it's my fervent hope that these pages will help you to do exactly that!

The Monster in the Lake

Lake Griffin, Lake Apopka, FL –August, 1999

Have you ever read a headline that gave you a bad case of "the creeps?"

Let me tell you about a recent Saturday morning when I picked up a just-published copy of the *Florida Game and Fresh Water Fish Commission Newsletter*—and came across a news report that positively made my flesh crawl.

Printed in 36-point **Boldface**, the headline on the story ran as follows:

SCIENTISTS PROBE ALLIGATOR DEATHS ON LAKE GRIFFIN

Leesburg, Fla.—Wildlife scientists from a variety of state agencies are trying to figure out what is killing alligators on 9,000-acre Lake Griffin. At last count, at least 40 gators have died of unknown causes.

Meanwhile, adult gators are producing few viable eggs.

"Since the spring of 1997, we've had low hatch rates and high mortality of adult alligators in Lake Griffin," said Dr. Perran Ross, a University of Florida biologist who has been hired by the state to study the mysterious alligator deaths. "Eggs are dying during incubation, or within five to ten days of being laid."

According to the expert, only four percent of the lake's alligator eggs are hatching, even as the recent die-off continues to accelerate.

Although the exact cause of the deaths has not yet been pinpointed, researchers are focusing their efforts on four possible explanations:

- *Cylindrospermopsis*, a form of blue-green algae that can discharge toxins into fresh water under some conditions;
- a disease, so far unidentified, that has attacked the alligator population;
- chemical contamination, possibly from nearby citrus processing or farming operations;
- poor nutrition among the alligators, who may have been deprived of some of their food supply (fish and small mammals) in recent months.

• • •

Why did this particular story send me into a sudden, fullscale attack of the heebie-jeebies? Well, for starters, long experience had taught me that this kind of highly visible public health issue usually brings on a major attack of the Appearance of Good Science (AGS), as described in the preceding chapter!

At Lake Griffin, all of the factors were present for full-speed-ahead whitewash. Let's face it: in *this* dramatic scenario, we were dealing not with some abstract concepts about possible mutations in microorganisms—but with prehistoric carnivores that appeared to be dying at the height of adulthood.

Of course, they were also floating aimlessly about on the lake, while failing to evade passing boats . . . a state of affairs that was certain to bring the newshounds sprinting to the scene of the "eco-disaster." *Alligators on drugs? Alligators on poison? And what about the overnight disappearance of all those trophy bass and brine shrimp?*

Somehow, one of Florida's most famous and photogenic ecosystems had managed to collapse almost overnight. How could the marvelously complex, 9,000-acre aquatic environment that was Lake Griffin have come apart at the seams like this . . . in a period of less than three years? Was it any wonder that photos of the lake's dead gators and dead pelicans were now appearing on front pages all across the Sunshine State?

Send in the AGS troops! Maybe I've grown cynical, but the truth is that whenever I hear how an environmental or public health problem is to be "studied by many different groups of scientists," the hair immediately begins to stand up along the back of my neck. Why? It's simple: during more than two decades as a public health activist, I've learned that when government and academic organizations start "helping out" with a problem, less and less tends to get done!

But the bureaucrats of Lake Griffin hadn't counted on the presence of a very bold and very courageous Florida woman whom you're about to meet. Her name is Ann Griffin—and the threatened lake where the alligators wouldn't stop dying was named after one of her ancestors.

Ann Griffin grew up around the lake that bears her name, and she fell in love with its stunning beauty as a child.

Ask her to describe the world she knew as a kid—the gently rolling hills and the gleaming lakes of the *Ocklawaha* watershed —and Ann Griffin will tell you about lazy summer afternoons when she climbed the Spanish moss-draped branches of the live oaks along the water's edge . . . or sat on her family's rickety pier and fished for bass with a cane pole . . . or hiked among the gurgling marshes of this astonishingly beautiful region, in search of ibis and the osprey and the majestic bald eagle.

"That's all gone now," Ann told me. "It's all been poisoned. Now the lake is full of toxic algae, and the copper from the muck farms has ruined the sediment. After all these years . . ."

She paused for a moment, and I could hear the anger bristling in her voice.

"Dr. Shoemaker, can you imagine how it feels, to wake up one morning and find your lawn littered with poisoned, dying pelicans?"

• • •

In this chapter, you're going to get a disturbing look at how chemical pesticides can team up with a voracious, one-celled predator—a frighteningly single-minded life form known as *cylindrospermoposis*—to create an ecological disaster that Ann Griffin and her neighbors now call: "The Monster in the Lake."

She isn't exaggerating, either.

After spending months working with some Florida doctors to treat sick patients and conducting research on this spoiled paradise, I can tell you for a fact that toxic algae have now become an ecological threat—not just to the Ocklawaha chain of lakes, but to all of central Florida, including the Orlando area. At the same time, the algae are now threatening to move north and east, via the St. Johns River, toward distant Jacksonville.

Unfortunately, the story of what went wrong at Lake Griffin is also being duplicated in dozens of lakes and rivers throughout the region . . . and especially at nearby Lake Apopka, where animals, fish and human beings alike have apparently been poisoned by a microbe created by mutation—or perhaps a series of mutations—that inhabits pesticide-polluted lake sediment. Spooky? You bet. I'm convinced that the story of modern Lake Griffin could have provided the script for a 1950s sci-fi flick, "The Algae That Ate Orlando!" (starring Raymond Burr, of course), if only Hollywood had known about it.

Already tragic, this saga of dead alligators and pelicans grew even darker in late 1999, when several human health studies revealed that the new poisons in the watershed are also taking on a toll on thousands of Hispanic, Haitian and African-American farm workers. Add to those accounts my own study of local patients who have developed signs of chronic, neurotoxin-mediated illness (including symptoms, positive FACT, and response to CSM treatment), and you can see that this scenario has all the makings of a full-scale environmental disaster.

Cylindrospermopsis is a *common* topic in central Florida. Lots of people are talking about it, but nothing is being done to come to grips with the problem. Is anybody out there really listening?

A similar theme in environmental disasters involving *Pfiesteria* and cylindro begins to unfold when wetlands are drained and farmed. That's because bad things can happen when ag chemicals (they're advertised as being perfectly safe on land) manage to find their way into the water column—whether estuary, river, lake, or even ocean.

Muck farming provides a classic example of how to concentrate biology-altering chemicals with biologically altered organisms. When the wetlands of central Florida are drained by pumping water into the nearby shallow, diked and slowly flushing lakes, the rich soils that result can be planted. These wetlands are simply loaded with organic material. Remember, however, that all crops must be protected from pests, including other plants, insects and fungi.

This system of farming calls for the wetlands to be flooded again after the harvest, protecting the soils from oxidation. Lake water is thus mixed with ag chemicals and silts. Now repeat the process, mixing drainage from wetlands with the mother lode of aquatic species that inhabit the lakes.

Add a few more chemicals (say, from an old Super Fund site —such as the DDT—and copper-manufacturing plant on the south shores of Apopka), and watch natural selection begin. Now flush lake water downstream, from one lake to the next, via an elaborate system of canals.

If a few colonies of cylindro become resistant to normally lethal algicides such as copper, imagine how quickly the new strain will begin to dominate the water column. Every time it rains, or a strong wind stirs up the fluffy lake sediments (silty loams), a new pulse of algae-killing chemicals will be re-suspended, leaving only cylindro behind to reproduce.

Now "arm" cylindro with a toxin structure eerily similar to the dinoflagellate and fungal toxins, and the results will seem obvious.

Some of these toxin-forming blue green algae species have
been extensively studied by researchers, such as Wayne Carmichael, Ph.D., at Wright State University in Ohio, who has shown
that CSM binds powerfully to blue-green algae toxins. Is it any
surprise, then, that the human illness caused by such algae toxins
can be treated effectively by the same CSM protocols I use for
other neurotoxin-mediated illnesses?

But who will be able to prescribe CSM for the pelicans and
the alligators?

•   •   •

Disaster Strikes the White Pelicans

Intent on obtaining the highest-possible crop yields, the
"muck farmers" around Lake Apopka spent several decades
pumping various pesticides, herbicides and fungicides into the
jet-black mud that they had reclaimed from the edges of the
lake . . . and especially from its contaminated north shore,
where heavy metals have been playing havoc with wildlife in
recent years.

What the muck farmers didn't realize, however, was that the
DDT-like chemicals they were pouring into the ground—along
with tons of copper sulfate and other fungicides aimed at knock-
ing out several strains of crop-attacking fungus—would settle
permanently into the sediment along the lake bottom . . . with
major consequences for all life-forms that had once flourished
in this wetland habitat.

The first dramatic sign that Lake Apopka and her sister-lakes
(Griffin, Dora, Beauclaire and several others) might be in trouble
appeared in the mid-1990s, when the State of Florida purchased
a series of former muck farms and then flooded them with lake
water with the intent to create a wild bird sanctuary. (The state
also hoped to encourage the construction of new town houses on
some of this reclaimed land—a highly risky strategy, given the
obvious sediment-contamination.)

Instead, of a sanctuary, they created a slaughterhouse for white pelicans.

"What they did, they bought some of the big farms on Lake Apopka," remembers Ann Griffin. "And the farms along that stretch—it's only a few miles from Disneyworld, remember— were all discharging DDT-type stuff and copper and other fungicides directly into the lake.

"After they bought those farms, the folks who were creating the bird sanctuary decided to flood them. In the past, these fields had been drained each year by the farmers. But now they were full of shallow water. The fish became concentrated there —and as a result, all these migratory birds flew in.

"They can spot fish [in shallow water] from the air, you see? So we got all these American white pelicans, thousands and thousands of them. And they started gorging themselves on the fish in the shallows.

"And they started dying. Hundreds of them. They collapsed on the shoreline and they went into convulsions. In the end, more than a thousand of these beautiful birds died horribly, right in plain sight on the edge of Lake Apopka."

As later laboratory tests would suggest—but not prove—the dead birds had been killed by toxins either contained in the fish or in the shallow water, itself. Had those lethal poisons been hatched by a new mutation of cylindro . . . a microbe whose DNA might have been altered during exposure to copper and other pesticides and herbicides from farming operations around the lake?

The official cause of death was listed as exposure to outdated, long-lived chemicals that were no longer in use, including organochlorine compounds and toxaphene. The State also announced that its survey team had found chemical evidence of dieldren and DDT. But the tests that had been performed for toxic chemicals produced contradictory results as to the possible presence of these chemicals—and another series of tests for "abnormal" substances also led to findings that were sharply at variance.

"Somehow, the fish had accumulated all these pesticides," says Ann Griffin today. "We know now that there must have been all kinds of reactions and byproducts in the soil from these leftover chemicals, and they produced all sorts of [mutated] microbes that may very well have been poisonous."

Horrified by the slaughter of the birds—whch triggered news-paper headlines all across the country—Griffin and her neighbors received more disheartening news a few months later, when the first signs of an "algae attack" on their once beautiful Lake Griffin began to materialize.

"There's no mistaking that particular algae [*cylindrosper-mopsis*]," explains the Lake County environmentalist, who has become something of a local legend in recent years. "It's a vivid green—so green that it looks like fresh new paint.

"It started showing up on Lake Griffin about two years ago, and it was so startling that right away, I called the Florida Department of Environmental Protection to report a paint spill!

"But it wasn't really paint. It was algae—with that character-istic 'pea-green' color that people in this region have come to dread."

Make no mistake: The people who live along the Ocklawaha chain of rivers and lakes have learned to fear that "pea-green" in recent years, and with good reason.

Also known as a "cyanobacteria," the one-celled invader has completely overwhelmed the watershed—to the point that it now accounts for *more than 95 percent of the total "biomass"* in key areas such as Lake Apopka and Lake Griffin.

Where did cylindro come from? A passing purple martin from Sao Paolo, Brazil? Did it emerge from a passing ship's ballast, or ride to Florida aboard an exotic species of fungus that was re-portedly brought from Brazil in 1987 to combat the U.S. fire ant population? (The Institute of Food and Agriculture Services of the University of Florida studied that particular issue in 1987.) If ten years is the typical amount of time required for a mutant species to show effects (see the discussion of *Aphanomyces* in

Chapter Three, "Clear As Mud"), it's conceivable that one of Florida's many exotic species of plant and animal and microbe was already resistant to copper before it got to the lakes.

But how can a single organism become so totally dominant in a previously diverse and mature ecosystem? What if its "secret weapon" turned out to be the simple fact that the algae could survive—could thrive, even—in an altered habitat where chemicals were wiping out all other forms of aquatic life? In that thoroughly alarming situation, no other organisms in the watershed would be able to compete.

For normal blue-green algae, growth is limited by the availability of nitrogen, phosphorus and sunlight. But those limiting factors don't apply to cylindro. It can "fix" its own nitrogen, merely by absorbing it from the surrounding air. Cylindro requires very little phosphorus, and it grows happily in both low- and high-intensity light.

Already blessed with these advantages, cylindro reportedly owns one other huge asset for survival: a biochemical "secret weapon." For reasons that remain unclear, the organism puts out a virus-like cyanophage that activates at temperatures above 77 F. and then becomes an efficient killer of other algae species. Given all of these strengths, mighty cylindro clearly belongs in the company of other "Cell From Hell" organisms such as *Pfiesteria*!

Like a massive army outfitted with a weapon that could not be stopped, this pea-green predator in recent years has been marching non-stop along the entire Ocklawaha waterway, altering every water-based ecosystem in its path.

Ask Ann Griffin to describe the impact on her own 9,000-acre lake, once routinely described as one of Florida's "most beautiful bodies of water," and she doesn't hesitate: "This area used to have a quality of life that couldn't be matched anywhere! Every day meant another wildlife adventure, if you wanted to take the time to enjoy it. The bass fishermen used to come here from all over the state, and the water was an absolute delight. But not now.

"You see, the alligators are now dying on Lake Griffin. And they found all these toxins in their systems. And experts think it was produced by all this cyano-bacteria. But they refuse to talk about neurotoxins. Do they think the problem will go away if it isn't discussed?

"We've lost 180 alligators so far. Ten died last month, alone. And we were just out in the boat the other day, and we saw another one. They're continuing to die. And those alligators, they dig down into the sediment, where all the pesticides are."

But what about the people? How significant is the threat to human health throughout the watershed, where the State of Florida currently operates several major parks and camping and fishing facilities for unsuspecting citizens?

Note well: According to several recent worldwide health studies, *cylindrospermopsis* in drinking reservoirs has caused outbreaks of severe human liver-disease (hepato-enteritis) in Australia, Brazil and China during the past few decades. (Interestingly, the Brazilian form of the organism turns out to be resistant to copper!)

The human illness caused by cylindro is largely undocumented so far. Still, the first verifiable reports of this frightening ailment are beginning to trickle in. Here in Maryland, for example, I've been keeping close tabs on nearly 20 patients who were treated for algae-linked illness by two local physicians who prescribed CSM therapy. It should not be surprising that these patients with typical neurotoxic symptoms (including CS deficits and exposure only to the lake) improved rapidly with CSM therapy.

I should also point out that cylindro toxins appear to be effectively bound by CSM. And that fact is further supported by evidence showing that one of the major chemicals with the ability to transport the toxins inside cells is taurine, a "close cousin" of bile salts bound by CSM.

What struck me as especially interesting about my cylindro toxin-patients was that none of them had abnormalities of the liver. Was I seeing a brand-new species of cylindro, and if so, what was its chemical makeup? Unlike the symptoms caused by liver ailments, these complaints left patients struggling with "fatigue and dullness," which usually means a neurotoxin is involved rather than with the kind of jaundice that has killed several cylindro victims in Australia in recent years. But this Florida illness looked similar, but less intense than the disease outbreak that had occurred earlier in Brazil, in which toxins invaded dialysis machines and sent the patients attached to them straight to the grave. And indeed, the dialysis catastrophe shows how low-molecular weight toxins are able to move through even the most delicate and sensitive artificial membranes.

In another unusual twist, this form of cylindro exerted its powerful effect only on patients with direct water contact. In fact, none of my patients was struggling with an illness caused by vaporization or aerosolization of toxin.

Given this pathogenic background, it's easy to imagine Ann Griffin's consternation—and that of her neighbors—when officials at her local Water Management District recently unveiled plans to tap the same Lake Griffin for drinking water for tens of thousands of area residents!

"I went to a meeting of the District just the other day," said the dedicated environmental activist, "and I told them about the foolish risks they were taking with everyone's health. I read them a study that talked all about 'acute hepatotoxicosis,' which is a medical term for acute poisoning as a result of cylindrospermopsin or microcystin (another blue-green algae toxin). And I read them a key section of the study, which pointed out:

"'Reported hazards to human health include gastro-enteritis, asthma, eye irritation, blistering around the mouth and nose and toxic injury to the liver. Hepatotoxins damage liver tissue and cause pooling of blood that can lead to circulatory shock and liver failure.

"'It has been documented that *cylindrospermopsis* is responsible for an outbreak of severe hepato-enteritis in Australia in the 1970s. But the effects of cylindro aren't necessarily limited to toxic illness; increasingly, there's evidence that they may include cancer. The strongest current evidence for a link between human cancer and cyano-bacteria in water supplies comes from research by the Department of Epidemiology at Shanghai Medical University. These studies were motivated by a very high incidence of primary hepato-cellular carcinoma—liver cancer—in particular regions of southeastern China. There is circumstantial evidence for a possible role of cyano-bacterial toxin.'"

When Ann Griffin testified at hearings held before the St. Johns River Water Management District in March of 2000, she described how an outbreak of cylindro had caused widespread human illness in Australia in the 1970s:

"The problem is that all of this is fairly new in Florida, and the scientists don't know what these toxins will do here. They have no guidelines, and they know very little about the toxic aspects of *cylindrospermopsis raciborskii*. There's no way to tell whether it's safe to drink the water from Lake Griffin. They don't know enough about this toxin!

"And I didn't even tell them about neurotoxins made by cylindro, such as anatoxin-a and anatoxin-a(s)."

Ann Griffin's fears about potential health hazards outside Lake Griffin in the Ocklawaha watershed were quickly confirmed, when area farm workers near Lake Apopka began to display the classic symptoms of toxin-mediated illness. Eventually, I wound up working with Florida doctors to treat 40 of these migrant laborers with the by-now-standard FACT, followed by regular doses of toxin-dissipating cholestyramine.

These clearcut cases of human illness related to blue-green algae toxins including cylindrospermopsins have so far received little public attention in Florida, since no systematic health study of the cylindro problem has ever been conducted.

Nonetheless, one voice has broken the silence—loudly and frequently—about the health risks that now face several hundred thousand migrant laborers throughout the region. Poorly organized and barely literate in some cases, the Hispanics and other minorities who live in the migrant labor camps have received very little support in their struggle to protect their health.

Yet they have been heartened again and again by the determined advocacy of social activist Jeannie Economos, who has worked long and hard to defend the migrants through the local chapter of The Farmworker Association of Florida.

While the growing concern for the alligators and white pelicans of central Florida is entirely understandable, not enough attention has been paid to the plight of these migrants, who must work daily in fields laced with the same pesticides that have poisoned nearby lakes. Today there are increasing reports of "toxin-mediated illness" among these hard-working seasonal laborers—the men and women who pick all those oranges, melons, tomatoes, carrots, grapefruit and more for which Florida is justly famous.

It's not a pretty picture, of course. But there's also some good news to report, on this front . . . starting with the fact that my new CS test has already proved itself to be a powerful diagnostic tool when it comes to measuring the impact of neurotoxins on brain functioning.

"It is important to note," Economos wrote in a recent letter to the Florida Health Department, "that in the wake of the discovery of the bird deaths, and the disclosure of highly toxic chemicals found in bird tissue, none of the [Florida] agency officials involved in the investigative collaboration were making mention of any correlations to possible human health effects from exposure to these same chemicals, and/or from eating fish caught in the lake or the drainage canals of the farms.

"The Farmworker Association of Florida (FWAF) has long been concerned about the consequences to farmworkers' health from their repeated, close and sometimes direct contact with highly dangerous pesticide chemical compounds."

Sounds pretty awful, you say? But there's more: according to Ann Griffin, the worst part of the entire story may be the way in which most local residents of the Ocklawaha have refused to fight back against this documented poisoning of their own landscape.

"There's no question but that the abuse is still going on," she says angrily. "Many of the homeowners, themselves, are doing it!

"The homeowners who live on the lake are spraying herbicides and pesticides and fungicides right up to the waterline. They're just more interested in having grass that grows up to the edge of the water, and they're killing the lake as a result.

"It's pretty sad, the way the chemicals have ruined these lakes," she will tell you with a weary sigh. "Because these pesticides they're using do not go away. They get down in the sediment, and then they attack the reproductive systems of these creatures. [The scientific term for them is 'endocrine disrupters.'] Just last year, for example, the University of Florida was doing a study on the alligators . . . and they found that some [were] half-male and half-female."

Ann Griffin also points out that the increasing attacks by the cyano-bacteria have damaged her own health: "A few years ago, I started getting sinus infections and colds much more often than I used to. And I was trying to associate that with being around the lake. I had been wading out into it, planting things or taking exotics out. So I was in the water a lot, and I kept getting sick. It just seemed like my immune system was down.

"During the same period, my son was living in a cottage on Lake Griffin, not too far from here, and he was starting to get very sick. I mean, it just seems pretty obvious to me that anything that affects the wildlife has to affect humans.

"And now they're starting to talk about *drinking* the water out of Lake Griffin—but what about all the herbicides and copper sulfate in that water? I'm worried that when they drain the lake, they'll expose all these toxins in the sediment to the wildlife, and we'll have another situation where thousands of pelicans die from eating toxic fish.

"You know, I've got a friend, Mitzi, who's a wildlife rehabilitator. And she's pretty tough. She has a farm where she keeps all these hurt animals and birds, and it's almost like a zoo.

"Well, they called on her, when all these pelicans were dying. And she tried to care for them. She told me: 'It's never gotten to me before, but this has really gotten to me: the pelicans all dying.'

"It was just a terrible tragedy, and it affected her deeply."

Ann Griffin shakes her head, then gazes off over the shimmering expanse of pea-green water. "We don't want to see any more disasters like that here, Dr. Shoemaker.

"We've got to get these lakes cleaned up, before it's too late!"

• • •

Shoemaker's "Mutation Theory": The Only Logical Explanation?

How serious a threat do the neurotoxins produced by this genetically mutated version of cylindro pose to human health along the watershed?

Here's a brief summary of the health hazard, as analyzed by the St. Johns River Water Management District, after extensive sampling of the waters of Lake Griffin:

ABSTRACT

Cyanobacteria blooms are common in many of Florida's most important lakes, rivers and estuaries and threaten water quality, surface drinking water supplies, public health and aquatic ecosystems. In 1998, following the formation of the Florida Harmful Algal Bloom Task Force, a collaborative investigation of cyanotoxins in Florida's surface waters was initiated by the St. Johns River Water Management District, Florida Marine Research Institute, Florida Department of Health and Wright State University.

Project objectives include: (1) identify surface waters that experience extensive cyanobacteria blooms; (2) collect and identify potential toxigenic species; (3) screen samples for the detection and isolation of algal toxins; (4) characterize algal toxins present in water and animal tissues.

Approximately 135 water samples have been collected from 125 surface water bodies throughout the state and analyzed for the presence of cyanotoxins, including microcystin, cylindrospermopsin, anatoxin-a and paralytic shellfish poisons (PSPs).

Results indicate that *Anabaena, Microcystis* and *Cylindrospermopsis raciborskii* are the primary bloom forming cyanobacteria in Florida. The statewide distribution of C. raciborskii and recent development of severe blooms and dominance by this species in many of Florida's lakes has raised concerns for ecological and human health.

Surface water samples dominated by C. raciborskii were found to be toxic (italics mine) by mouse bioassay with HPLC results suggesting the presence of a compound similar but not identical to cylindrospermopsin identified from Australian waters. (Of course not—it's probably a new species!)

Relationships between surface water quality and the production of cyanotoxins, and the concerns for present and future drinking water supplies will be discussed in terms of specific management actions required to reduce the impact of harmful algal blooms in Florida.

Did they really take only 135 samples? If so, that isn't sufficient. There should be that many samples from each lake. Who analyzed what, where, and when?

If a problem is severe enough to wipe out an ecosystem, it's severe enough to do the studies right!

The reality of environmental testing includes the final rate limiting steps in science: money and politics. The Florida Harmful Algal Bloom researchers don't volunteer their time or pay for tests themselves. If the State doesn't fund a study, no research is done. If only we had a clearinghouse to channel private money into public health oriented research (private foundations have trouble finding worthy beneficiaries of trust money that must be spent). We don't, of course.

The final hurdle would be permission. If the Secretary of the Department of Health says no water samples will be tested for chemicals used by landowners living adjacent to a site, no tests are done. If the public demands "something be done," then a policy might change. But there really isn't much academic freedom for scientists working on projects subject to political pressure.

What else can we learn about cylindro and the mysterious deaths along the Ocklawaha chain of lakes?

For starters, these horrific events must teach us that any small change we make in our habitat can have enormous consequences. Unlike physics, in which every action must produce an equal and opposite reaction, biology is a world dominated by "unpredictable cascades." Example No. 1: Use antibiotics extensively to control illness in a human population, and you may very well stimulate the growth of competing bacteria which gain a "selective advantage" when their neighbors are wiped out by the powerful antibiotic.

Example No. 2: Use long-lasting pesticides such as copper sulfate to control fungi on cropland that adjoins warm-water lakes, and you may wake up one morning to find your entire watershed covered with "pea-green" algae. Once again, "selective advantage" worked to promote the health and growth of the resistant blue-green algae, by killing off competing organisms.

It's complicated.

And maybe this is the time for a little old-fashioned, intellectual humility.

Maybe it's time to remember that some of these environmentally caused health problems are beyond our intellectual grasp. We can make models of illness and ecology—but no model can hope to match a much richer and more detailed observation of what actually occurs. When we see illness, we don't always see obvious causation.

Perhaps the best strategy is to continue struggling to understand how our own behavior is altering the habitat, and then to stop acting in ways that cause dangerous mutations.

As for myself: More and more, I'm convinced that we *can* figure out ways to behave more responsibly, in terms of our daily interaction with the environment.

And a good place to start, surely, is by listening to the Ann Griffins of the world . . . to the people who have witnessed— "up close and personal"—the human devastation that ensues whenever we fail in our duty as responsible stewards of our own habitat.

The Argument against
The Public Health Departments

It didn't take long for the Lake Griffin Saga to begin sounding like a broken record that played the same phrases again and again. Should we worry about sick patients? No, of course not . . . the lake is safe! Neurotoxins wiping out life-forms? Not at all . . . we must perform more tests!

Once diagnosed, the symptoms of toxin-mediated illness can be effectively treated with the same cholestyramine regimen that works so well on other toxic illnesses, such as chronic Lyme, sick building syndrome, ciguatera and *Pfiesteria*-related human illness syndrome.

My discussions with patients in central Florida showed the same familiar patterns and symptoms. Once again, I found myself charting predictable Contrast Sensitivity deficits with FACT; once again, I witnessed considerable improvement in patients who took regularly prescribed doses of CSM.

I also treated several "cured" patients who had quickly reacquired the telltale symptoms of neurotoxin-mediated illness, after being re-exposed to pathogens. Although the toxin-forming organism and the environmental disaster that created this epidemic were new to me, the symptoms involved were all too recognizable. And so was the "official response" by the government and the medical profession. Once again, I found myself watching indifferent politicians and health bureaucrats dismiss an obvious health threat—even as they issued solemn bulletins and consensus reports that bristled with "AGS" (also known as

Strategy No. 1 in the "Appearance of Good Science").

The facts spoke for themselves, however. Lake Griffin was full of alligators which exhibited markedly abnormal behavior . . . along with reduced nerve conduction velocity and particular lesions in the central nervous system. Remember, too, that these animals were swimming through an identified neurotoxin in the water, every time they went nosing through those thick clumps of copper-resistant, pea-green algae.

The State of Florida responded to the crisis in typical fashion —by promising to "study the problem" (AGS, Level Four). Moving with glacial slowness, the state bureaucrats set about the task of analyzing this system of slowly flushing basins. During the next few months, numerous public meetings were held and the State Legislature debated the issue endlessly. In the end, however, nothing got done.

The Florida "paradise" had been destroyed by this scenario, perhaps forever, and yet the state environmental officials hadn't done anything except to "study" the problem. Wasn't it obvious to these scientists that microbiological testing should have been done, early on? Why hadn't they asked themselves—soon after the arrival of the cylindro—if this voracious, fast-growing organism might not be resistant to copper?

In order to conduct the lab tests that might answer those questions, I worked with Lake Griffin property owner Skip Goerner—the founder of a local citizen-action group—who sent me 24 samples of water from Lake Griffin; each had been collected and carefully documented at a different lake-site. At first I was fearful that I might not be able to find the cylindro in these samples. But there was no need to fret: The water Skip had sent along was a "monoculture" of algae. Unlike the great Dutch scientist, Anton van Leeuwenhook, who confronted a universe of swimming microbes in his drop of pondwater, I found myself peering through the lens at a single family of fast-multiplying blue-green algae.

Next step: I subdivided the samples and started adding copper to some of them in varying amounts.

The algae didn't die. I then added a fungicide to different subcultures of the algae—and still the organism wouldn't die. Finally I combined the fungicide and copper and fed it to the organism, which continued to grow and thrive. What did these developments mean? For comparison purposes, I subjected a mixture of species of algae from our ponds (no copper or fungicides ever used), to the same exposures . . . and felt some vindication for my theory when both the copper and the fungicide, while acting separately and together in extremely low combinations, quickly wiped out all of these microorganisms.

I don't pretend to be running a blue-green algae diagnostic laboratory, but my simple experiments made it clear that we *need* such a facility to take a long, hard look at the impact (or rather, *non*-impact) of these lethal chemicals on cylindro. The EPA grades the poisoning-potential of chemical substances on a scale from I to V—and there you will find copper listed in the "Class I" (or most lethal) category of biocides.

Was this a changing ecosystem? Would it diversify on its own, as the forces of natural selection inevitably introduced a blue-green algae-eater into the environment to harvest this "standing crop" of toxin-forming microbes? Not anytime soon . . . because the new algae predator would have to withstand a lot of poison. Could a dinoflagellate survive the toxins? *Pfiesteria* and its cousins *love* to eat blue-green algae. What a twist of fate that would be: the new Cell from Hell is eaten up by relatives of the *old* Cell From Hell!

Of course, the era was long gone in which the farmers had flooded their muck farms in winter and then drained them before the planting season . . . which meant that the "pulse" of wetland water with its load of pesticide and fertilizer residues would no longer contribute to the process of natural selection taking place around the lake.

Lake Griffin had become an "ecologically stable ecosystem," and it now seemed likely that the blue-green algae were going to be with us for a very long time. And that fact was frightening to contemplate. At this point, it seemed clear that cylindro had become so utterly dominant that it could be stopped only by the sheer, crushing weight of its own ubiquity.

Although it was true that even the most successful organic populations sooner or later "crash," this particular organism had now become so huge that waiting for it to poison itself with its own wastes was certainly a long-term ecological proposition! Pondering the grim reality, I asked myself a number of tantalizing questions, including these:

• Why had the cylindro turned out to be resistant to the copper-based pesticide residue that was almost certainly filtering into the lake from ag land, including the nearby orange groves? Had it really come from Brazil?

• Was the algae also resistant to the fungicide that had been sprayed for many years now on nursery lands, carrot farms and other agricultural operations? Was there any proof that fungicides also kill algae?

• Why had so many ornamental nursery men reported "crystal-clear" water in their drainage ponds until the early 1990s . . . after which swarms of algae began blooming at runoff sites?

• Why were similar blooms of algae growing so profusely on the copper piping of air and heat pumps? Was that the warning of a copper-resistant organism?

• And finally: How had a blue-green algae gained a foothold in local greenhouses and ferneries? Was it cylindro? Or had the algae actually come from the land—and would it eventually become known as "A Cell From Hell," like *Pfiesteria* and *fusarium*?

Although I knew I couldn't prove it, the facts all pointed to a single theory which would account for the algae outbreak of the early 1990s: Somehow, this organism had become resistant to copper! Even worse, the organism was resistant to the fungicide. Was the latter being washed into the water, then breaking down into isocyanates and carbendazim? What did I know about the mechanism by which fungicides caused genetic changes in algae?

Of course, the idea of copper- and fungicide-resistance in algae was a *truly* alarming possibility . . . because it suggested that it might already be too late to turn back the tide of cylindro in these lakes, over-burdened as they were with copper in sediments. If Lakes Griffin and Apoka had been so damaged that they could no longer change, then the toxin-spewing invader was here to stay—the chief resident in a mature ecosystem that had been distorted by years of silent poisoning.

Once again, it now seemed clear, the "alligator in the coal mine" warnings had been ignored—until suddenly the alligators were no longer able to hatch their eggs, even if they did survive to breed. (At that point, of course, "environmental awareness" became the buzzword of the day among corporate managers and politicians and private citizens alike.)

Remember that while the alligator may be the symbol of the primordial ooze that rules the Florida swamps, these creatures are reptilian predators. They certainly aren't warm and cuddly creatures. And when they eat golden retrievers or a three year old child, the stark relationship between predator and prey suddenly jumps into clear focus.

Somehow, the death of an alligator isn't as dramatic—or as affecting—as the death of a manatee. In Florida these days, "saving the manatee" amounts to nothing less than a statewide passion. And when cylindro finally begins to invade the manatee habitats, so that these lovable "sea cows" are dying painful, neurotoxin-mediated deaths, then the cry will go up everywhere: "Fix this ecological problem, and fix it *now!*"

The proliferation of cylindro is not limited by geography. There's no reason why the manatee won't be another "threatened species" adopted by the mass media—once the sea cows begin to swim around aimlessly, while failing to avoid the propeller blades and sand bars and entangling mangrove roots that can wipe them out. The state will study the problem, of course; you can be sure that there will be "consensus statements" and "expert statements" galore. The passionate speeches will thunder all across Tallahassee, as well as Washington. "Save The Manatee!"

If the invasive *hydrilla* species of water-based vegetation can't survive in cylindro-infested water (and it can't), what will happen to the unfortunate manatee—which depends for its daily sustenance on this once-flourishing plant? What will happen when the cylindro begins to dominate every waterway in central Florida?

Unfortunately, we don't have the luxury of taking several years to "study" that question. Unless we act now, we're going to watch the sea cows of the Sunshine State face extinction in front of our eyes.

Faced as we are with the formidable problem of blue-green algae domination of the central Florida lakes, what realistic solutions can we hope to find? Given the presence of so many long-lasting environmental poisons in the lakes, can anything be done?

One especially creative approach calls for dredging the six feet of fluffy, toxic chemical-enriched sediments at the bottom of the lake. But that operation will only guarantee the most efficient re-suspension of toxics to the water column . . . even if we somehow manage to find a suitable disposal site for the dredged soils. Also: won't dredging simply speed the proliferation of cylindro, as runoff from the digging adds even more toxins to the mix?

A second strategy—and a potentially disastrous one, in my view—would require the lowering, or "drawing down," of the level of water in the lake. That approach, however, will rapidly create a perfect environment for growing more blue-green algae, as wet, sunlight-exposed areas are greatly expanded. And where will these drained waters end up? In Jacksonville?

A third approach would be to attempt to restore the prior ecological integrity of the surrounding wetlands, so that they might once again filter the waters that flood into these stressed-out lakes. This solution makes sense—but it means that houses and marinas won't be built in the area, and that farms will not be allowed to flourish, despite the political and economic demand to "use the land." Once again, won't filtering wetlands simply provide more habitat for cylindro?

And each of these emergency tactics could easily trigger *other* environmental problems that might prove even more troublesome than the ones we already face. For that reason, I advocate a different approach: know the enemy. Know everything about cylindro. Instead of rushing into all of sorts of frantic activity, why not form an "action-team" that would carefully examine the local ecosystem (including, especially, those sick alligators and birds) . . . and then begin thoughtfully interviewing area residents and studying a cohort of sick patients from the area?

I have just such a cohort of patients in mind, of course: some neighbors of my index cases. Their numbers are fairly small . . . but all that would be needed is to spend a few hours going door-to-door, in order to add to their ranks. The FACT would be quite helpful in conducting the screening process for new patients—and the diagnoses could then be fine-tuned by a team of skilled physicians who could not be manipulated or dictated to by public health officials. In this way, they could build a policy consensus that would not be controlled by the politicians, and local citizen-action groups could help to generate a powerful political demand for action.

Is there any doubt that a strategy of this kind would meet with shrill objections from federal and state regulatory agencies?

I can hear the howls of outraged protests already. "Yes, but your findings aren't validated yet, Dr. Shoemaker. There may be confounding variables waiting down the road! What we *really* need is a 'biomarker.' After all, your treatment isn't proven yet. And besides, we all have bosses who will make the decisions: It's out of our hands!"

Do you wonder why sick patients often find it difficult to trust their public health officials? These suffering people don't want to be "evaluated"; they want to feel better! They want to know that the medical establishment places their interests before everything else. But they also understand fully that in most health departments, "filling out the paperwork" comes first— and that it usually overwhelms the desire to care for individual patients. Besides, the Health Department only exists to help people with baby-planning, venereal disease and mental illness clinics, right?

When it comes to the "biomarker" issue, the situation seems even more frustrating. How can you use a serological (blood) test for a toxin that circulates outside the blood? Answer: The FACT measurement of Contrast Sensitivity quantifies the impact of organic toxins on neurons . . . which makes it a powerful physiologic biomarker for the presence of the poisons that cause many forms of chronic illness.

Like the rifling on a bullet, or the track of a neutrino in an atomic accelerator, the identifying marks left behind by toxins can be clearly observed—simply by scanning the results of a patient's FACT.

Now, there's no denying that many variables affect the FACT. Yet the test contains several built-in features that allow it to sort out and evaluate these same variables. In addition, taking a careful medical history and scrutinizing it vigilantly can also help to pin down these confounding variables. This is the kind of diagnostic work that physicians do every single day, as they go about such routine, repetitive tasks as sorting out the causes behind a patient's chest pains.

Instead of turning cases of toxin-mediated illness over to a 24-year-old graduate student armed with a five-page checklist, physicians need to learn how to use the latest medical tools—such as FACT—to identify the actual environmental culprit.

But what if the diagnosing physician can't be sure about the ultimate cause of the symptoms and the FACT deficit that he or she is seeing? Is the source of the ailment cylindro, or maybe sick building syndrome? In those cases, it's important to remember that you *can* go ahead and treat the illness, even if you can't be sure about its environmental source. (And the good news here is that CSM therapy is quite benign.)

When the health department says, "No, treatment may cause side effects, and more importantly, it may also alarm the public, so don't tell them that there is a treatable illness at work out there," I can feel my pulse quickening: "But our entire profession is *based* on the principle that says the patient must be informed. If I don't inform you about the risks of Lyme disease vaccine or gallbladder surgery, I run the risk (and properly so) of being sued for negligence."

In the same way, when the local or state health department willfully withholds information about risks from environmentally acquired, toxin-mediated illnesses that could affect the quality and quantity of life (not to mention the rate of learning disability in our children), then the health administrators are also guilty of negligence. The point here is that withholding evidence of health risk—or distorting the evidence of that same risk—significantly restricts freedom of choice among patients.

The deliberate withholding of evidence is frowned upon by our judicial system . . . and if you doubt that, just ask the U.S. tobacco companies about the possible consequences of such stonewalling!

Consider the biological perspective. Am I just over-reacting?

Ask yourself: what therapeutic choices would those syphilis patients in the notorious "Tuskegee Study" have made, if they'd been told that they were actually suffering from the debilitating illness? Wouldn't they have "taken a chance" on penicillin, whether or *not* it had been studied in large clinical trials? Is CSM treatment of cylindro poisoning in an affected high school sophomore really any different?

A large part of my work consists of patient-based observational studies (case/control studies) in which the patients are actually sick. I think I know how *they* would feel about the ongoing debate in academic medicine over the scientific value of "observational studies" versus "prospective, randomized clinical trials!"

In the end, of course, that debate comes down to the "unit of practice." Isn't the best way to care for society as a whole to make sure that we give each individual our very best attention and concern . . . rather than breaking populations down into statistics and then making judgments on the basis of "1.25 units of care?"

The saddest aspect of this spirited and passionate debate emerges when one faction or another—usually with utter disregard for humanitarian ideals—decides that the health department should not become engaged in the quest for truth, and should not release important medical information to patients, or to the patients' doctors.

I can't tell you how many times I've found myself enraged and also powerfully energized by the arrogance of a public servant who has just explained to me: "We can't tell the public what we know; there would be panic in the streets!"

Sorry, but I'm not buying that. Fear is always conquered by facts! Remember the great panic over *Pfiesteria*, and the early refusal of public health officials to even discuss the epidemic of illness that resulted from it? These days, the State of North Carolina actually announces the *Pfiesteria*-count in key watersheds on its website. Does that public information strategy create any more fear than announcing: "The risk of forest fire is high in this area today?" Of course not.

Let's tell the public the plain old truth—the first time and *every* time. They can handle it! And while we're at it, let's tell parents how to go about the important task of getting their kids tested for chronic, neurotoxin-mediated illness (See Chapter 26: "Why Johnny Can't Read").

Let's shine a cleansing and healing light into the murky depths of America's public health system—by finally giving our patients access to a new approach to diagnosis and treatment!

"Fad Medicines"
For America's "Fad Diseases"

Pocomoke, MD –July, 2000

Step right up, ladies and gentlemen: It's time to meet Prilosec, the best-selling American drug of the late-1990s!

The pitch sounds pretty familiar, doesn't it?

Have you noticed that there's a definite pattern in the diseases—as well as the medications—that seem to dominate the American health care marketplace year in and year out? And have you *also* noticed that, one way or another, most of these different ailments and their chemical antidotes also seem to be blamed on . . . *stress?*

It's a proven fact: During the past ten years or so, the top spot among U.S. diseases has clearly belonged to "reflux esophagitis" —a highly unpleasant condition, made worse by stress, that leaves its victims gulping back gallons of fiery stomach acid each day. How many heart catheterizations or gall bladder tests are performed annually because of the doctor's concern that the pain of reflux might actually be coming from somewhere else?

A powerful symbol of the hectic, high-speed society in which it occurs so often, "Reflux" (along with its older, more prosaic stress-cousin, the ordinary peptic ulcer) helped to make "Tagamet" the pharmaceutical star of the "Me Decade" (the 1970s) and Zantac the headliner of the "Junk-Bond Decade" (the 1980s).

These powerful biochemical antacids (remember the innocent days of "No acid, no ulcer!" and "Tums for the Tummy?") undoubtedly became major drugstore players because of the way they can "turn off" the scalding product of the stomach's acid-manufacturing machinery.

Unfortunately, *that* over-worked mechanism—a well-documented response to stress—has now become such a common feature of holding down a job (or driving in freeway traffic) that millions of Americans find themselves paying $3-per-pill (or demanding that their *insurance* company pay $3-per-pill) for the chemical fix that will help them get through each jagged-edge workday, while no doubt asking themselves: *Will I be able to sleep tonight without being awakened by heartburn and chest pain?*

Of course, there are still a few acid-sufferers out there who insist on gobbling calcium carbonate by the tubeful, even as they hope against hope that the "extra calcium" they're ingesting will also save them from the ravages of osteoporosis!

Too bad . . . but the reality is that the chalk (or maybe the oyster shell) product they're devouring won't be absorbed very efficiently, and it probably won't help their bones at all. Is it any wonder that Prilosec and its proton pump-inhibitor cousins continue to nail down the Big Pharmaceutical Bucks year in and year out? Another big part of the reason for its success is that proven-bad-guy-bacteria, *Heliobacter pylori*, which directly attacks the stomach by burrowing into the lining and causing lots of gastritis/ulcer problems. As long as the ulcer-causing bacteria remain alive, you can be sure that stomach acid will be doing its dirty work at the site where the protective mucous layer of the stomach was breached by the bacteria. (Sounds a bit like *Pfiesteria*, doesn't it?)

Antibiotics for ulcers: amazing!

And true. Put all of these stomach-facts together, and it's easy to see why millions of patients don't think twice about taking at least one—and often *two*—of the hard-hitting Prilosecs and Zantacs each and every day. As long as our society runs on equal parts of anxiety and aggression, there will always be a stomach acid-market!

Like Prilosec and its acid-blocking competitors, that ubiquitous antidepressant, Prozac, has also enjoyed a sales boom in recent years. After leading the pack for some time, Prozac has lately lost some of its merchandising punch, having been replaced in many bathroom medicine cabinets by the newer SSRI meds that are all the rage today.

We all have heard of the link between the Prilosec-promoting acid disorders and the kinds of psychic disturbances that have fueled the Prozac boom. The names of the illnesses, "post-traumatic stress disorder" or "dysthymia" or "situational depression" (to say nothing of the more impressive "limbic system dysfunction") might be new but the mind-body link is the same as it always has been.

For all of these conditions, the Prozac 20mg tablet has often been the solution-of-choice (even though 5 mg would probably serve as well, while also saving on cost). And don't forget the unrest that so overtakes women who are struggling with pre-menstrual syndrome. Should we really be startled to discover that half the women age 20–50 in the U.S. now are likely to own a prescription for Prozac that will be taken on a cyclical monthly basis?

And how about Bestseller No. 3: Xanax? It really is the best medication for treating "chronic panic disorder," another popular new diagnosis. I've said it, myself, many times: if depression and anxiety are the result of a chemical imbalance in the brain, there's no reason to suffer endlessly—not when simple, safe, effective medications can help. Unfortunately, however, this syndrome often gets tagged with the catch-all moniker of "chemical imbalance" . . . when it actually occurs as the result of a chronic, toxin-mediated illness.

Surely we should be diagnosing such illness properly—and not merely covering it over with a mood-altering drug.

Do you have to face an angry boss? Give a speech? Wedge yourself into an MRI machine? Drive across a flimsy-looking bridge? Go ahead . . . pop your pill and say goodbye to the major psychological complaint of our era: runaway anxiety!

On reflection, it really doesn't seem very surprising . . . the way in which our popular diagnoses have become so vague and fuzzy during the last two decades. Put yourself in the shoes of the overburdened primary care physician. Look at the patient with trigger-point pain and lots of other symptoms . . . then think about that recent article in a widely circulated "throw-away" medical journal on Fibromyalgia.

"You've got fibromyalgia!" That ringing declaration takes place hundreds of times each day in doctors' office scattered all across America. Remarkably, the victims of stress-related illnesses often seem to present with every symptom in the diagnostic manual. Is there any doubt that diagnosing disorders such as fibromyalgia, depression and Reflux have become the Standard of Care in the "Chemical Decade?"

Here's a case in point. Just yesterday, a vigorous, 80-year-old man visited my office for Lyme treatment. His daughter had been wrestling with chronic Lyme for years, and had responded well to CSM (See Chapter 13: "Healing Chronic Lyme Disease"). This concerned woman had spotted her father's ECM rash and had sent him to me immediately. And I couldn't help noticing how his medical record contained a very typical-sounding comment from his cardiologist:

"Mr. Jones is caring for his wife, who has Alzheimer's. He clearly is straining under that load. I feel his symptoms of fatigue, muscle ache and shortness of breath are more typical of depression, and I've prescribed Prozac for him. He vigorously resisted the recommendation—but I think if you suggest the diagnosis to him as well, he'll be more likely to start taking the medication. At any rate, his shortness of breath isn't from congestive heart failure or a pulmonary embolism."

This man's cardiologist is a caring physician, and his comments were obviously heartfelt, but wrong. Mr. Jones had six of my eight categories of neurotoxic symptoms and a positive CS test. He did well at first with antibiotics (although they didn't reduce his symptoms), and then much better with CSM therapy.

Like fibromyalgia, "chronic pain," "chronic fatigue" and "trigger-point" pain are also being diagnosed with ever increasing frequency these days. By now you probably know that those are the symptoms of a chronic, neurotoxin-mediated illness. But which particular one is it . . . or is it more than one? I remember the Lyme patient who worked in the sick building next to Lake Griffin. Here was a man struggling with three neurotoxic illness at once: chronic Lyme, sick building syndrome, and blue-green algae-related human illness!

Could there be a more compelling example of how this new family of diseases is taking a growing toll on the populace at large?

Last but not least in our rogue's gallery of fad drug-fixes is an often-used pain medication—Hydrocodone—which now ranks No. 4 on the list of popular prescription drugs. Hydrocodone is extraordinarily effective, providing relief for patients with chronic pain syndromes. Just half a tablet at night . . . and you can feel confident that that you'll awaken fully rested in the morning, without returning to the endless cycle of muscle spasm followed by more pain. Habituation is a problem with this narcotic, of course. But when experts in chronic pain management say, "Keep a constant level of the medication in the bloodstream for control of pain," that's exactly what we do.

Pain can't be measured, and chronic pain is a formidable foe. How many patients pay the price of habituation in exchange for less pain?

What would it mean . . . if that chronic joint pain, chronic muscle pain and chronic abdominal pain could be better managed —starting with a clear neurotoxic diagnosis?

To answer that question, start by taking a moment to look at the symptom complex of these fad illnesses: fatigue, muscle ache, joint pain, muddled thinking, headache. See any patterns? Here's one: the physicians who diagnose such vague ailments as

fibromyalgia rarely take a neurotoxin history. Why not? For one
thing, the specialists—the cardiologists and the pulmonologists
and the orthopedists, among others—are all focused first and
foremost on their own specialties. So we usually wind up hearing
a lot about "mitral valve prolapse" in fibromyalgia, and "hyper-
ventilation," and even "costochondritis," respectively. In the end,
if we can *name* it (even without a convincing test to prove it), it's
a diagnosis that most patients will accept.

"You have fibromyalgia, Mrs. Jones. Here is your antidepressant prescription." Don't take it Mrs. Jones!

So here I stand—insisting that CS is a useful test, and that
CSM is benign therapy. Contrast that with the expert witness
from the insurance company who says: "There's nothing wrong
here, Your Honor. We took x-rays in our office and ordered
physical therapy for the patient from our affiliated PT office.
We also asked our chronic pain associate to inject those trigger
points and set up epidural blocks. No problem at all! I also prescribed a bit of Prozac, sir. Right now, we're wondering if some
chiropractic might also help."

Nothing was wrong . . . because the *right* tests weren't done!

And while we're on the subject of fads . . . you've read in this
book that the big medical buzzword today, whenever research-
oriented physicians talk about the key mechanism involved in
illness, is "cytokines."

It's true. "Inflammation," "pro-inflammatory cytokines," and
"interleukin I-XII": these are among the very hottest new biochemical terms in the world of modern medicine. And whenever a new one is discovered, simply add a Greek letter to it, as
in: "interleukin I-beta!" That's because, more and more, the
ability of longer-living "monocytes" (white blood cells) to make
and release powerful chemicals has become a major element in
defining and diagnosing medical conditions.

Cytokines are real; they aren't just a fad. But with so much
having been written about them in the medical journals in recent years, its almost too much. Everything in medicine doesn't

involve cytokines. Or does it? Still, I have a somewhat different take on the "cytokine world" . . . since the chronic, neurotoxin-mediated illnesses that I often treat usually include low-molecular-weight toxins which trigger a TNF-alpha response (a cytokine, remember) by stimulating the production of that substance through the activation of TNF genes.

I honestly believe in the power of molecular biology to answer our fundamental questions about health and illness. Yet the primary care- and people-oriented approach in me cries out for some balance and perspective.

The physiology of disease remains mind-bendingly complex, of course. But you don't need to do graduate work in biochemistry to understand that many of today's "fad diseases" are simply the result of the increasing prevalence of chronic, neurotoxin-mediated illnesses. Indeed, the problems just seems to get worse by the year.

Ask yourself: given the fact that money has replaced morality in so much of our public life, is it any wonder that the incidence rates for such medical illnesses as ulcers, depression, anxiety, and chronic pain are rising faster than the Dow Jones average? What came first—the sick building or the job stress?

"Doctor, I know my job is the problem. The stress from working there is unbelievable. My high blood pressure, reflux, headaches and depression are from my job. But you know I can't quit because of the benefits! In just five more years I can have my pension and go do what I want to do."

It's a pity . . . but when an individual willingly trades his health for "benefits," despite the added tax of job-stress, why should we be surprised to discover that our state or federal public health agency also "trades" the health of human beings for political gain by concealing the magnitude of toxin-mediated illness?

So what's the best cure for the "fad illnesses" that continue to erode our quality of life in this society?

Instead of popping more pills—whether for excess stomach

acid or for out-of-control anxiety—shouldn't we begin working on the *real* sources of the pathology that increasingly threatens us . . . namely, those deleterious changes in our society, along with the toxin-linked illnesses that are now being triggered by our changing environment?

chapter 13

Event

Healing Chronic Lyme Disease

Pocomoke, MD –May, 1999

"Until now, I felt like I was facing a life sentence of imprisonment, with daily bouts of torture, but now I have been given a chance for parole."

—Diane Stephenson, 53, Cleveland, Ohio

"I am so thrilled, because I'm getting my brain back. I've always been an intelligent person, and to suddenly become dopey, and *know* that you're dopey—that's the scariest thing. I can't even tell you the horror of it."

—Marie Moore, 51, West Milford, New Jersey

The stories you are about to read are real, and so are the struggling, suffering human beings who lived through them.

After treating hundreds of chronic Lyme disease patients in recent years, I'm convinced that their disease represents the most debilitating—the most fatiguing and agonizing—form of neurotoxin-mediated illness now at work in the United States and the rest of the Western World. It's also the most neurologically diverse, because it mimics virtually every neurologic disease in the world.

Make no mistake: contracting chronic Lyme is always a horrific and tragic event in the life of the victim. This disease takes away normal life, destroys family relationships and makes the ordinary activities of daily living (such as standing unaided at a sink to brush your teeth) exhausting ordeals in which the sufferer struggles to get from moment to moment.

One of the most maddening aspects of Lyme is the way it masquerades as so many *other* illnesses—often leaving the clinician feeling baffled and the patient without even a name for the disorder that is slowly destroying his or her life. Sir William Osler delivered a brilliant insight into the dynamics of disease, when he said that "to know syphilis is to know medicine."

To confront chronic Lyme disease, on the other hand, is to begin to realize just how *little* we know about the mechanisms that cause disease. That's because Lyme is always more than just an "infectious disease"; it's also a toxin-mediated illness that evades most of the weapons contained in the human immune system.

Experience shows that chronic, neurotoxin-mediated illness is a painful experience for everyone who struggles with it. Yet chronic Lyme patients frequently must endure an additional layer of misery—namely, the indifference which their ailment so often provokes in the medical community. Chronic Lyme sufferers know they are sick, and they know they *became* sick after being bitten by a tick (or after exposure to areas where others have been bitten). Afflicted with an obvious and multi-symptom disorder, they suffer even more when they discover that all too often, the medical community doesn't even consider their illness to be real.

Here is the *real* tragedy of Lyme disease. Take a look and you'll soon discover: Lyme disease is all around us. It's found in nearly every state in the Union, and it usually presents with a specific, distinctive group of symptoms. Yet many physicians (probably the majority, in fact) refuse to acknowledge its reality! (For a compelling example of how that refusal affects patients, see the tables in Chapter 16, "100 Weeks In The Medical Wilderness." In this chapter, the numbers tell the story of chronic Lyme sufferer "Jill," who consulted 32 different medical practitioners over an 18-month period and obtained virtually no relief.)

In some ways, the tragedy of modern Lyme disease parallels the tragedy of the U.S. Civil War. In the contemporary version, however, the saga consists of "medical brother against medical brother" in a heartbreaking struggle that leaves thousands of tormented Lyme patients undertreated or untreated each year. Another remarkable parallel: the way in which well-entrenched, "institutional" physicians—who typically deny the existence of chronic Lyme and leave its victims untreated—control most of the financial resources in the ongoing debate. Like General Grant's endlessly re-supplied Union Army, these institution- and government-linked practitioners are able to rely on their huge financial advantage (in the form of endless government and industry grants) . . . while the isolated ranks of those doc- tors who *do* treat chronic Lyme patients are mostly cut off from the research support necessary to prove the validity of their approach.

Today the battle over the reality of chronic Lyme rages un- checked, even as staff physicians from institutions such as Yale and the State University of New York at Stony Brook continue to insist that, "No, it isn't Lyme if we *say* it isn't!"

Armed with an endless stream of Big Science research dollars, the well-connected defenders of the "Chronic-Lyme-Doesn't- Exist" school are able to publish the same scientific "findings" over and over again in the nation's leading medical journals. All too often, their strategy sounds like the Consensus Approach of the Appearance of Good Science: Repeat the conventional wisdom on this subject often enough, and people will eventually believe it.

Meanwhile, many of the same physicians from the "Learning Centers" are busy testifying as expert witnesses at insurance hearings where patients are denied long-term health insurance benefits because their disease doesn't exist!

Tragically, much of the suffering caused by chronic disease doesn't have to continue, year in and year out. Remember that old saying: "It's amazing how much can get done when it doesn't matter who gets the credit?"

In the case of chronic Lyme, unfortunately, it *does* matter—because the grants and the academic advancement and the expert witness fees and the royalties all flow toward the Upholders of the Conventional Wisdom at the Lyme bastions.

But you can be sure that these Big Science Dollars rarely translate into helping chronic Lyme patients ease their suffering, when the truth of the illness is denied. All too often, when the "expert" says the disease isn't present, no treatment will be prescribed. At that point, the patient gets left behind.

In most situations, of course, the chronic Lyme battle lines are drawn around two key issues:

FIRST: What *is* Chronic Lyme disease, anyway? What is its etiology? During earlier studies, I defined "Chronic Lyme disease" as a constellation of symptoms that persist following antibiotic therapy—with all of these symptoms being related to a tick bite or exposure to areas where others had tick bites.

In order to justify a diagnosis of chronic Lyme disease, patients must display four of eight symptom categories—and they must also show a deficit in Contrast Sensitivity. The symptom categories, which are found in all diseases that cause chronic, neurotoxin-mediated illness syndrome, include the following:

- fatigue, weakness;
- headache, confusion, vertigo, difficulty in word-finding;
- memory impairment, disorientation, impairment of concentration, reduced task completion;
- hypersensitivity to bright light, night blindness, conjunctival injection, tearing, blurred vision;
- muscle ache, cramp, joint pain;
- secretory diarrhea, nausea, anorexia, abdominal pain;
- sinus congestion, cough, sore throat;
- shortness of breath, asthma-like symptoms.

It should also be pointed out that this syndrome is *not* defined by a blood test, nor by such arbitrary criteria as "producing five bands on a Western Blot Test," as currently defined by the CDC. The key point here: we can identify chronic Lyme as a clinical syndrome that triggers a deficit in human Contrast Sensitivity. *This deficit can be measured and quantified.*

SECOND: After you concede that the illness *does* exist, what's the most effective treatment for the thousands who have contracted it in recent years? Here the answer is complex. While some patients do require prolonged antibiotic treatment (whether intravenous or oral), we must recognize that such treatment will always be inadequate in cases of chronic, neurotoxin-mediated Lyme. Antibiotics do not kill toxins! Toxins aren't alive.

We must also understand that many chronic Lyme sufferers will end up with co-infections, also from the bite of an infected tick—in addition to those produced by *Borrelia*—and that the most devastating of these will be from a protozoan called *Babesia*. (In recent years, there has also been an explosion of an unusual, rickettsial species called *Ehrlichia*.)

Experience shows that many of today's chronic Lyme patients are carrying *Babesia* and *Ehrlichia* and several other bacterial strains in addition to *Borrelia*. More than 10 percent of Lyme patients nationwide are recognized as being co-infected with *Babesia*, for example. Has anyone diagnosed *Anaplasma* yet?

These qualifications only serve to trigger another series of related medical enigmas. Among them: Does anybody out there really know an easy, reliable way to diagnose the disease? If it *can* be simply and safely diagnosed, is there a way to effectively treat it with appropriate antibiotics?

The answers to these Sphinx-like questions probably lie deep within the body of the Lyme vector . . . inside the spirochete bacterium, *Borrelia burgdorferi*, that is, which spends its life riding around in the mid-gut of the ordinary deer tick. (Remember that similar spirochetes cause a number of other painful illnesses —such as syphilis, relapsing fever, and leptospirosis, along with yaws, pinta, and other tropical diseases.)

Of course, these are hardly your "ordinary" bacterial infections, in which a one-celled pathogen invades tissue, causes some local cell destruction and then perhaps emits a few toxins . . . before finally entering the bloostream and setting off an "immune response" that either kills the invader or ceases when the host is killed by the bacterium.

The spirochetes described above (and especially *Borrelia*) move best through skin tissue outside of blood vessels. These organisms are nicely equipped to crawl alongside blood vessels, inching past un-alerted, blood-borne defenders, even as they corkscrew themselves into every unprotected area of the body.

You won't often find these microorganisms in the bloodstream, because they simply can't move very well against the kind of current found inside rushing veins and arteries. Their locomotions, like those of the earthworm, require pressure to be exerted against the firm edge of a surface.

Safe from blood-borne antibodies, the Lyme bacteria creep through body tissues in search of a sanctuary—such as those found in brain, skin, heart, bone and joints (the list is quite long, actually)—where they can "dig in" and settle down to begin the next stage in their life-cycle. In many cases, they seem to be quite content to make a quiescent cyst. Given our current knowledge, however, no one can identify whether or not the Lyme spirochete actually causes the symptoms of illness when housed in one of these cyst-sanctuaries.

When a spirochete makes its way into a sanctuary, where the body's immune system cannot quickly annihilate it, the odds are high that it can live for an extended period. Spirochetes have been demonstrated in synovial lining cells of joint, heart muscles, special skin cells called "fibroblasts," meninges (the covering of the brain) and other regions. But does the presence of a living spirochete in a sanctuary mean that it is actually causing an active infection? Perhaps not. After all, research shows clearly that the body often manages to seal off tuberculosis (TB) germs in patients, forming a small wall (known as a "granuloma") that encases the still viable TB germ.

Surely the existence of the granuloma suggests that invasive microorganisms can live for extended periods in the body without setting off the warning bells of infection?

We now know that the TB germ responds to changes in the environment provided by the host by switching its food source from carbohydrates to fatty acids. This shift allows "persistent survival" of the germ, even though the symptoms of infection may not be present. And that particular metabolic change requires "differential gene activation" . . . a biochemical event no different (at least in concept) than the event in which a Lyme spirochete shuts down its production of antigen OspC, then switches to manufacturing antigen OspA as soon as it senses blood in the mid-gut of its host-tick.

Another way to explain this phenomenon is to say that as soon as the tick's blood-meal begins, the spirochete replaces one type of antigen with another on its cell surface in order to feed and breed properly. The Lyme spirochete can change its life form (to a cyst) when faced with starvation. In similar fashion, the one-celled *Pfiesteria* organism changes its life-form in response to its changing food supply. Amazingly, however, this microscopic quick-change artist can complete the transition to a completely new form in only four hours! In the same way that Lyme activates and suppresses genes in order to feed and propagate, *Pfiesteria* adopts a new costume via gene activation and suppression.

Obviously, these concerns lead to a searching question about Lyme diagnosis: What should we do if the Lyme organism is just alive enough to make an antigen or cause a DNA PCR test to become positive? If the patient is healthy, when do we stop therapy? And what if the immune system doesn't pick up the presence of the spirochete? If the patient is sick, do we withhold therapy?

The Contrast Sensitivity test gives us a simple answer to these questions. Remember: living Lyme organisms make neurotoxins. And toxins cause a deficit in CS. If the CS deficit appears, treat with antibiotics first, then with CSM. If patients don't improve,

look for undiagnosed co-infection—or question the Lyme diagnosis altogether.

Remember, also, that your next walk through somebody's
backyard shrubbery might be enough to create a new exposure
and perhaps a new Lyme infection. That's because the body
doesn't always manage a killing immune response to the spirochete the first time around. Recurrent symptoms in the absence
of a new exposure must mean reactivation of the latent organism. Yes, it's complicated! Entire volumes have been penned on
the subject of "reactivation of TB" . . . but not about a similar
awakening of the pathogens that cause Lyme.

More background: *Pfiesteria*, ciguatera and many dinoflagellates make a cyst-form as part of their life cycle, and it isn't
unusual to find protozoans making cysts, either. (As a matter
of fact, some researchers have argued that spirochetes actually
behave more like protozoans than bacteria.) The cyst permits a
viable organism to remain dormant for years, like a seed slum-
bering in the desert. Later, when the proper environmental conditions finally appear, the organism rises from the cyst like a
blossom rising from the Kalahari.

In spite of our vast knowledge of many living systems, science
actually knows very little about the factors that influence the
life-cycles of spirochetes. And indeed, the scientific debate over
these aspects—like the debate over the existence of chronic
Lyme, itself—continues to escalate from year to year. (Sounds a
little bit like the wrangling over *Pfiesteria*, doesn't it?)

To make matters even more difficult, however, you sometimes
will find several *different* types of *Borrelia burgdorferi* present
whenever a patient is struggling with chronic Lyme. (How many
different strains can co-exist within the same tick?)

In the United States, the *sensu stricto* strain of the *Borrelia
burgdorferi* spirochete gets the lion's share of the publicity,
and is usually identified as the key culprit in outbreaks of Lyme.
But at least 25 other strains of *Borrelia* have been identified.
Do these operate to cause disease in the same way that *sensu
stricto* sickens its host? And if so, how can we identify them

with an antibody test that can *only* confirm the presence of *sensu stricto?*

Already confusing enough, the process of diagnosing Lyme becomes even more muddled when you consider the often variable responses of the immune system to these extravascular (and sometimes intravascular) organisms.

Given all of these factors, is it any wonder that patients whose immune systems don't produce antibodies (or at least, antibodies that we can measure) often wind up being told that they "aren't sick" by a physician who insists on a positive blood test in order to make the diagnosis? And is it any wonder they come out of such medical consultations feeling frustrated and enraged by the resulting indifference to their painful symptoms?

Interestingly, one major spinoff of the widely publicized Human Genome Project has been the development of new technology aimed at identifying the genome of the Lyme spirochete. (Forget for a moment that there are probably several.) But the task is huge; one recent study in *Nature*, in which 1,283 Lyme genes were so identified, only serves to point up the staggering complexity of the problem.

Among the genes that were carried on plasmids (tiny bits of DNA shared by one bacteria with another), fully 85 percent were found to be "novel," or newly created. These were brand-new genes! As if we didn't *already* have enough to be worried about, regarding the subject of "antibiotic resistance" conveyed from bacterium to another by plasmid genes!

The great variability introduced by DNA-sharing via plasmids raises yet another provocative problem: the possibility that in the past, Lyme spirochetes might indeed have been routinely killed by three weeks of antibiotic therapy . . . but that as the DNA-sharing among the bacteria continued, the disease-causing agent evolved into forms increasingly resistant to even our most powerful antibiotics.

And what role has chemical alteration of the human habitat in recent years played in *that* particular evolution?

Indeed, one has to wonder if the dynamics of this illness would change all that much, should we decide not call it "Lyme disease"—but instead simply referred to it as a "tick-borne, chronic, neurotoxin-mediated illness!" Would the civil arguments about Lyme finally be laid to rest at the "Appomattox Court House" of this bold new concept?

When it comes to Lyme disease, after all, the vector simply happens to be ticks which play host to various strains of *Borrelia*. And this problem of nomenclature points up the central theme of *Desperation Medicine*—the idea that with rapid chemical alteration of our human environment, the entire concept of "diagnosing disease" has to be thought of in a new way—as broad-based and holistic and requiring a "systems approach" in order to achieve true reliability and accuracy. Look at everything!

All right, what about treatment? What should a caring physician do for a patient with an illness caused by a tick? Some history, first: in recent years, the vast majority of American physicians have learned about Lyme from Allan Steere, M.D., who was the first to publish extensively on the subject of diagnosing Lyme disease. Today, Dr. Steere is generally regarded in the American medical community as "The Father of Lyme Disease."

Starting in the mid-1970s, Dr. Steere worked for many years as a researcher on Lyme, along with countless other physician-colleagues and physicians-in-training. As a Fellow in Rheumatology at Yale University, he came upon the startling realization that a group of cases of "juvenile rheumatoid arthritis" (JRA) found in patients living around Lyme, Conn., actually involved a pathogen other than the ones responsible for JRA.

The discovery that the illness was actually caused by a spirochete, by Dr. Willy Burgdorfer, treatable with antibiotics, changed Dr. Steere's career forever. Recognizing that work, the National Institutes of Health gave him a "career award" for outstanding scientific achievement.

There's no doubt that Dr. Steere made valuable contributions to our knowledge about Lyme. But we should also remember that he and his disciples now steadfastly maintain that any symptoms which return to a patient after three weeks of anti-biotic treatment *must* by caused by something other than Lyme. Apparently, the NIH agreed with him—hence the award.

But what about the hundreds of sign-carrying picketers *outside* the hall who protested that award, while contending that their *chronic* Lyme had gone untreated for many years—largely because of Steere's refusal to acknowledge the long-term version of the illness and because of his perceived participation in what eventually resulted in denial of insurance benefits to thousands of patients with chronic symptoms from Lyme.

Indeed, the published record offers considerable evidence for the existence of chronic Lyme. Example: it's interesting to note how early scientific papers on the topic pegged the rate of "persistent" Lyme cases at 10–20 percent of the total, only a few decades ago. By the early 1990s, however, there had been a major shift among the "institutional" Lyme physicians, and the term persistent was heard far less often.

Suddenly, that 20 percent group of long-term Lyme patients was determined to be suffering from "fibromyalgia" by many physicians. (And this all-inclusive diagnosis seemed even more likely in situations where the patient happened to be a woman!) But other institutional doctors came up with such familiar-sounding—and difficult-to-pin-down—ailments as depression and chronic fatigue syndrome. Here is the classic tactic that forms the very heart of the Appearance of Good Science: "The Smokescreen!"

As the years passed and our knowledge about the disease in-creased, a few non-institutional physicians around the country became known as "Lyme-literate." These practitioners were intimately familiar with the scientific literature. But they also treated thousands of patients who struggled from minute to minute with the disorder. These doctors in daily clinical practice often saw patients with chronic or cyclically recurring tick-borne infections, and they wound up prescribing large amounts of anti-biotics—whether intravenous or intramuscular—over prolonged periods of time.

214   Healing Chronic

In many cases, the results of these lengthy antibiotic regimens were beneficial. But many other patients simply did not improve, regardless of the amount of drugs they were given.

Incredibly, the debate over the cause and treatment of chronic Lyme soon deteriorated into all-out attacks on the medical licenses by proponents and opponents of the various schools of thought. As a result, many Lyme-literate physicians were literally hounded out of practice or away from treating Lyme patients. Dr. Steere now faces challenges to his own licensure in his home state of Massachusetts. So who will win the Lyme Civil War? In the end, it's the *patient* who loses.

Of course, I had never imagined that the violent assaults on credibility and character I'd witnessed during the *Pfiesteria* battles (See Chapter Two: "The Showdown") would ever be repeated in American medicine. Wrong! As a matter of fact, the debate over the "Cell From Hell" soon began to look like mere squabbling among siblings, compared to the vicious medical warfare over chronic Lyme.

Still, I had high hopes that the Lyme in-fighting might come to an end in April of 1999, when a Lyme researcher—Dr. Sam Donta of Boston University—announced that a crew of investigators from his shared lab led by Dr. Mark Cartwright had isolated a neurotoxin manufactured by *Borrelia*.

As you might imagine, I was delighted to hear about this discovery. Of *course* Lyme makes a toxin! How else could you explain the Jarisch-Herxheimer reaction? Doctors have known for many years that treatment of spirochete-linked illnesses (such as syphilis with penicillin) often was followed within a few days by a powerful syndrome that included fatigue, headache, a speeded-up heart rate, rises or falls in blood pressure, chills, sweats and more.

Most medical experts long ago agreed that those symptoms are due to the release of toxins from within the dying bacteria ("endotoxins"). Many bacteria release such endotoxins, and the syndrome is well studied and well documented.

This discovery was a huge advance, as far as I was concerned. Remember: if I could be certain that Lyme manufactured and released a toxin while still alive (an "exotoxin"), then I could be sure that Lyme was a chronic, neurotoxin-mediated illness. And once *that* fact was established, I knew I could detect the impact of Lyme toxins on visual functioning with Contrast Sensitivity testing and then treat the disorder with cholestyramine.

It took me a year to generate the kind of data I needed from 71 FACT patients who had presented with classic chronic Lyme symptoms following a tick bite or exposure to areas where there had been such bites. These patients all shared a few characteristic traits: they were all refractory to antibiotic therapy, and they were all without a confounding medical diagnosis. (They also shared, to a patient, a FACT deficit that clearly responded to CSM therapy.)

As it turned out, the patients who warranted a clear Lyme diagnosis—either by displaying the characteristic "Erythema Chronicum Migrans (ECM) Rash," or via an indisputable positive blood test—were no different, neurotoxicologically, than the groups of patients who displayed symptoms following a tick bite but did not present with a rash or have a confirmatory blood test.

When compared to control patients (this group displayed one symptom each), the known Lyme patients averaged eight symptoms each from the Neurotoxic Illness Chart and the "Test Negatives" averaged six symptoms. (These were patients who would never have been told they had chronic Lyme disease. Yet their illness was clearly documented by CS.)

In a study conducted by Steve Nostrom, R.N., a Lyme activist located on Long Island, over 600 of his 1,000 patients did not have a positive blood test. Nostrom had not recorded specific symptoms . . . but isn't it time we put the "blood test argument" where it belongs, on the barely simmering back-burner? Especially when the CS test is so much better?

No wonder Allan Steere and his followers had been so eager to say that their chronic Lyme patients had something else. They simply had failed to acknowledge the existence of the chronic, neurotoxin-mediated syndrome that Lyme creates. Nor had they seen that fibromyalgia, depression and fatigue are also among the symptoms caused by Lyme—or that they can also be alleviated by CSM therapy after diagnosis via FACT.

As it turned out, a patient's FACT score proved to be far more effective at determining the presence of chronic Lyme than any blood, urine or other Lyme diagnostic test. Although few physicians realized the value of these approaches in the early going, interest in this new diagnostic tool skyrocketed after I gave a presentation on diagnosing Lyme at a regional meeting of the American Society of Microbiology in April of 2000.

Still, treatment experience showed that there were some significant problems with the Herxheimer Reaction, and that about 10 percent of the patients were not improved (see Chapter 15).

Nevertheless, being able to help 90 percent of the desperate patients was a major breakthrough in the struggle to improve treatment for chronic Lyme.

The stories you're about to read provide a key theme for *Desperation Medicine*, in which "any improvement is a godsend and any cure is a miracle!"

As Pat Smith of the Lyme Disease Association has often reminded me, we cannot use the word "cure" when discussing reduction of symptoms in patients. That's because it takes only one awakening cyst—or maybe the breakdown of a protective sanctuary—in the body of an affected patient to begin the process of chronic infection all over again.

Dr. Mitch Hoggard of the Chico, Calif., Hyperbaric Chamber facility heard about my work and then brought together a group of referring physicians to explore it. Quite generously, Dr. Hoggard began referring patients to my protocol, performed in his office, instead of using his hyperbaric chamber—once he recognized the effectiveness of FACT and CSM in diagnosis and therapy. Other physicians followed suit, to the point that my protocol has now spread to 25 states and five foreign countries (See Chapter 29: "Struggling Toward The Light").

After several years of treating patients and researching the problem, I can tell you that, yes, the chronic, neurotoxin-mediated illness from Lyme is real.

I can also tell you that the "institutional" physicians and researchers will soon have to revise their easy dismissals of this chronic disease. It's time to begin educating the American public and also the American medical community about the facts.

We need to pull together at this point, in order to protect the treating physicians and their patients. We do that best by making sure no one gets lost in the endless conflict between different Lyme ideologies.

We can learn a great deal from the three women whose stories follow. Marie Moore, Rhonna Smith and Diane Stephenson show great courage in their continuing quest for health—in spite of years of disabling Lyme. They can inspire us all.

One of the greatest rewards for a treating physician is to help a patient return to normal functioning, and in that regard, I always think of a fourth woman: a dedicated mother I know named Susan Blemlek. Her son Mike not only overcame a brutally disabling case of chronic Lyme that had lasted nine years . . . he was even able to finish college and then get married, soon after FACT and CSM therapy helped him to begin a new, toxin-free life in which he seems to have abundant supplies of energy and enthusiasm.

I was thrilled to receive an invitation to Mike's wedding, and I still get goose bumps every time I read the card of thanks that his mother sent me:

It's been three months [without painful symptoms] and my son is smiling! How can I ever put into words how I feel? He's well, he's teaching and he's planning his life! Thanks for giving me my son back!

—Linda Blemlek

MARIE MOORE: Life Inside the "Twilight World"

Ask Marie Moore to describe the agony of chronic Lyme disease, and this 51-year-old writer and theatrical designer won't hesitate.

"It was a nightmare," says Moore, a West Milford, N.J., resident who struggled with the devastating illness throughout most of the 1990s. "I was so sick that I could not function at all. I just couldn't. Headaches, fatigue, aching joints, fever . . . most of the time I just lay in bed and cried.

"I took seven or eight naps a day. I was sleeping 20 hours out of 24, and I could not function. I could hardly say sentences, and my thoughts were all muddy and jumbled."

Like many Lyme patients, Moore has no memory of ever being bitten by a tick. "I had never even seen one until three years ago," she says. "But I think I probably picked it up in my own backyard.

"At the house next door, the father had Lyme, also. But he had the rash [a common symptom] on his face, so he was treated early. It was surprising to see—in just a couple of weeks—how horribly it affected him."

The mother of two teenagers (one of whom also contracted the disease), Moore had been extremely active and productive until the symptoms of Lyme erupted in late 1994.

Like so many other victims of the disease, she sank quickly into a twilight world of crippling headaches, nagging fever and fatigue so overwhelming that she could barely lift her head from the pillow.

Even worse than these symptoms, however, was the treatment she began to receive from friends and family members . . . along with several medical doctors who seemed to have no clue about the actual nature of her illness.

"This disease tears apart couples, tears apart families," she will tell you with a mournful sigh. "And that's because it's such an unpopular thing to get. Lyme disease is what you get when you don't want to go to work or school today! That's how the world treats it. It's a joke. It's funny.

"You know, it's right up there with Sunlight Deficit Disorder, as far as laughability. People do not realize the horrible extent to which this disease can go."

While she struggled to hold her family together, Marie Moore spent endless hours in consultation with medical specialists . . . most of whom wound up telling her that her agonizing illness was entirely in her head!

"The treatment I've gotten from the medical profession is almost as bad as the disease," she says angrily. "It started right when I first got sick—and was misdiagnosed as having Lupus. And I was treated for that, instead of Lyme.

"Other doctors would listen to me and then run a bunch of psychological tests, and then tell me I was nuts."

Until the fall of 1999, when she showed up in my office in Maryland, Marie Moore had bounced from one physician—and one antidepressant—to the next. Endlessly patronized by the hurried physicians who routinely under-diagnosed and over-prescribed tranquilizers for their patients with multiple, vague complaints, she had grown accustomed to being told that her excruciating symptoms were sheer fantasy. Late in her treatment she finally began to obtain compassionate care from some Lyme-literate physicians . . . even if her illness didn't improve much under their supervision.

Marie Moore needed a miracle.

As she wrote in her journal shortly before our first visit together:

> At times it seems that all my dreams
> Are pigeons made of clay,
> Targets for the guns of fate,
> Victims of uncaring hate,
> Shattered as I watch and wait
> For one to get away.

• • •

From the Public Health Department of Colorado to the research labs of California (where the disease officially doesn't "exist") to the ivy-covered campuses of Yale and Tufts (where it's always "cured in three weeks"—or else it was "caused by something else"), the U.S. medical profession seems to be caught up in a epidemic of denial about chronic Lyme.

Simultaneously we are inundated by endless research on tick-borne diseases—along with a surging growth of "alternative medicine" treatments, some of which amount to little more than mere hucksterism.

Some of the highly dubious remedies find many takers, and why not? Long-suffering patients, desperate for relief, will experiment with anything and everything in order to feel better. Cost is no object for many of these victims. But you can be sure that money *is* the object of unscrupulous practitioners who measure human suffering in dollars and cents.

Here is the cultural and economic backdrop, then, for an illness that has quietly invaded backyards in nearly every section of America and Canada. (I base that sweeping statement on the "sites of acquisition" that I've charted among my many patients.) Sure, the epidemic of chronic Lyme is partially the result of building homes in remote regions where animals like woodchucks and red squirrels should be the most numerous residents . . . but these changing demographics don't tell the entire story.

What we have to realize now is that we've gradually been changing our habitat in a thousand different ways, in recent years —and many of these alterations have been ideally suited to the proliferation of deer, mice and their accompanying ticks.

• • •

Before we find out what happened to Marie Moore when she opted to battle her chronic Lyme disease with cholestyramine, let's take a quick look at how—and why—this ailment makes people so sick.

Inside the Toxic World of *Borrelia burgdorferi*

Ever stared at a pile of tangled spaghetti hanging from the side of a plate? That's an easy way to picture the *Borrelia burgdorferi*, the nasty bacteria that triggers the complex set of reactions known as "Chronic Lyme disease" in human beings.

A worm-like spirochete, *Borrelia* makes its home inside the mid-gut of the ordinary deer tick, where it gets along quite contentedly with its ugly-looking host. But when the bacteria-infected tick attaches itself to a human, bad things start to happen. As the tick feeds on its victim's blood, the spaghetti-shaped invader begins to move.

While some experts say this migration takes 24 hours, I know otherwise from watching how quickly some of my patients got sick. (Or else our Maryland Eastern Shore Lyme spirochetes are zipping around on jet skis!)

Gliding invisibly through the tick's saliva, the bacteria soon move into the tiny wound in the host's skin . . . where they quickly take up residence and begin to thrive.

The symptoms that sometimes follow—the "bull's eye rash" and the flu-like headaches, fever, joint and muscle aches—have been catalogued by health researchers at such national medical institutions as the Centers for Disease Control in Atlanta, Georgia and the National Institutes of Health near Washington.

According to these nationally accepted authorities, Lyme is an "easily curable" form of bacterial illness and can be eradicated within a few weeks, simply by administering antibiotics.

What the authorities so far have failed to grasp is the crucially important long term (or chronic) component in this fast-spreading disease. In fact, many victims of chronic Lyme never do fully recover from their confrontation with *Borrelia*: Their debilitating symptoms continue year after year, and their lives deteriorate to the point that many become near-invalids or invalids. They are walking shadows, with hollow eyes who struggle endlessly with fatigue, fever, headaches and arthritis-like swelling and aching of the joints.

Why can't America's practicing physicians take better care of patients like Marie Moore? Why can't they seem to understand her complex, challenging illness? Perhaps it's because so many of them simply haven't been trained to take a "systems approach" to diagnosing and treating such ailments. Instead of thinking about disease pathogens as ceaselessly evolving organisms in an ever-changing habitat, many of today's leading disease-researchers tend to treat them as static, motionless entities that can be analyzed like a problem in trigonometry or calculus. In the end, a phrase like "Lyme disease can be cured in three weeks!" sounds like the same mantra we heard over and over again during the *Pfiesteria* epidemic: "The river is safe!"

Burdened with the rigid logical structures required for the deductive reasoning approach to epidemiology, these institutional scientists seem unable to demonstrate (or maybe they aren't *allowed* to demonstrate) the kind of intuitive, creative thinking that can lead to authentic new discoveries.

Breakthrough

A unique direction for treatment of chronic Lyme Disease came into focus back in the late 1990s, when Environmental Protection Agency (EPA) neurotoxicologist Ken Hudnell, Ph.D., joined me in a new study of dozens of patients who were suffering from chronic Lyme.

Our approach to the disease was different from the mainstream of conventional medical thinking. Instead of swamping our Lyme patients under another tide of antibiotics, we decided to try to pinpoint the effects of biological neurotoxins that were actually triggering the symptoms. We soon discovered that those Lyme neurotoxin symptoms fit the model of other neurotoxin-mediated illnesses such as *Pfiesteria* and *Ciguatera*. We *also* discovered that the impact of the Lyme neurotoxins on brain activity can be effectively measured, using the same, simple test of Contrast Sensitivity that monitors how well the brain and optic nerve distinguish the patterns of gray, black and white during ordinary vision.

The CS test once again became the key tool in our new approach to diagnosis.

After testing dozens of Lyme patients and coming up with accurate, solidly verifiable results, we knew that we were on the edge of a huge breakthrough. If we could accurately identify patients at the bedside, we knew we'd be able to confirm my theory of how *Borrelia* makes people ill for years at a time.

In May of 1999, we began CS-testing patients with a prior diagnosis of Lyme disease. In the end, we administered the FACT to 71 of these Lyme victims. We found that they displayed the impaired visual contrast that is a clear marker for this disease. And measurable visual impairment—a sure sign of damage caused by neurotoxins—was taking place long after most of the patients had undergone extensive treatment with antibiotics.

This successful verification of the CS test meant that we had finally nailed down a foolproof method for identifying chronic Lyme patients . . . since the quantifiable degree of contrast-impairment (now called the "Hudnell Sign") serves quite nicely as an accurate measuring stick for the impact of neurotoxins on brain tissue.

Next step: now it was time to find out if the same neurotoxin-binder I'd already been using on many of my *Pfiesteria* patients (our old friend cholestyramine, or CSM) would serve us equally well in the battle against the ravages caused by *Borrelia.*

So far, so good. After undergoing rigorous physical exams, the patients who had scored low on the CS test were given prescriptions for CSM, in the form the drug "Questran."

While taking this medication, the patients were tested at intervals of two, seven and 14 days, and until they were symptom-free.

The results were astonishing.

In patient after patient, the cholestyramine regimen produced a dramatic improvement in FACT scores, along with a rapid reduction (beginning within 36 hours, in most cases) of the painful symptoms of chronic Lyme.

All at once, Dr. Hudnell and I were looking at clearcut data proving that treatment with a neurotoxin-binding medication powerfully diminishes the misery of this chronic ailment! And indeed, for many of these patients, the elimination of such painful symptoms as brain fog, blurred vision, joint aches and fatigue currently appears to be virtually complete. The good news is that relapse in the absence of re-exposure did not occur often, if at all. Time will tell if the absence of relapse persists.

Still, it's important to remember that in our present state of knowledge no chronic Lyme patient can ever be described as "fully cured." Although they often refer to themselves as "symptom-free," they know that relapse is an ever-present possibility, in the same way that patients with a "cancer cure" usually fear the next unexplained symptom.

Because of the impossibility of achieving a "final cure" for Lyme, I remain very cautious in my forecasts for patients who have improved greatly under my protocols. And my caution is especially pronounced in the case of Marie Moore, who is much better these days—but who nonetheless faces a significant possibility of relapse.

Almost from the beginning of her treatment, I knew that Marie was struggling with *Babesia* as a co-infection, and that her symptoms could return. Still, I promised her that I would not rest until I had "wrestled the co-infection problem to the mat!"

•   •   •

Like many of the patients in the CS-cholestyramine experiment, Marie Moore found that the combination of the vision test and the medication dramatically changed her life.

"It's been wonderful," says Moore, while describing her "new life" as a writer, theater set-designer and part-time river kayaker. "I suspect that I will always have some residual effects, but I'm getting my brain back!

"I'm also thrilled to see how my skin has improved. I no longer look like a leprosy victim. Before, my skin was so bad that I was deadly afraid to go out of the house. I didn't want anybody to see me.

"I started on the cholestyramine back in September of 1999, and I have seen dramatic improvements. Dr. Shoemaker is not entirely happy with my progress, however, because he seems to want a total cure. I'm not yet completely symptom-free, but the improvement has nonetheless been fantastic. I am so thrilled!"

RHONNA SMITH: "I Couldn't Finish a Sentence"

Her name is Rhonna Smith, and she is a remarkably courageous high school computer science teacher whose story about living with the horrors of chronic Lyme disease will leave you shaking your head.

"The fatigue was so severe," remembers the 42-year-old Smith, "that I was sleeping 18 hours a day. I could not go into school; all too often, I couldn't even finish a sentence. One of the things I teach my kids is how to diagnose computer problems—and I couldn't do it, myself!

"I would sit there in front of the computer and try to figure out what was wrong with it, and I didn't have the first clue. The fatigue is so overwhelming that you almost feel like you've got 30-pound weights around your arms and legs."

A veteran teacher at the Olmstead Falls High School near Cleveland, Ohio, Rhonna Smith says she is convinced that she caught chronic Lyme from a deer tick: "I don't remember ever being bitten, but we've got a garden in my backyard, and we live in a wooded area. The deer come right up in the yard and eat out of my garden.

"At this point, I'm absolutely convinced that I've had Lyme disease for the past nine or ten years."

According to this dedicated teacher, the most dreadful aspect of her disease was having to raise three children (they were 12,

10 and eight years old when the disease first struck) in spite of overwhelming fatigue that haunted her day and night.

"I just don't know how I managed," she says today. "I really don't know how I raised those kids. I think I'm a pretty strong-willed person, and I know I've been a fighter all my life. But it finally caught up to me, back when the children were little, because I finally reached a point where I simply could not function.

"I was treated with antibiotics for years and years, and I also spent a great deal of time in the hospital."

She pauses for a moment, then reflects on her years of suffering with a weary sigh: "You know, my disease was so bad in the early years that I had to go through a period of grieving. A period of mourning for *myself*, believe it or not. I was forced to admit that I'd lost my life . . . or at least, the life I'd hoped to be able to live.

"Everything just fell apart. And at one point, I remember how I had to take an entire quarter off from school. They knew I wasn't going to be there for the whole nine weeks. And I remember sitting on the floor of my kitchen and crying, on the first morning that I didn't go to school. Because I really wasn't sure whether or not I'd ever be able to go back."

But she did.

In the end, after consulting a dozen different doctors and spending tens of thousands of dollars on prolonged intravenous antibiotics, she wound up calling my office to ask some questions about the new Contrast Sensitivity testing and cholestyramine therapy that are just now beginning to attract medical attention in the Midwest.

In her own words, here's what happened next:

"Well, I took the visual contrast test [FACT], and I tested highly positive. And right away, Dr. Shoemaker said he wanted me to try his cholestyramine on me, to see if it could help clean the toxins out of my system.

"Within a day or two, I started going through a pretty severe Herxheimer Reaction. For a while I was so dizzy I couldn't stand up, and my joints ached like they hadn't ached in several years. I went through that kind of misery for two or three days, but then things started to get better, *much* better!

"Soon my strength began to return and my headaches and dizziness abated. My joints felt better and I just seemed to have a whole lot more energy than I'd felt in years. After a few months, I found that I had enough energy to resume my teaching—and I can't tell you how wonderful it feels to finally be back in that classroom.

"Because of these wonderful new tools for fighting chronic Lyme—I'm talking about CS testing and CSM therapy—I have been able to pick up my life where I left off. And I really think I'm a whole lot better teacher because of what I went through.

"I've learned a little bit about compassion, for one thing. And as I shared some of my problems with my students, I could see how they were beginning to develop some new feelings of compassion and sensitivity, themselves.

"You know, it's very interesting . . . when you begin to realize that the lessons we learn at school aren't restricted to the ABCs and Xs and Os. This experience taught me how to value people more. How to appreciate my own children, and my own students, and to be grateful for the time I've been allowed to spend with them."

Smiling warmly, Rhonna Smith summed up the agony and the ecstasy of her ten-year battle with chronic Lyme disease:

"I never thought I'd be able to say this, but as horrible as my disease has been in many ways, I actually think I've gained some positives from it.

"I'm convinced that Dr. Shoemaker is totally determined to help his patients overcome their health problems—and that he'll stop at nothing to achieve that!"

• • •

DIANE STEPHENSON:
"This Isn't Lourdes—It's a Journey through Hell"

The nightmare began innocently enough. She felt a "tickling sensation," that was all, located just above her right knee. Then a momentary pin prick. Then a slow, steady pinching . . . as if some tiny, sharp-edged claw had burrowed its way beneath her skin.

Diane Stephenson hurried into the Ladies Restroom.

It was May of 1987, on a college campus located just outside Corpus Christi, Texas.

Stephenson had journeyed to this crowded auditorium to watch her daughter, Sandra, graduate from Texas Christian University with a degree in psychology. But now, as the audience filed slowly into the great hall where the diplomas would be awarded, she found herself marooned in the Ladies Room, struggling to pull what looked like a "hard-bodied spider" from the soft flesh of her lower thigh.

Alarmed by the tickling, the 45-year-old Stephenson—a healthy, active woman who loved to hike and canoe through the forests around Lake Erie, in her native Ohio—struggled frantically to brush the "spider" from her leg.

No such luck.

Incredibly stubborn, the tiny insect clung to its perch, while the increasingly panicked Stephenson struggled to "brush it off."

"I was rather hysterical because I hate spiders," she would re-call later. "But I couldn't seem to brush it off. It finally just kind of backed up and crawled slowly down to my knee, and I flicked it off my leg and hurried back to the auditorium."

Although Stephenson didn't know it at the time, she'd just been bitten by a southern arachnid species known as the "Lone Star Tick." (Back then, the CDC didn't know that Lone Star Ticks carried Lyme. Had she been bitten earlier too?)

Dismissing the seemingly trivial incident, she applauded her daughter loudly, then enjoyed a champagne reception at a downtown Corpus Christi hotel. The next day, accompanied by her husband of 26 years, she began the long journey back to her home in a Cleveland suburb.

She was thoroughly startled, 15 days later, when a "great big red circle" suddenly appeared on her right leg, just above the knee. At the center of the circle was a tiny, painful indentation —at the very same spot where the Lone Star Tick had attached itself to her skin.

Very strange.

And there was more. Within 24 hours, Stephenson was startled to discover "ten smaller circles on my right leg, reaching all the way down to the top of my foot."

Her voice shook with fear as she described what happened next.

"I was pretty worried, so I called a dermatologist. But I couldn't get past the gal on the front desk. She asked me: 'Does it itch?'

"'No.'

"'Are you sick?'

"'No.'"

The receptionist thought for a moment. If the patient wasn't suffering any discomfort, how serious could her condition be? The "red circles" were probably nothing more threatening than a mild skin rash. . . .

"Ms. Stephenson, your symptoms don't sound that bad. Why don't we schedule an appointment with the dermatologist for next week?"

Diane thanked her, and hung up.

It was an all-too-common mistake.

Three days later, she began to experience flu-like symptoms: muscle aches, a bad headache, blurred vision and a low-grade fever. She also felt light-headed, dizzy. Was the flu affecting her sense of balance?

But the red circles on her legs were receding: they were nearly invisible by now.

It didn't occur to her that there might be a hidden connection that linked the tick bite, the red circles, and the flu-like symptoms that were now making her miserable.

Unaware of what was happening to her, she waited patiently until the day of the appointment with the dermatologist. He took a quick look at the fast-vanishing red circles, then listened sympathetically while she described the "bout of flu" that had wiped her out.

He saw no connection, either. After prescribing a mild rash medication, he smiled cheerfully and sent her on her way.

Within a few weeks, the nightmare had begun. Starting in July, Diane began to suffer from massively debilitating health problems—including "fatigue and eye discomfort and aching joints and a stiff neck. And then I started having lots of skipped heartbeats.

"I felt like I was going to pass out. I felt light-headed and I had all these other symptoms. Something was terribly wrong and I knew it. So I went to a cardiologist at Grandview Hospital. I told him how my joints were hurting, and that I was having problems thinking, and I was forgetful and I had all these headaches. And I'd been hearing a few things about this new disease that people could get from camping, if they got bitten by a tick. . . .

"So I asked the doctor: 'Do you think this could be Lyme disease?'

"And he laughed. He said: 'Limes, lemons! Honey, you've been down to Mexico, and up to Canada [traveling]—you could have gotten anything!'

"And then he turned around to dictate my story, and he made it sound ridiculous. He said: 'Well, she got bitten by a bug when she was down in Texas, and then she couldn't hear. She couldn't see, and everything started hurting. And she pretty well went to heck in a handbasket!'

"And he was laughing about it . . . and there I was, feeling extremely ill right then, and watching him laugh at me."

• • •

As unbelievable as it now sounds, Diane Stephenson would spend the next 13 years in an agonizing, futile quest for medical help. Frequently ill, she would spend months at a time restricted to bed . . . while feeling so weak and dizzy and feverish that she could barely lift her arms over her head.

During this long, nightmarish odyssey, Stephenson would consult with 30 different doctors, most of whom would listen impatiently for a few minutes to her long list of painful symptoms, then quickly prescribe a tranquilizer designed to calm her down and ease her anxiety, without examining her symptoms in detail.

While spending several hundred thousand dollars on medical specialists, she would gradually discover that most of the physicians she was depending on had very little time for—and very little interest in—the medical enigma that her case represented.

The breezy, half-hearted treatment she was receiving from these "pillars of the medical establishment" became painfully clear during a shocking episode with a neurologist, back in mid-1990s.

"The neurologist basically wanted me to take Elavil," Diane says scornfully today, and I said: 'I won't take that; I've been offered that so many times.' So then he said, 'Well, how about amitriptyline?'

"I stopped going to him that very moment. Does he think I'm stupid? Amitriptyline *is* Elavil! No, I haven't had very good experiences with doctors. Now, you know how when you're sick, you pray constantly that you'll get well?

"Well, when I was sick, I'd pray constantly that I'd die in my sleep. But sometimes I would also pray that I had a disease that would be acceptable to the medical establishment, so that they would treat me. I would pray that I had diabetes, or congestive heart failure, or even coronary heart disease. Anything that's in the book, anything that's considered acceptable.

"Why is there a prejudice against my disease? Is it because they don't know much about it?"

• • •

Like many of the patients in the CS-cholestyramine experiment, Diane Stephenson would one day find that a combination of CS testing and CSM had the power to change her life.

Before that happy hour arrived, however, this softspoken and gentle homemaker would be forced to endure 13 years of "living hell"—years in which she struggled to make dozens of medical specialists pay attention to her *symptoms*, instead of automatically prescribing tranquilizers for her.

"I'll never forget the day I visited the famous Cleveland Clinic," says an angry Stephenson today. "They did a psych test on me and they told me I was suffering from anxiety. The Cleveland Clinic doctor said I needed to take a tranquilizer.

"He also said I had symptoms of irritable bowel [syndrome], and that Metamucil would probably take care of it.

"So I left there quite depressed, because I was having all these problems and they just wanted to give me Elavil and Metamucil! Still, I told myself: 'The Cleveland Clinic is supposed to be the best,' and I decided to try a different avenue there. I went to a cardiologist. But that doctor got me into his office and he said, 'I see *sick* people here! What are *you* doing here? You are not sick —you have a severe anxiety neurosis!'

"And of course, he wanted me to take tranquilizers, but I never took any of them. I told him, 'If I take drugs, I won't be thinking clearly.'"

As the months turned into years and the tormented Stephenson could obtain no relief for her symptoms, her mood approached despair. Meanwhile, the "medical experts" kept dismissing her case with off-the-wall diagnoses.

Ignoring her comments about the tick bite (and the swelling that had periodically recurred around the area of the bite over the years), the specialist recommended immediate surgery for a hernia in her groin.

Stephenson declined.

Imagine her shock, a few weeks later, when yet another doctor suggested that she was actually suffering from "pelvic inflammatory disease," and suggested yet another round of antibiotics. But how could they help? She'd already taken huge doses, they had failed to make a dent in her symptoms!

More than two years after being bitten by the tick, Stephenson still hadn't been diagnosed as having Lyme disease.

But then she got a lucky break during a visit to the Wright State University Medical School, when a sympathetic intern agreed to "read an article" that Stephenson had run across. The subject of the article: Lyme disease.

The article provided a dramatic insight: the realization that the symptoms caused by *Borrelia*—the headaches, the muscle and joint aches, the low-grade fever, the blurred vision and the memory loss—were precisely the same symptoms which had been tormenting Stephenson for months at a time. The doctor "rolled his eyes" when she requested it . . . but then finally relented and agreed to give her the "ELISA Lyme Antibody Test."

Ten days later, Diane remembers, "He called me up and said: 'I am so sorry to tell you this.' And I knew exactly what he was going to say. He said: 'Your test was highly positive, and not only that. You've had it [Lyme disease] a long time.' And he said he was sorry.

"But I was happy. So happy! You see, I'd been sick for two years, and now I was going to get treated. We knew what it was . . . and that I wasn't just struggling with anxiety and neurosis!"

But Diane Stephenson would not have been so joyful, if she had known what lay ahead. During the next decade, she would receive thousands of doses of high-powered antibiotics (while spending hundreds of thousands of dollars) in a quest to eliminate "the bug" from her system.

Because her doctors had no way of knowing that her excruciating symptoms were actually being caused by the *toxins* in her system, and not the bacteria, they continued to prescribe IV

antibiotics for her. But antibiotics can only operate in the bloodstream, where they attack and destroy microbiological invaders
like any other blood-borne pathogen.

The years passed one by one. And Diane suffered. Listen to
her describe the hell of chronic Lyme, and especially the hell of
the dreaded "Herxheimer Reaction" that would set in each time
antibiotics killed large numbers of spirochetes.

"I thought I was dying. If I tell you that I'm weak . . . well,
I'm a hundred times weaker with a Herxheimer. I'm lying in
bed, and I feel like my heart is not going to beat, because my
heart is too weak. I feel like I can't breathe, because my lungs are
too weak.

"I lost a lot of weight, because I couldn't even lift my arms to
feed myself. I'd try to get dressed, but I couldn't. I'd have to
hold onto things, just to walk into the bathroom. And I'd stay in
bed for three months at a time. I could not even go out to eat
because I was so weak. I would get dressed and get in the car
and my husband would drive me to the restaurant. And I would
get inside, and then run out of energy. I had just enough energy
to get there, and then I could not eat. I was exhausted.

"And I would go out to the car. We had these seats that would
recline, and I would go back there and lie down. . . ."

After 13 years of this agony, Diane Stephenson rang my
telephone in Maryland in the winter of 2000.

What happened next was an extraordinary event—the event
that Diane Stephenson now describes as her "life-changing adventure."

The first thing I asked Diane to do was to take the Contrast
Sensitivity test. She did, and within a few minutes, it was clear
that she was truly suffering from the neurotoxin-mediated illness that is chronic Lyme disease. One by one, she described
the classic symptoms of the disease: the pounding headaches, the blurred vision, the muscle aches and the short-term
memory loss. All this, along with the CS deficit, confirmed the
diagnosis.

Without hesitation, she agreed to start my new protocol, so that we could begin leaching the *Borrelia* toxins from her exhausted body.

Like most patients, Diane was frightened by the thought of starting this new program and for good reason.

Before she could benefit from the drug therapy she was about to receive, I told her she'd have to "run the gauntlet" of an intensification reaction—much worse than the Herxheimer—which occurs when the body's high tide of toxins finally begins to ebb.

The Herxheimer is universally dreaded, because it can last up to several weeks. But the intensification reaction multiplies the misery of the "Herx" at least tenfold. This sometimes excruciating response to the cleansing of tissues usually *intensifies* the very symptoms it's supposed to relieve, at least during the early period of healing.

In the following chapter, I'm going to tell you exactly what happened to Diane when she hit the whirling turbulence of the Herheimer. (I'll also explain how we drew up a strategy—based on taking preventive doses of pioglitazone—that would help her successfully manage this potentially agonizing reaction.)

But first, the good news. After less than 72 hours, this courageous battler found the symptoms of chronic Lyme beginning to leave her. Stunned, she could hardly believe her good fortune. Where was that blaster headache? Why wasn't her neck "killing" her, as it usually did upon awakening?

"There are no words to express the feeling I've got right now," she said just the other day, describing the exaltation she felt as she began to recover her health after 13 years of illness. "Getting well is a life-changing event! It's like when I gave birth to my baby girl—there were no words for that, either.

"I feel like I'm well on the road to a cure. Just a few days ago, I would go up a flight of stairs and become profoundly short of breath. I'd have to hang onto the rail and recuperate, because my legs were so shaky and painful, like they could not carry me up the steps.

"Yesterday I went up a flight of stairs and I stood at the top, and I *wasn't* short of breath. I didn't have profound pain. I'm almost afraid to say it's gone for good, but right now, I'm just feeling effervescent about it all!"

•   •   •

DIAGNOSING CHRONIC LYME: Why Does the Stonewalling Continue?

Mention the term "chronic Lyme disease" to most American physicians, and the odds are high that you'll be met with skepticism, sarcasm, and maybe even some outright disdain.

"Right," says the typical U.S. "institutional" doctor, "this is a case of chronic Lyme! What classic American medical journal did you get *that* out of—the National Enquirer?"

I've always believed that facts are the best antidote for gratuitous criticism and closed-mindedness. And yet the arrogance of some of our most highly placed physicians and health researchers seems to be so great that even the light of hard, cold facts cannot reach it.

It's difficult to believe that most of these chronic Lyme-denying physicians cannot be moved by the endless reports from patients who describe symptoms that range from severe joint pains to stiffness to "lightning-like" pain that explodes deep in muscles and then jabs like white-hot needles into every nerve along their pathway.

It's also difficult, as a practicing family physician, not to respond to these descriptions of searing sensitivity to bright lights (and especially to blue tones), along with the harrowing reports of nightmares full of death, blood and dismemberment. And what about the patients who complain so often of two-day bouts of exhaustion—merely after completing such simple chores as vacuuming the living room rug?

It's an embarrassment to the medical profession, but the blunt fact is that the majority of U.S. physicians remain vastly uneducated about chronic Lyme symptoms such as memory impairment, shortness of breath and sensitivity to bright light.

For many of us who practice family medicine day in and day out, however, listening to disturbing descriptions of chronic Lyme long ago became part of the routine at the office . . . once we began to see how common chronic Lyme really was. Like many family doctors, I had no clue about the dynamics of this fast-spreading ailment—until my experience with *Pfiesteria* threw open a window on the entire world of chronic, toxin-mediated illnesses.

Physicians like me have been able to work with these patients, in most cases, because we've taught ourselves how to *listen* to them. In the best tradition of Sir William Osler, we've "taken the trouble to elicit a careful medical history, so that the patient, himself, can tell us what the problem is."

Let me give you an example of what I mean by describing a recent incident that shows how "listening to patients" can pay huge dividends.

Only a few months ago, my esteemed colleague Dr. Arthur Raines (See Next Chapter, "Lion Fish"), asked to accompany me to a chronic Lyme clinic at Mitch Hoggard's Hyperbaric Oxygen Chamber facility in Chico, Calif.

Art explained en route that he has long been intrigued by my ideas about the chemistry at work in chronic, neurotoxin-mediated illnesses. He was fascinated, he said, by the way low molecular-weight toxins might impact on nuclear receptors, and how they appear to activate genes that trigger the production of such powerful, genetically linked toxic agents as tumor necrosis factor alpha.

Dr. Raines listened very carefully as I interviewed each of our Lyme patients that day, and as I asked each one detailed questions about his or her disease symptoms . . . such as "a lightning-bolt pain that explodes deep in the large muscle groups or the back of the neck."

As patient after patient described similar histories, Art's polite skepticism began to change to excitement. "I think that if one of my interns started talking about a pain that bores like lightning into a large muscle group and then explodes," he said at one point, "I'm sure I'd assume he was crazy!

"But I've heard that symptom described so often today that I can't help wondering: how did you ever come up with *that* question?"

I nodded at him. "Art, the first time I heard a Lyme patient tell me about it, I didn't believe it, either. But I always ask the question . . . because if a patient knows that I understand the unusual symptoms he has, he'll immediately know that I've grasped the reality of his illness. Most physicians lose the chance for instant rapport with Lyme patients by not asking about the unusual symptoms. Like skin pain made worse by water droplets in a shower.

"Trust me: that kind of confidence makes all the difference in the world."

Then the very knowledgeable and empathetic Dr. Raines pointed out: "You know, about 20 years ago, they did a study on schoolchildren in my county. And it turned out that about 40 percent of the kids had scored positive on a test for the presence of Lyme disease. I still do consults for the local school district . . . so maybe we could dig out that old study, find the folks who had positive scores and who stayed close to home, and then do some testing of our own. We could ask them how they're doing —and maybe learn something new about the reality of chronic Lyme. That wouldn't be too difficult a task, do you think?"

Art's attention to the symptoms being described by my patients, already keen, really perked up when I started interviewing a cattleman from Chico who had been struggling with chronic Lyme since 1984.

The weary cattleman's wife also had chronic Lyme, and yet they'd recently been blessed with a daughter, after 15 years of miscarriages. (The child seemed to be growing normally, so there was no way to know if she was suffering from congenital chronic Lyme.)

As always with a new patient, I started by asking the cattle-man some key questions that might reveal the presence of a neurotoxin-mediated illness.

"Oh, yes," he said in answer to Question No. 4, "we use a *lot* of chemicals in the cows. I don't rightly **know** what's in them, to tell you the truth. But I think I might **have** gotten sick in the foothills—or maybe it was back a few **years** ago, when we were baiting coyotes.

"It's pretty bad for the cows out there, you know? I've gotta keep the heifers out of them foothills! If they get pregnant back there, they'll abort just about every time.

"They keep coming down with this disease . . . we all call it *tick fever.*"

Foothill tick fever?

Question: Was the cattleman describing classic ***Brucella abortus*** . . . or was his halting narrative actually pointing the way toward a diagnosis of *babesiosis*, in which trans-ovarian passage of the parasites causes spontaneous abortions in cattle?

And what about the cattleman's *wife's* own miscarriages?

I told Art about the fabulous scientific detective work that had been done by Theobald Smith, who had conducted such brilliant studies on *Babesia* carried by ticks on southern cattle. More than 100 years had passed since the great "Chisholm Trail" cattle drives from Dallas to Abilene, during which the southern ticks had transported *Babesia* halfway across North America.

Smith's painstaking discovery was a classic example of rigor-ous field science that defied the "standard scientific practice" of the day. His work showed that the cause of anemia, fetal loss and death in southern cows moving along the Chisholm Trail was actually an intracellular parasite, *Babesia.*

Unlike its distant relative, *Plasmodium* (which causes malaria), *Babesia* can cross the placenta into unborn calves, where it con-tinues its life-cycle without participation of an intermediate vector—even though it often kills the adult host. (See Chapter 18: "Escape From Nashuon Island.")

"You know, Ritchie," said Art at one point, "we should have learned more about ticks and human illness during all those years."

Case closed!

Flying home to Pocomoke from Baltimore a few days later, I was left to reflect on how much we still *don't* know about tick-borne illness, and especially about chronic Lyme disease.

Question: Is the "foothills tick fever" actually a brand-new human disease? (I can't tell you how many state health departments—including the health department of the Lone Star State —continue to insist in the Year 2000: "We don't *have* any Lyme disease in this state!")

But the facts say otherwise, and it's time we stopped ignoring them.

As my airplane soared above several new housing developments on Maryland's Eastern Shore, I looked down on a landscape punctuated by darkly sinuous rivers and green foliage. There were many cul-de-sacs with homes in various stages of construction. I gazed at several ball fields, some older housing units with more mature plantings, and a wide greenway separating the developments from a nearby expressway.

Then I caught a flicker of movement 3,000 feet below, and suddenly I was watching two small groups of deer work their way back toward the woods, after munching on some of those brand new shrubs in some of those brand-new backyards.

It wouldn't be long, I knew, before the first reports of a new disease—*chronic Lyme disease*—began to trickle in from these habitat-altering housing developments.

Final Question: Will our rapidly expanding knowledge about the relationship between neurotoxin-mediated illness and our chemically altered environment permit us to build an adequate defense against the certain epidemics of toxin-linked illnesses that are headed our way?

No one can answer that question with certainty.

But one thing is sure. If we continue to avoid this issue . . . if we allow the climate of medical disinformation to continue hiding from the stark reality of such accelerating illnesses as chronic Lyme, we will have almost no chance to prevail against them. The epidemic is here.

We need to look around us. We need to listen to the sick people and really hear their despair. We need to become healers.

The hour of Desperation Medicine is at hand!

Lion Fish . . . or *Lyme* Fish? An Essay on Comparative Toxicology.

Santa Barbara, CA –February, 2000

"Good morning, Dr. Shoemaker. This is Sonny, from Santa Barbara!"

The voice was thickly accented: Vietnamese. Sonny had emigrated to this country at the height of the Vietnam War, and he'd worked long and hard to build a successful career as a California restaurateur.

"I want to thank you, thank you from the bottom of my heart. I'm feeling so much better, for the first time in so long. Thank you, thank you! You were wonderful to help Dr. Art and me. Now I can work again, without pain. So thank you very much. If you're ever in Santa Barbara, come see me. I love you, thank you, thank you!"

How's that for a "good morning" on a rainy Monday in April?

Sonny Nguyen was the number-one "fish man" in Santa Barbara. If you want the freshest sea trout or rock lobster in all of California, Sonny's Surfside Restaurant and Market is the only place to go. But the seafood chef's medical history turned out to be even more interesting than his adventures as a Vietnamese refugee who had taught himself how to thrive in a totally new culture.

In recent years, Dr. Art Raines, a distinguished pathologist and bariatrician from Dallas, Tex., has participated with me in discussions about the best way to help Knoll Pharmaceuticals market their weight-loss medication, Meridia. Many of those very interesting talks have taken place at meetings of the American Society of Bariatric Physicians (ASBP).

I admire Art greatly, and I especially enjoy talking with him about "the physiology of fat." He's a charismatic medical man, and everybody seems to like and trust him right away.

Anyway, I thought I had some good ideas (with accompanying supportive data) on obesity, and I was convinced that the best results for Meridia use could be obtained by my protein-sparing, low-amylose diet. (Meridia hasn't agreed with me yet, but Art has been hard at work, subtly selling the protein-sparing concept to the corporate bigwigs.)

Art had phoned me in February of 2000: "What are you up to, Ritchie?"

I'd already sent him a summary of the lecture I was sched-uled to present at the next ASBP meeting in Portland, Oregon, scheduled for the following May.

"Art, this talk is gonna be wild! I've got a pile of references to back up my theories about environmental acquisition of diabetes and obesity. I'm also going to present data on about 30 patients who've been cured of abnormalities in insulin receptor physiology caused by biological toxins."

"Oh, really?" Art chuckled out loud. "Good luck getting any-one to agree with that! But you know, Ritchie, I did hear that Vietnam vets exposed to Agent Orange were coming down with diabetes in unusual numbers."

I mulled that idea for a few moments. "There may have been mycotoxins in Agent Orange, Art. Remember 'Yellow Rain?' And they added a lot of spermicides to the mix, as well. It looks like we were dropping everything we could find on Vietnam."

"Interesting," said Art. "But tell me more. Which toxins can cause diabetes?"

"Well, chronic Lyme patients are the worst. Lots of them come down with diabetes about three months after they first get sick from the Lyme bacteria. But by binding toxins and treating them with diabetes medications—called 'glitazones'—I can show that the insulin receptor defect caused by the toxins is corrected."

"No kidding? The diabetes goes *away?*"

"Sure does. Meet CSM, Art—the new weight-loss drug!"

• • •

I hung up, then shook my head ruefully. While Art soaked up the rays in sunny Santa Barbara, I was running after Lyme patients in dear old Pocomoke! Some guys have it all figured out.

But then one morning a few weeks later, Art rang me back. Brilliant or not, he said he was stuck and he needed some help.

Talking fast, the Texas physician outlined his treatment problem. His long-distance patient, Sonny Nguyen, worked all the time; the Vietnamese entrepreneur didn't travel and he didn't take vacations. But in recent days, this human dynamo seemed to be exhausted from morn to night.

Suddenly, he couldn't manage to work four hours a day, let alone 14. And that was a real problem, because Sonny's fish restaurant was all he had to feed his immigrant family.

About two years ago, Dr. Art explained, Sonny had accidentally brushed one hand against the side of a lion fish in his aquarium. A fish fancier, he had been raising these exotic swimmers for years, as it turned out, and he'd never been envenomated before.

Too bad. Sonny's arm hurt, and it had begun to swell almost immediately. Moving quickly, he'd plunged the affected hand into hot (105-degree) water, and he'd kept it immersed for 90 minutes. The heat had knocked out the protein-like, high-molecular-weight toxin, so that both the swelling and the pain gradually diminished.

Unfortunately for Sonny, however, the same poisoning-scenario was repeated two months later. This time his hand had slipped in the aquarium, and the spines of the lion fish had broken the skin. But luck had seemed to be with him, at first—no pain, no swelling, nothing. He'd soaked his arm again, however, just to be on the safe side.

Thirty-six hours later, though, Sonny's muscles had begun to ache. Soon his head hurt badly. He felt exhausted . . . maybe he was working too hard?

The next day the small joints in his hands felt a little stiff. Aspirin didn't help . . . and neither did green tea, acupuncture, or aroma therapy.

Still, Sonny did not become alarmed. He was getting a little older, after all; surely these recent memory-lapses were merely the result of aging?

A few more weeks passed, however, and nothing had improved. As a matter of fact, his memory seemed to be getting worse. And when his knees suddenly began to swell up, Sonny knew it was time to see a physician.

His workup was unremarkable. The rheumatologist in L.A. declared himself to be baffled—and so did the team of specialists from Stanford. Sonny was missing more and more time from work, by now, and he kept telling the doctors that all he wanted was a week's worth of prednisone, so that he'd "have enough energy" to keep up with his life.

Sonny's doctors had done an excellent job, as far as I could tell. They'd used every weapon in their medical arsenal, but the patient hadn't gotten better. The prednisone helped, but only for a short period of time.

Then his hair started falling out. Steroids? Fatigue? Depression? You name it. A few more weeks passed. The doctors took turns draining the fluid from one knee or another, while frequently injecting his small joints. Sonny tried antidepressants, along with andro, ginseng and colloidal silver. But nothing worked.

Then one day, Sonny got a lucky break. Jay Ruskey—an exotic orchardist who grows chermoya, among other species of plants —dropped by the restaurant. After listening to the exhausted chef's litany of complaints, Ruskey arranged for a consultation between Sonny and his own longtime pal, Dr. Art. And within a day or two, the veteran pathologist was on the horn to me, asking for my opinion.

"Ritchie, I've got one for you. If you can fix Sonny, that would be good. He's really struggling."

Next step: I quickly e-mailed a CS Test to Dr. Art, who gave it to Sonny, right at his restaurant . . . as I listened in on the phone. Positive! "Start him on cholestyramine," I told Dr. Art. "If the Contrast Sensitivity test shows the deficit, he will get better. Only Lyme disease causes the Intensification Syndrome."

Two days later, a worried-sounding Dr. Art phoned me again.

"Ritchie, Sonny is a lot worse. It's like all his symptoms have multiplied. Are you sure you know what you're doing?"

"Art, get him another Vision Test, right away. He's having an Intensification Reaction. If the CS is falling, start him on pioglitizone and he'll be better in 36 hours."

Looking back on it now, I find the Sonny Nguyen case to be incredible. Paul Auerbach, M.D., one of the U.S. leading authorities on Wilderness Medicine, knows a great deal about lion fish and such related marine toxin-bearers as scorpion fish and stone fish.

"This should become a Case Report, Ritchie," said Auerbach, when we discussed Sonny's bizarre toxin-history. "No one is doing much in treatment of marine toxins that I know of, except you. Call Jay Burnett at the University of Maryland; he's written a book chapter on lion fish."

I did as instructed. But Dr. Burnett had not heard of a chronic neurotoxin-mediated illness caused by lion fish. "Let me call my colleagues in Australia, Ritch, and I'll get right back to you."

No such luck. As it turned out, nobody in the world of medicine has seen this pathology before. Was the Fish Man's illness actually the result of the lion fish stings? Sonny didn't have any other exposures that could account for his syndrome, so where were we? His long (and expensive) workup had provided no better explanation.

All at once, the situation seemed clear: This was a case of "Chronic Lion Fish Envenomation" acting like "Chronic Lyme Disease!"

Obviously, it's going to be important to document the structure of the lion fish toxin in the days up ahead.

Meanwhile, we also needed to make sure that Sonny got through his Intensification Reaction with the help of pioglitazone. (He did and went on to complete his recovery with cholestyramine.)

The next chapter in this exciting medical saga will occur in about three months, when we learn whether or not Sonny develops diabetes. If he does, the link between Lyme and lion fish toxins will be established beyond a reasonable doubt.

Not to worry, however: If Sonny *does* start to develop high blood sugar, I've got a treatment for that, too.

Last Question: Does Sonny Nguyen know any Agent Orange victims—American or Vietnamese—who are also struggling with diabetes?

Come to Pocomoke, guys, and let me introduce you to the CS Test!

chapter 15

Event

Lessons from
Solving the Herxheimer

Pocomoke, MD –March, 2000

Diane Stephenson has a wonderful name for the painful re-action that usually sets in, soon after the human body begins cleansing itself of the Lyme toxins that cause chronic illness.

She calls it "The Wild Beast."

"When the dreaded Beast arrives, you go through agony," says the courageous Stephenson, who endured many years of chronic Lyme disease but is now on the road to recovery. "You wake up one morning, and it's like your symptoms are suddenly so much worse than before you started antibiotic treatment. It's torture, believe me. I can't tell you how many times I went through the process, over the years.

"Day after day, I'd lie there in bed, struggling with this pro-found feeling of doom. This profound feeling of exhaustion! My heart felt too weak to beat. I'd be hot and cold, all at once. Faint and dizzy. I had a desperate feeling of needing to do something, but I was unable to discern what it was.

"What did I need to do? I was agitated, and just profoundly sick. In some ways, my symptoms seemed like those described by drug addicts when they go through detoxification. I was faint and perspiring, then ice-cold. And so shaky. It seemed like my insides were at war. And there I was, trapped inside this twitching, painful body. And my mind remained in a foggy state —a sickening, confused, trance-like state.

"It was like you'd been on some terrible, gyrating ride which leaves you disoriented and nauseated, unable to regain your bearings."

• • •

Along with her gift for words, Diane Stephenson has a rare ability to look pain and discomfort in the face and not blink. Her journal descriptions of the "Intensification Reaction" that takes place whenever the human body rids itself of chronic toxins (after therapy with CSM) have opened a window on one of the least understood mechanisms in human physiology: the intensely uncomfortable symptoms that together make up what medical sciences now describes as "The Herxheimer Reaction."

Remember that the Intensification Reaction follows therapy with CSM, while the Herxheimer Reaction (much less severe) often occurs in the wake of antibiotic therapy.

Question: Why is it that the vitally helpful and health-restoring process of "binding" and then removing toxins so often triggers an accentuation—the "Intensification Reaction"—of such debilitating symptoms as fatigue, muscle aches, headache and confusion?

ᵀn this chapter, we're going to take an up-close look at a strange paᵣadox that usually emerges during the healing of chronic Lyme disease.

The paradox: "Before you can get better, you'll have to get worse for a while!"

In order to understand why the "Herx" is such a problem for folks who are battling particular (but curiously, not *all*) neurotoxin-mediated illnesses, we're also going to take a very brief—and very simplified—course in organic chemistry. While exploring the wild, wonderful worlds of the polymerase chain reaction (PCR) and "extravascular circulation of low molecular weight ionophore toxins," we're going to chase the Wild Beast into his lair and de-claw him. How? It's simple. Once we understand what really goes on inside the body during "detox," we can design a therapy (sometimes featuring the drug "pioglitazone") that will allow us to reduce the severity of these painful symptoms, even as the healing continues.

Key point to remember: Organic ionophore toxins make people sick by circulating outside the bloodstream, through fatty tissues. (Remember that fatty tissues are not restricted to fat cells.) The toxins are low molecular weight, and they cause symptoms through two different mechanisms. First, they attack cells directly, by attacking their electrical or food supplies. And second, they cause destructive distortions in cell chemistry by attacking and activating genes, and causing those genes to send harmful "chemical messages" that produce destructive enzyme reactions among cells.

• • •

Taming the Wild Beast

Ask any chronic Lyme patient—or any other neurotoxin-afflicted patient, for that matter—to recite his or her symptoms, and you'll probably find yourself listening to the same litany of endless, mournful-sounding complaints, as follows:

- "I get these pounding headaches . . . worse at night, when I see headlights. But sometimes I get them just from the fluorescent lights in my office. And when I take aspirin, they only seem to get worse!"

- "The muscles in my arms and legs ache like there's no tomorrow. I feel good when I work out, but I don't recover for two days afterwards. Am I just getting old?"

- "I made myself go to work this morning, but I couldn't remember my own computer password! What's wrong with my memory?"

- "My vision keeps getting blurry, and my thumbs go numb. Then my stomach goes into spasm, too. My doctor says I'm depressed."

• "Why am I dozing all the time? Even at work, when I used to be hustling, I usually feel so weak and tired that it's an effort to keep concentrating, ignoring the ever present brain fog."

During the last several years of treating neurotoxin-mediated illnesses—Chronic Lyme, Chronic Fatigue, Sick Building Syndrome, *Pfiesteria* and all the rest—I've heard those symptoms repeated so often that I recognize the pattern, even when the patient's major complaint consists of a single symptom.

While treating thousands of patients suffering from these chronic symptoms, I soon realized that although I felt I understood the biochemistry involved in their discomfort, I had no proof that confirmed my model. What is it about these organic toxins from multiple species, I soon began to ask myself, that produces the commonality in symptoms among so many of the people I treat?

For some time, I'd been struck by a peculiar fact. Regardless of whether the illness involved was Lyme disease or *Pfiesteria* or chronic fatigue or ciguatera, the symptoms were strikingly similar. Did that mean that the biochemical structure of all these toxins might be the same?

In order to attack that question, I had no choice but to employ the "inductive method" of reasoning that I've often talked about in this book. Although I soon learned that there was a commonality in *part* of the structure of all the different toxins, their remaining chemical structures were widely divergent. Their similar effects on my patients were also painfully evident. Instead of endlessly asking the analytical question "why" (a "deductive" approach that quickly narrows your field of vision to a few endlessly repeated observations), I asked "how?"

Unlike "Why," "How" is an "open-ended" question that allows the thinker to take intuitive "leaps" of logic in search of answers. Of course, it also makes the investigator vulnerable to critics asking "Why?" So how was I to figure out the Herxheimer? I started by asking a few questions that would have made Francis Bacon proud:

- What do I already know about these organic toxins?
- What do I know about my patients' symptoms?
- Based on what I know, can I make any generalization about how toxins work to make people sick?
- What chemical compounds are involved, and how do they interact with human cells to cause symptoms of illness?
- Do toxins produce both "direct effects" and "indirect effects?"
- And finally: How does a non-absorbable powder stimulate the sudden worsening of symptoms related to intravascular events? What causes the human body to experience the Intensification Reaction of symptoms—Diane Stephenson's "dreaded Herx"—even as disease toxins are being cleansed from the system by CSM? In other words: why did my patients suddenly get ten or 20 times worse, before they could start to get better . . . so that I always wound up urging them to "hang on through the Herx, because there will be a soft landing on the other side?"

That last question on the "dynamics of the Herx" sent me off on a month-long literature search performed by Russel Kujan of the Maryland Medical and Chirurgical Library. Russ remains a treasure to me. Every time I call him and ask for another search on another abstruse topic, he dives into the work and provides me with the references I need.

After settling down with a stack of articles, I read everything I could about the *Borrelia* bacterium that makes Lyme toxin. Studying the files, I recalled that a key component of the bacterium's cell membrane was instrumental in triggering the release of a compound called "Tumor Necrosis Factor Alpha," or "TNF." This powerful cytokine has become increasingly prominent in recent research on multiple disease processes. It has also been pinpointed as a "chemical trigger" that contributes to environmental acquisition of diabetes and obesity by disrupting the body's sugar-processing insulin receptors.

That observation made me stop and scratch my head. As I thought back on my lengthy research with insulin receptors, I remembered that part of the mechanism of action of a diabetes drug (pioglitazone) is to reduce—or even remove—the effect of TNF on the receptor.

With growing excitement, I asked myself: "If TNF can be blocked at the insulin receptor—and TNF also seems to be deeply implicated in the Herxheimer reaction—might it be possible to use the same insulin-modifying medication to help block TNF in the Herx?" If so, would this explain why chronic Lyme patients and other chronic, neurotoxin-mediated illness patients often develop obesity problems (without a corresponding change in eating habits, that is) . . . and why they never seem to respond to standard weight-loss techniques?

At first glance, the proposition looked absurd. Talk about an "inductive leap!" With no proof that a toxin was involved, I knew I needed more research before I could feel comfortable about my idea. Yet the exhilarating possibility remained: If TNF turned out to be a key factor in both insulin disorders and neurotoxin-mediated illnesses, it might be possible to use that insight to get a better handle on how the substance actually caused damage to cells in disorders such as chronic Lyme disease.

Example: Did TNF change the way white blood cells aggregate in small blood vessels, through a process called "margination?" Was it also the key component in apoptosis—the "programmed death" of cancerous or inflamed cells—by activating a whole series of enzymes with jaw-breaking names, including nitric oxide synthase?

All at once, I began to sense that I was on the edge of a startling new discovery about how disease-causing toxins attack cells.

That new direction would be based on the fact that the body has two main kinds of switches that turn on or turn off genes.

When patients are given a new diabetes medication in the glitazone family, the drug switches on a positive and health-protecting group of genes controlled by a number of "super-family nuclear-receptors" known as PPAR-gamma. In situations where the PPAR-gamma receptors are not triggered, however, and a TNF-producing gene is instead switched on by its own super-family of nuclear receptors, the outcome will almost certainly be destructive attacks on enzyme reactions in healthy cells.

Our body has many levels of checks and balances; this is only one of them. Activating PPAR-gamma turns off TNF production, and activating TNF turns off PPAR-gamma activity.

As I struggled to understand the process of cell disruption that causes the Herx, I realized that the key question was whether or not I could be sure the Lyme toxin switches on the gene for manufacturing TNF. And the answer was no—at that point in my research, I simply didn't know. (Other small molecular weight biotoxins like okadaic acid, nodularin, and ochratoxin do turn on the TNF genes.)

This mechanism, found in dinoflagellates, blue-green algae and fungi, surely *could* apply to spirochetes. Once again I reminded myself that I didn't fully understand the biochemical structure of the toxin. But neither did anyone else!

I refused to become discouraged, however, because I had long understood that when you're breaking new ground in science, absolute certainty is a luxury to which you're rarely entitled. Regardless, I decided to go ahead and attempt the "leap."

And it worked! As you'll see clearly later, exploring this genetic aspect of chronic, neurotoxin-mediated illness eventually opened a window on the crucial role played by particular enzymes, including phosphatases, in the inner workings of an entire family of little-understood diseases. Destroy or disable the phosphatases, and you'll also destroy the checks and balances essential to cellular homeostasis based on glucose metabolism. (If that theory sounds too complicated and too simplistic at the same time—it is!)

After an extensive review of these problems, I was struck by possible parallels between my research on the factors involved in obesity (especially as related to defective insulin receptors) and the biochemistry of toxic illnesses.

Two key facts seemed to provide a good starting point. First, as every biological researcher will tell you, the *structure* of an organic compound will usually determine its *function*.

Second, it soon became evident that although each of the toxins involved in the various neurotoxin-mediated illnesses is manufactured by a different organism, the symptoms they cause are remarkably similar.

Looking more closely at the organic chemistry involved, I soon discovered that a particular part of the structure of the toxin-attack was always the same, regardless of the particular poison involved. In every case, the toxin molecules worked by configuring themselves into three-dimensional rings of atoms that shared negatively charged atoms. It didn't matter if the negative charge was shared by oxygen (dinoflagellates and fungi), nitrogen (blue-green algae), or possibly sulfur (spirochetes).

In scientific terms, this toxic structure is known as a "molecular dipole," or "ion ring."

The ion rings vary slightly in terms of overall molecular structure, based on the species that is synthesizing the toxin. In the case of the dinoflagellates, for example, you get a ring of six or seven oxygens (a polycyclic ether) . . . whereas the blue-green algae (*microcystis*) have a cyclic peptide structure creating a ring of nitrogen atoms.

The fungal organisms, on the other hand, make a ring of oxygens from the carboxylic acid ether backbone of their molecules.

Regardless of the particular configuration, however, the bottom-line result is always the same: each one of these toxin molecules holds the potential for creating an "ionic sink" containing these shared electrons at its central core. This core develops a net negative electrical charge.

The point is that this special configuration, or "ion dipole," is the electrostatic trigger for moving positively charged ions —such as the vitally important potassium—against the "electrical gradient," or basic electrostatic energy field, of the healthy cell.

The result is that these toxic dipoles disrupt the electrical gradient of potassium inside the cell (and sodium outside) by hooking one end of their molecular support system into the fatty part of cells, the membrane, and then dragging potassium into them, where it quickly disrupts the electrical potential of the gradient. (I recognize that this simplified model may not include some other factors involved in cell damage by toxins, in addition to corruption of the gradient. Those factors include disruption of sodium and calcium channel receptors, as well as many other "downstream" factors.)

To picture how the process works, think about static electricity. What happens when you run a comb through your hair on a dry winter day? Your hair rises to meet the comb . . . because the oppositely charged particles involved attract each other with great force. But what would happen if you diluted the tension of those opposite charges, by overloading either the negative or the positive energy flowing through the system?

That's exactly what happens when these molecules, or "ionophores" (each includes a "fat-loving," or "hydrophobic" end attached to a "water-loving," or "hydrophilic" end) drag potassium across cell membranes. Suddenly, because of the potassium overload, the powerful electrical imbalance between potassium and sodium cannot be discharged in order to allow nerves and muscles to function normally.

And when that happens, the cell loses its normal electrostatic potential. Suddenly, it can't rely on electrical tension in order to move substances around the cell, or power electrical-chemical reactions. Like a car battery with a huge positive terminal but only a tiny negative input, the cell has lost a great deal of its ability to deliver a strong charge and cannot provide enough power to sustain normal life processes.

Like the defective battery, the cell that has been poisoned in this way still puts out a small amount of "juice"—but it isn't nearly enough to accomplish all of the metabolic tasks required for healthy homeostasis. In scientific terms, it can no longer "propagate an effective action-potential" in order to achieve adequate electrical transmission.

Put in a nutshell, we can say that the fat soluble, low molecular weight ionophore neurotoxins (but there are also many other kinds of neurotoxins, remember) usually work in the same way: they create chemical reactions in which too much potassium enters the cell, fouling the "electrostatic gradient," and thus crippling the cellular electric generator on which living tissue must rely. Metaphorically speaking, poisoning a cell with potassium in this way is no different from running a lawnmower with the choke fully on. Could the poison be a sodium molecule? Or something else? (Researchers will surely tell us later.)

So far, so good. At this point in our "Biochemistry 101" adventure, we can see clearly how organic toxins work to shut down electrical functioning in the cell.

Next problem: how does our old friend, the cholesterol-lowering drug cholestyramine, work to neutralize the impact of these toxins on fat-containing tissue?

The answer is simple. In order to remove the toxins from a patient's system molecule by molecule, we must find another molecular sink—another atomic structure that will lock onto the toxin's ionic ring in the same way that the toxin locked onto the potassium atoms before dragging them into the poisoned cell.

Obviously complex, the chemistry is nonetheless easy to describe. In order to prevent the toxin molecules that carry the ion sink-lock from being reabsorbed in the small intestine (their usual fate, as they circulate throughout the body's system of fatty deposits before ending up in bile), our toxin-fighting friend, the CSM, presents them with an ion "key" structurally similar to—and essentially the same size as—the potassium molecule.

As the toxin molecules move through the gut, they encounter a different positive charge that fits into the molecular sink. This charge is derived not from potassium, but from the similarly sized (and similarly positively charged) quaternary ammonium contained in the CSM. Once again, the key fits into the lock.

But this time, something different happens. Because the toxin molecules are being held by the uniquely configured atomic structure of CSM, with its long, polystyrene backbone, they cannot be reabsorbed back through the intestinal wall.

Fortunately, the ion dipole-CSM link has already been studied by a major U.S. pharmaceutical company, Aventis. Designed to treat rheumatoid arthritis, their new drug—Arava—breaks down in the human liver, producing the active metabolite "M-1." As it does so, that particular compound has been documented to circulate from the bile into the intestine, in association with the bile salts glycolate and taurine.

Normally, M-1 will be reabsorbed in the last section of the intestine as part of enterohepatic recirculation, after which it is transported via the portal vein of the liver back into the rest of the body, where it operates to reduce the pain caused by RA. Most of the time, a portion of the compound diffuses into bile and the cycle will then be repeated.

Documented studies show that treatment of M-1 patients with CSM reduces the steady-state concentration of M-1 by binding the latter (perhaps with other bile salts). CSM thus prevents the distribution of M-1 from the liver back to the body. In this way cholestyramine can dramatically lower the body's burden of M-1 in only 24 hours . . . in spite of the fact that the M-1 would otherwise persist for weeks in blood, bile and instestine.

The good news here is that the chemistry of M-1 allows it to create a molecular dipole of precisely the size that will allow CSM to act as a kind of "electrostatic sponge." And indeed, the research record shows clearly that CSM provides this benefit in test after test, based on its chemical structure and its ability to bind molecules of a particular shape.

When toxins, such as those produced by *Borrelia* or drugs such as Arava—an FDA-approved substance remember, collide with CSM—they fall into a "molecular bear trap," and they can't escape. Since they aren't being reabsorbed through the lining of the gut, they must be excreted with stool. And thus they end up exactly where they belong—at the bottom of the toilet!

In a delightful twist of biochemical irony, what we've done is used the toxin's own molecular weaponry to trap it. And every time we trap a toxin molecule and excrete it, that's one less molecule to worry about.

For the patient, the result can be summarized in a joyful exclamation: "Good-bye, neurotoxin-mediated illness!"

With our vitally important CS Test in one hand and our cholestyramine (CSM) powder in the other, we can rid most patients of their *Pfiesteria* symptoms in only ten days. Chronic Lyme patients, on the other hand, may require more than six weeks of treatment before their health is restored, sometimes completely, but not always. The Lyme improvement rate of 92 percent says "improvement": it doesn't say "cure."

Such wide differences in the amount of time required for healing can tell us a lot about the different chemical makeup of these organic toxins, and about the speed of their movements within the human body.

Once we understand how organic toxins disrupt and weaken the cell's electrical gradient, it's relatively easy to comprehend the dynamics involved in the two-pronged (or more!) attacks by some of these toxins on enzyme reactions in glucose-processing. What happens here, first, is that the toxins attach themselves to enzymes involved with normal functioning of insulin receptors, and thus foul up the cell's sugar intake and processing plant, which effectively knocks out its supply of energy. The toxins also play havoc with key enzymes, called "phosphatases," that act like the graphite rods in the "nuclear reaction chamber" of glucose that has been released from glycogen-storage to be burned for energy.

Under normal circumstances, when a glucose molecule is released by enzyme action from glycogen, the chemical reaction of glycolysis is shut down by opposing and controlling enzyme systems—in those situations, that is, where it has obtained enough energy to regulate itself. That reaction is the main function of the phosphatases. Inhibit the action of those enzymes, as happens when blue-green algae toxins attack a neighbor, and the cell will continue to chew up its glycogen one glucose molecule at a time until all reserves are depleted.

If you want to make a living cell mortally tired and phlegmatic, simply devour its glycogen without control by disrupting the phosphatases that are designed to prevent just such runaway wastage of this vital food storage. To understand the process, imagine an exhausted Olympic marathon runner staggering across the finish line, with his glycogen reserves totally depleted.

Go ahead: ask him to remember the last two paragraphs of *The Great Gatsby*, or *War and Peace*. Of course he can't do it; there isn't enough energy left in the tank to perform the memory feat!

So much for the two major mechanisms in which toxins attack and disable cells in the human body.

As it turns out, however, these two weapons represent only a portion of the enormous firepower wielded by neurotoxins.

What I did not grasp until much later in my investigation was that many of these toxins also *possess the ability to attach themselves onto specialized segments (called "nuclear receptors") of the cell's DNA. After they attach to these major groups of controlling genes, they then "turn on"—inappropriately—other genes that then "transcribe" the DNA message into mRNA. The mRNA is then translated into normal biochemical processes at the wrong time.*

As you might expect, this action soon cripples or destroys cells, rather than helping them to maintain homeostasis.

I learned this key lesson about the marvelous complexity of the toxins by watching many patients struggle through the mysterious Herxheimer Reaction, in which their toxin-illness symptoms would be enormously multiplied over the space of a few days. The Herx always began only a day or two after patients began their CSM treatments.

Defeating the Herx soon became my primary research focus, even as some other Lyme physicians were just beginning to recommend rudimentary forms of my CSM treatment to their

patients . . . but *without* the protective protocol. I was delighted
to see this early acceptance of CSM therapy getting underway
—although I couldn't at first help wondering why some doctors
were employing only part of the therapy. They were reluctant to
use the safety net of pioglitazone for unknown reasons.

As you might imagine, given the ongoing struggle to understand chronic illnesses such as Lyme, studying the molecular
biology of the toxins soon gained my full attention. Grappling
with the huge complexity of these problems, I did my best to ignore the political battles that continued to rage over conflicting
protocols for treating Lyme. (Ironically enough, it soon began
to seem almost as if my approach to the problem gave the "institutional" physicians a place to hide—while shrugging their col-
lective shoulders and wailing helplessly: "Gee, we didn't *know*
about neurotoxins!")

While these battles unfolded, of course, the Lyme-literate
practitioners continued to fight the good fight . . . doing everything they possibly could to accomplish a very simple goal:
helping patients get better. I worked hard at disseminating my
new knowledge to them—but I knew it would take the medical
world a few years to begin recognizing the existence of this new
family of chronic illnesses.

The next step in my campaign to understand the physiology
of these new diseases required a clearer understanding of toxin-
chemistry. Obviously, these harmful substances had learned how
to "sneak past" the protein-defenders (antibodies) who stand
eternal watch along the cell walls, or membranes. Was there any
doubt that such subterfuge requires some enormously complex
maneuvering, and even a bit of "biochemical trickery" at times?

In order to evade the antibodies, remember, the toxins must
appear to be benign organic substances going about the helpful work
of assisting in the thousand and one tasks of cell repair, message
transmission and metabolism that take place from moment to
moment inside every cell. Simply stated, the toxin cloaks itself
by taking the form of an ionophore, like a stealth fighter that
knows how to become invisible to its enemy. Regardless of the

"disguise" chosen by the attacking toxin, the basic gambit never varies: one way or another, the invader must circumvent the guards. (Remember that in the world of infectious diseases from bacteria—as opposed to toxin-mediated illnesses—being spotted by the antibodies usually means quick, certain death.)

When the raid on the cell membrane is successful and the toxin manages to breach the cell barriers, it can then carry out its search-and-destroy mission without much opposition. (Most of the protein-powered cell-defenders are still cruising along in the bloodstream—outside the cells—looking for "aliens" to attack.)

Once inside the cell, organic toxins will hone in on their targets in the nucleus.

The effects of such attacks on cell functioning can be devastating. For the individual whose body is experiencing these assaults at the cellular level, such reactions as fatigue, muscle ache and mental confusion are perfectly consistent with the havoc taking place in the micro-world of enzymes, DNA and toxin molecules.

I know this part is complicated, but stay with me. The physiology and chemistry may get a bit thicker for a few pages . . . so take a deep breath and enjoy!

The bottom line: although I knew I'd made some good progress at drawing the chemical portrait of the disease mechanism, my neurotoxin theories still left the $64 question unanswered.

$64Q: If countless toxin molecules are being driven out of the body ("chemically bound" and then excreted by the CSM), why do the patient's symptoms get dramatically worse? Clearly, the toxin particles must be doing something *else* as they circulate throughout the body of the suffering patient.

Another way to pose this same problem is to ask again: How can a non-absorbable, toxin-biding agent, CSM, cause Lyme patients (most of whom have experienced the Herxheimer before, while taking heavy doses of antibiotics) to suddenly get much worse?

Mulling the problem, I suddenly asked myself: what if the toxins didn't just attack the electrical and metabolic systems inside human cells? What if they *also went after the "command and control" centers of the cell—the genes and their all-important deoxyribonucleic acid, or "DNA"*?

What if the toxins did more than just shut down the sugar and electrical factories in the cell? What if they went after the cell's "brain," as well? *Let me look again at what I already know.*

Starting, of course, with the key fact that this same DNA-attacking mechanism had *already* been proven to be at work in other diseases, previously. Example: the latest research has recently documented how dinoflagellate toxins—such as okadaic acid—are quite adept at "turning the switch" that sends cellular DNA into high gear, releasing the dangerous compound, TNF.

Investigators in the lab and out in the field have also shown that fungal toxins can attack DNA in the same manner. Couldn't Lyme toxins—along with the poisons produced by other disease agents—be capable of the same scenario?

Picture the scene. Like generals perched on hilltops high above a great battle, the genes issue a never-ending series of coded messages to the troops below. These blueprint messages —chemical instructions, actually, for the necessary steps in building the proteins and enzymes required to maintain healthy metabolism, while also fending off enemies—are conveyed to their cellular recipients by special couriers, the "Messenger Ribonucleic Acid," or "mRNA."

Remember that the mRNA couriers are exquisite copies of the DNA. They pass the DNA-message on to the cellular troops, who need their marching orders.

Enter, now, the dastardly organic toxins (from a Lyme-infected tick, let's say), which have just been driven out of millions of cells through the power of the relentless CSM. How would those toxins respond to this sudden attack from out of the blue?

In order to answer that question, we must remember that there is a continuous circulation of toxins migrating from nerve to muscle to fat cell. And the key elements in the fat cells, "adipocytes" are the sections of DNA that contain the majority of receptors which turn on the TNF.

The process is simple to understand. It begins when the toxin enters an adipocyte and migrates into the DNA, where it turns on the switch that will force the fat cells to make TNF. After that, the TNF is free to wreak havoc in millions of cells and millions of blood vessels throughout the body.

The specific switch for TNF is activated by the low molecular weight toxin, and the switch will be turned on as long as the toxin is bound to the receptor for it on the DNA. Measuring TNF in serum can give us an idea about how many toxin molecules are activating DNA transcription, but the correlation isn't 100 percent. Research shows clearly that the rise in TNF-mRNA in the bloodstream following CSM dosing is a better measure of toxin activity on nuclear receptors.

Remember, also, that the switch is turned off when the toxin spontaneously dissociates itself from the molecular receptor . . . or when a different switch, the PPAR gamma, is turned on by an activator ("agonist") of its own, such as pioglitazone.

As long as the Lyme organism is alive and manufacturing toxin, the TNF load can continue to rise. And indeed, the longer patients suffer with chronic Lyme, the longer it takes to clear the toxic residue from the illness.

When the toxin dissociates from its nuclear receptor, it moves from cell to cell, where it will often act to disrupt electrical function. In many cases, however, the invader will end up impairing phosphatase activity, or even binding to a nuclear receptor in a *different* cell. This model posits an equilibrium of toxin-distribution in the body . . . but that equilibrium is obviously disrupted when CSM triggers the drainage process, thus pulling the plug on the circulating toxins.

Question: Does this sudden disruption of the toxin-equilibrium make the poison move faster . . . thus activating more TNF genes than normal in a given period of time? That hypothesis dovetails nicely with the clinical image of the "TNF storm" precipitated by CSM. As Dr. Thomas Tosteson explained to me (regarding ciguatoxin), "The point is not that the dissociation constant is low, but rather that there *is* a dissociation constant! That means that if you bind soluble toxin, the neural tissue releases more.

"The point here is that CSM-binding will bring about a dissociation of toxin from its tissue-binding." (Here was the mechanism I had been looking for: disruption of dissociation equilibrium continually releases new toxin molecules from their binding sites or receptors, resulting in the blizzard of symptoms even though the total amount of toxin isn't changed.)

I like the elegance of this explanation, but how can I prove its accuracy? Since a sudden shift in the TNF dissociation constant seems highly unlikely (such radical transformations just don't happen in chemistry), it may very well be that some other factor (or factors) play a role in the rapid surge of TNF. I'm eager to see what the next round of research will tell us about this problem. Models of biological activity are made to be disproved, but this model fits the current accumulated data exactly.

Surely the most destructive weapon in the arsenal of the toxins is this ability to turn on TNF in the human body—so that it will target the wrong cells, and then only half-kill them, leaving behind wounded, disorganized entities that can no longer maintain their cellular integrity.

When that happens in an optic nerve, the result is light sensitivity and blurred, fuzzy vision. When it happens in the sensitive nerves along the spinal column and skull, the result can be killer headaches.

And when it happens deep in the brain, in the centers that control feeling and memory, the result is sometimes the inability to remember what you needed to do in the afternoon (or even worse, how you feel about yourself, your anger or your loved ones).

After treating hundreds of chronic patients with CSM and then doing my best to help them through the agonies of the

Herx, I'm convinced that this kind of synchronous, intense onset reaction is caused by TNF and chemicals like it that are released from adipocytes after the toxins turn on the switch.

Delayed reactions, on the other hand (such as the later-phase reactions experienced by asthmatics after sudden attacks), are usually generated by white blood cells derived from monocytes, such as macrophages, and to a lesser extent, mast cells. These cells signal each other to move in and provide help (recruitment). They are also summoned to the battlefront by increased production of a causative compound, when genes coded to make that compound are turned on.

Why is TNF so powerful? One reason is that when it's released into the bloodstream, it causes white blood vessels to travel toward the target area. There they slow down (marginate) until they begin to form a kind of sludge, which occurs after TNF stimulates the local release of a special chemical, adhesin, released by lining cells of the blood vessels.

Once formed, the result is reduced blood flow, or hypoperfusion. The sludge soon begins to deprive cells farther downstream of the precious oxygen and glucose products they need to maintain their biochemistry. If that condition were permanent, it would be no different than the reaction (ischemia) you'd expect from blockage, like a stroke or heart attack. But this kind of hypoperfusion changes from minute to minute and hour to hour, depending on changes in toxin-effects, TNF levels and adhesin levels.

Chronic Lyme patients often are shown to have hypoperfusion of larger vessels in areas of the brain; these findings are usually gleaned during special tests such as the SPECT Scan. But the CS test allows observers to spot early changes in the smallest blood vessels, the capillaries . . . which makes FACT a more refined physiologic test than the SPECT Scan. In Lyme, the first action is in the capillaries, not the larger vessels. Lyme disease potentially causes changes in every organ system of the body.

To know Lyme is to know how little we know about medicine!

What hasn't been understood until now is that variable hypoperfusion also accounts for changes in the variable *symptoms* of chronic patients from minute to minute and hour to hour.

The connection between hypoperfusion and the Herx stood out clearly for me one recent afternoon, after I received a visit from Tom Judy, an executive for Stereo Optical Company. Judy was interested in looking at my CS data, and had made a special trip from Chicago to Pocomoke in order to do so.

After Judy examined the data I'd been gathering from my neurotoxin patients—but *before* we talked about my ideas regarding hypoperfusion—he declared that he'd "never seen CS numbers like those before!" He said he could hardly believe the test scores I had assembled. But when I showed him the confirmatory data, he was convinced. Then he added a few lines that solidified my developing theories:

"Those CS deficits you're finding in patients must be the result of hypoperfusion in the optic nerve head. They can *only* be caused by hypoperfusion. That's a problem resulting from reduced blood flow in the nerve, and we use CS to help diagnose glaucoma. In that condition, the extra pressure in the front part of the eye squeezes the blood vessels in the optic nerve, so blood does not flow normally.

"The result is reduced blood flow—which, if it were permanent, really, is no different than we see after a stroke. But the change you are showing occurs from minute to minute and hour to hour!"

Judy then pointed out that if you could "look directly at the optic nerve head, and show reduced flow in capillaries, then your model would make even more sense."

He had a good point. Listening to him, I also realized that I could completely confirm my model by accomplishing three key things:

- First, show how a rise in mRNA (specifically for TNF) preceded the reduced flow in the nerve head;
- Second, show that the subsequent rise in TNF coincided with the development of hypoperfusion in the nerve head and the

CS deficit;

*   Third, correlate improvements in CS Test scores with treatment and correction of hypoperfusion, reduced TNF and TNF mRNA.

One way to show the presence of hypoperfusion—the TNF Effect—in the optic nerve head would be with the use of a Heidelberg Retinal Tomogram Flow Meter (HRF), a tool capable of observing capillary flow. But these highly specialized devices aren't found in many ophthalmology offices. You won't find one at the Duke University Eye Center, for example, nor will you find more than a few of them on the East Coast.

At last count, there were only about 50 of these machines at work in the world, and for good reason, since they cost almost $100,000 each. Make no mistake, however: this machine has the technical ability to produce information that would convince even the most skeptical scientist of the vascular link to the biochemical reality that lies behind chronic, neurotoxin-mediated illness.

No, I didn't have $100,000 in spare change to buy an elegant diagnostic device such as the HRF. On the other hand, it was also true that the Heidelberg Company didn't realize the fantastic power of their new diagnostic tool. Someone needed to remind them that ophthalmologists all across American were buying the less expensive Heidelberg laser Doppler for diagnosis of glaucoma and cataracts (See Chapter Six: "Contrast Sensitivity.")

Tom Judy saw the point immediately and said he'd call Heidelberg for me to set up a meeting with Dr. Gerhard Zinser, President of Heidelberg Engineering. Scheduled for May 1, 2000, our discussion session would take place at the Association for Research and Vision in Ophthalmology (ARVO) convention in Fort Lauderdale, Florida.

It was to be a terrific meeting. Dr. Zinser instantly grasped the concepts of neurotoxin-mediated illness, cytokine response and hypoperfusion of the *lamina propria* (cells contained in a key layer of the optic nerve head). Even better, the Heidelberg engineer saw in a flash that my research, when published, would require other investigators to use his machine in order to study these problems further.

The result was that I ended up in possession of one of the world's most sophisticated ophthalmologic devices. After having it installed in my office, I received special training from an international retinal specialist Dr. Dirk-Uwe Bartsch, courtesy of Heidelberg. And the preliminary findings were nothing less than spectacular: this powerful tool made it crystal-clear that the deficit in blood flow is obvious. HRF was a direct indicator.

Just imagine what will happen in the future, when the trial lawyers begin to realize that an injury case can be adjudicated not on the basis of pain symptoms or immobility, following an accident—but by simply presenting their evidence in the form of physiologic correlates demonstrating how the client is suffering from a chronic, neurotoxin-mediated illness (caused by an *endogenous* toxin, no less)! (See Chapter 24.)

"Ladies and gentlemen of the jury . . . we ask you to simply look at the results of this 10-minute laser doppler ophthalmology exam, in order to see for yourselves the extent of the plaintiff's injuries!"

Is there any doubt that the HRF is going to have a major impact not only on chronic illness-sufferers—but also on liability lawsuits involving chronic pain, soft tissue injury and other forms of trauma caused by accidents?

Measuring blood flow is an important diagnostic tool, but it's not the only way to tell if a patient is suffering from a toxin-linked illness. Another effective approach is to measure the presence of the bacterium . . . either by pinpointing the presence of toxin-triggered TNF, or by analyzing the amplification of mRNA by the polymerase chain reaction (PCR). Invented in 1983, this Thomas Kuhn-like "leap" (See Chapter 22) in diagnostic technology resulted in the development of a device that would promote biomedical research by generating unlimited copies of DNA for study and manipulation. What better way to pin down the presence—or absence—of a spirochete than by assaying the local DNA?

Caring physicians (institutional or otherwise) who struggle to help Lyme patients would love nothing more than being able to determine—*conclusively*—when and if a patient should continue to receive antibiotic treatment, based on clearcut evidence of ongoing, active infection. No practitioner wants to treat patients needlessly with these powerful IV medications (or with unproven, homeopathic remedies, for that matter). Wouldn't it be nice to have diagnostic certainty in these cases . . . and to know for sure when the spirochete DNA is present? PCR gives us the tool to accomplish that very goal—because it can detect spirochete DNA in a blood specimen with unerring accuracy.

Even better, PCR can quickly tell us when a particular gene has been turned on, or transcribed, by detecting the presence of Messenger RNA. Of course, this terrific tool can also identify dinoflagellate DNA in a drop of water or a teaspoon of mud. It can pick up the presence of a mutated enzyme from a toxin-forming *E. coli* bacteria, or tell the archaeologist if his Inca mummy is genetically related to his Neanderthal mummy.

It can also help you separate the major types of Ehrlichia species, while also identifying the subtypes that cause diseases in dogs or humans.

In addition, many physicians are now diagnosing chronic Lyme disease based on the findings they obtain from PCR.

As always, however, there's a price to be paid for these wondrous, high-tech instruments. For one thing, they're enormously expensive. And the steep price tag on the machine, itself, is only the start of the problem—because after you've paid for the glittering hardware, you'll still need to find funds for lab space, quality controls, maintenance, tech salaries and continuing education.

(After only a few years, however, the "new machine" will be an "old machine," and therefore obsolete!)

That's one problem. Another is that these PCR assays are notorious for giving positive readings long after the organism being tested is dead. Noted authorities such as American Society of

Microbiology lecturer Kathleen Beavis, M.D., and J. Stephen Dumler, M.D., of the Johns Hopkins Microbiology and Pathology Laboratories have frequently warned in the past that PCR analysis is fraught with false positives.

And so once again, even with the use of the most advanced and accurate scientific technology, we find plenty of room for scientific argument. Remember that spirochetes rarely stay in the bloodstream . . . and PCR, like all related blood tests, can't tell us a thing about the Lyme organism that is resting comfortably in a fibroblast or a cartilage cell in a joint.

Fortunately for my patients, however, the diagnostic tool we've used throughout this book—the Contrast Sensitivity test—is far superior to all of these at confirming the presence of toxins in human brain tissue. Why spend $300,000 looking for an expensive diagnosis of Lyme, when you can spend five minutes taking an inexpensive test that has been correlated with the most sophisticated machinery in all of medicine and ophthalmology? The testing device, known as "FACT," costs only $500, and is available from Stereo Optical Company, Inc., of Chicago. (Call 1-800-344-9500.)

This is one of the key "Lessons of the Herx"—the fact that you don't need complicated diagnostic tools in order to confirm the presence of neurotoxic illness, or effectively predict the arrival of the Intensification Reaction that usually sets in when you begin to bind those toxins with CSM and flush them from the bodies of suffering patients.

Another key lesson is the new understanding that careful physicians can block the effects of TNF on de-toxing patients by pre-treating the latter with Enbrel, a soluble receptor (a kind of "micro-sponge," if you will) that reduces the impact of the TNF on the cells it targets. Used strategically, the sponge works effectively to shut down the effects of TNF on cells in blood vessels. Take away TNF, and you take away both the Herx *and* the Intensification Reaction!

Like Diane Stephenson, whom you met earlier, my patient "Jill" (See Chapter 16: "100 Weeks in the Medical Wilderness") somehow found the personal courage to take a CS Test daily for 12 days, even as she endured the worst agonies of a continuing Intensification Reaction. As her daily scores indicated, the alternate surging and ebbing of her symptoms correlated perfectly with the postulated neurochemical shifts along her retina and optic nerve. She needed Enbrel in order to continue her treatment . . . a fact which provided yet another example of this woman's personal courage. To her great credit, she hung on through some very painful symptoms, until the healing could begin.

Jill's case was especially instructive. As her physical symptoms worsened, I realized that all I needed was a laser-imaging that would allow me to show how these effects were occurring in her visual system . . . and thus to demonstrate the efficacy of the CS Test for even the most skeptical observer!

The physical challenge for Jill, of course, was that the TNF sponge speeded up the wave of CS change but didn't change its direction. Her serum levels of TNF had been high to begin with, which meant that as she went into the Intensification, her ordinary dreams were replaced by the horrible, dismembering nightmares that so many Herx veterans have described. (Be ready for that symptom when it arrives—because it's one you won't forget!)

But the good news for Jill—and for millions of neurotoxin-afflicted patients like her—is that we can now blunt the misery caused by the Herx.

Having finally untangled the molecular chemistry by which dislodged toxin particles manipulate the cell's DNA command centers, unleashing the blizzard of painful TNF reactions, I began to pre-treat patients with pioglitazone. This strategy worked effectively to strengthen the patient's PPAR-gamma defenses against the TNF nuclear receptor, as proven recently by physicians in more than 25 states in the U.S. and five foreign countries.

Now I knew that even if I couldn't prevent the Herxheimer, I could at least blunt its aggressive attack with this strategy of pre-treatment. In most cases, I could thus reduce the Herx to a pale shadow of itself. The TNF sponge was an ally of last resort.

As you're about to learn, that's precisely what happened to Diane Stephenson, who is living proof that Herx can be overcome on the long road that leads from the hell of chronic, neurotoxin-mediated illness back to thriving health.

• • •

Coming to "A Different View of the Herx"

When the Herxheimer Intensification Reaction struck Diane Stephenson in February of 2000, she was fully prepared to do battle with the "raging beast."

"I made it through the nightmare," she will tell you today, "because Dr. Shoemaker and I had already worked out our treatment plans long in advance. He prescribed pioglitazone and CSM for me, and he supported me by telling me that the medications manage the misery of the Herx.

"And that's exactly what happened. When the reaction to getting rid of the Lyme toxins arrived, I was prepared—if you can *ever* be prepared for such a thing, for this tornado that comes into your life!"

Although she was still fearful about the days of discomfort that accompany this unpleasant reaction, Diane also felt confident. "I did feel reassured," she said in a recent interview, "because I knew that I would not have to walk through that valley of the dreaded Herxheimer alone. I knew I could stop CSM any time, and that I wouldn't have to go to the point where it was unbearable.

"Anyway, I got started. I took pioglitazone for five days. I ate frequently, and my diet included lots of fresh vegetables, fruit and protein. But I stayed away from starchy foods such as bread, pasta, potatoes and rice, as instructed.

"Then I added CSM to the pioglitazone. And after just two doses of CSM . . . well, I must say I was a little unprepared! I didn't think the reaction would set in that quickly! But that's what happened. The Herx! I felt like I'd just gotten jerked into the dark side. And I was momentarily panic-stricken. And I was frightened that it would go on for days, or maybe even weeks, as it had in the past. I kept thinking about all those terrible days before, when I would lie in bed, too weak to even move.

"Well, I called Dr. Shoemaker, and his first words were: 'Don't panic.'

"He reminded me that he had prepared me for this terrible reaction, with the pioglitazone. And he was right. I endured a few painful hours—but when I woke up the next morning, most of the reaction had subsided. I almost felt like myself again! That raging Intensification beast had been tamed and I was feeling better."

"And things have been getting better ever since. Just yesterday, I went up a flight of steps and I stood at the top and I realized: I wasn't short of breath! I didn't have profound pain! It's like I've got a new baby again, and the baby is called: The Road To Good Health.

"I went through the worst attack of the Herxheimer on February 7th, 2000. (I still refer to it as the 'Herx,' even though I know I should call it the 'Intensification Reaction.') But the next morning I got up and I thought: It's a brand-new day. I feel like I've been half-dead with the flu for 13 years, and now I'm almost afraid to say that it's gone. I am just feeling effervescent about it all. It took 30 days for pioglitazone to keep the Herx away, but finally the reaction stopped and my symptoms disappeared.

"And you know what? I also have a different view of the Herxheimer now! For the first time, I see it as something that is controllable. And I'm just so thankful that Dr. Shoemaker has helped me get through it, so that I can start re-building my life."

chapter 16

Reflection

Jill: 100 Weeks in
The Medical Wilderness.

Long Island, NY –March, 2000

Table I
Age: 33
Occupation: Modern Furniture Design, Marathon Runner
Married 15 Years, Two Children
Disability Since 2/99: Sudden onset of cognitive loss. Had tick bite, 7/98, with intermittent episodes of dissociation, panic, thought disruption, but nothing sustained.

Table II
Symptoms:

Don't feel feet touch the ground when walking	Drop in blood sugar level
Floating, weightlessness	Head reeling
Extreme weakness, especially extremities	Uppity, giddy, zoomy
Can't feel own body	Tension
No weight to body	Unreality feeling
No memory of what I see	Disoriented
Feel like I am on a boat	Weird sensations
Woozy, dizzy	Weird perceptions
Lightheaded, extreme	Feeling like will pass out
Sense of no oxygen, glucose to brain	Endocrine way off
Spaced out, stoned	Forgetting everything
Out of body	So zoomy jumping out of skin
Brain is cross-wired	Have to hold on to walk
Tingling, numbness (non-anatomic distribution)	Sense of body being pulled up
Confusion	Urinary frequency and urgency
Visual hallucinations	Head draining
Panic	Phonophobia
Terror	Light sensitivity
No depth perception	Gapping in and out

Table III		
A Year of Lyme Toxin Hell **Jill's Doctors and Diagnoses in Calendar 1999**		
WHEN	**WHO**	**WHAT IS WRONG**
February	Holistic Center	allergies, stress on immune system
March	Allergist	Lyme, Babesia, allergy to mold
March	Holistic Allergist	Babesia, parasite, malabsorption
April	Private clinic	Entamoeba histolytica, candida, malabsorption
April	Internist	toxic
April	Nutritionist	Lyme disease
April	Neurologist	see a Lyme-literate physician (LLMD)
May	Acupuncturist	procedures
May	LLMD	Lyme and something else unknown
May	Endocrinologist	Rx Lyme and then see
June	LLMD	Lyme, Babesia, Dysbiosis, IV antibiotics
June	Tilt Table Test	low heart rate
July	Hematologist	CD4 Lymphocytotoxicity, unknown cause
July	Candida Expert	intestinal permeability
August	Clinic in Florida	detox with herbs
September	Psychiatrist	no, not crazy
September	Hyperbaric oxygen	dramatic worsening
September–October	Muscle Therapist	massage therapy
November	Hematology	Lymphopenia (Total WBC Count 1.3) Rx Neupogen

Table III continued . . .		
WHEN	**WHO**	**WHAT IS WRONG**
November	Hospital	Gram negative rod sepsis
November	Infectious Disease	Referred to Super-Specialist
November	ID/Hematology	auto immune disease, perhaps lupus
November	rheumatologist	not lupus, neurometric EEG
December	Epilepsy expert	not seizure, abnormal background, activity on EEG
December	Gastroenterologist	needs small bowel biopsy, too weak
December	Hematologist	drug toxic, parasites
December–March, 2000	Chiropractor/ naturopath	Lyme, Babesia, parasites, Allergy, stressed immune Syst. And opinion on IV Rocephin "Stay Away From Doctors!"
March–April, 2000	RCS	1. Malabsorption from tropical sprue acquired in Iran, 1979; 2. Negative nitrogen balance from protein-deficient diet; 3. Arsenic poisoning from one of many supplements, unknown which; 4. Neurotoxin illness; 5. Lymphocyte toxicity, unknown cause.

Table III continued . . .
Rx: Pioglitazone, CSM, Enbrel, B12, 1cc IM monthly, added protein in diet, stop supplements, stop confounding variables, stop antibiotics when LLMD agrees, manage intensification.
Result: Lean body mass increased 6 pounds, macrocytosis disappeared, lymphocytes no change. 4/28 had no symptoms, on 5/8/00 walked 5 miles, vision and thought clear, FACT almost normal. Still facing a few rough spots but life is returning to normal. Thanks.

Table IV			
WHEN	**MEDS**	**DIAGNOSIS**	
April	Nystatin	yeast	"bad reaction"
April	Biaxin	Lyme	nothing
April	Rocephin	Lyme	terrible Herxheimer for 3 weeks; In 7 weeks, relapse, worse
June	Diflucan	yeast	from Rocephin, no help
July	Valtrex	stealth virus	nothing
July	Claritin	allergies	hyper, speedy
July	Flagyl	Lyme/ entamoeba	terrible Herxheimer
July–October	Mepron & Zithromax	Babesia	better after 3 months
September	Hyperbaric chamber	Lyme	SLAMMED!
October	Klonopin	reduced blood flow to brain	terrible
November	Neupogen	WBC crash to 1.3	too late
November	Cipro IV	gram negative rod sepsis	almost killed me

Table IV continued . . .			
WHEN	**MEDS**	**DIAGNOSIS**	
November	Furazone	Giardia	nothing
November	Flagyl	Giardia	terrible
November	Mepron	Babesia	slight better
December	Thiobendazole	Giardia	improved
January 2000	NTZ	Giardia	terrible cognitive decline
February	Humitin	Giardia, entamoeba	weak, out of it, allergic reaction
February	Zithromax	Babesia	no help
March	Bicillin IM injections	Lyme	the final downfall
March	Xanax	counteract unbalanced Lyme chemistry	"Like a seizure"
March–May	Actos/CSM	protocol modified	intensification

From the Physician's Notebook . . .
Some Final Thoughts on the Treatment of Jill

How long will Jill's improvement last? I don't know. Her last two years have literally been a nightmare. Like most chronic Lyme patients for whom the brain is the target organ, her changes in cognition, sensation, position sense, smell, taste, consciousness and dreams varies from hour to hour.

In these cases, the patient's ability to think depends on what part of the brain isn't receiving blood [perfusion] properly. The wave of reduction in Contrast Sensitivity seen in Jill, as she tested herself daily in Pocomoke, provides indirect evidence that the deficits in perfusion suspected by Tom Judy and correlated with TNF-alpha levels truly do begin in the neurons that serve high-frequency, low-contrast function and then progress to low-frequency, high-contrast function. The improvement in CS seen in Jill mirrors the improvement of hundreds of patients with chronic, neurotoxin-mediated illnesses.

Her symptoms persisted at a high level despite reasonable efforts by reasonable health care providers using reasonable medications. The diversity of symptoms Jill recited continuously resulted in a number of reviewers of this account to discount her illness as purely psychiatric. In the sense that psychiatric symptoms may result from electrical and metabolic insults to the brain, Jill did have a psychiatric disorder, with a Lyme toxin as the ultimate cause.

Jill didn't list the number of physicians who listened to her briefly, then prescribed some psychoactive medication (Diane Stephenson has a drawer full of unfilled prescriptions) for antidepressants and anti-anxiety agents.

Part of Jill's problem was the sheer number of different opinions, prescriptions and therapies, foods and health substances she received, and the way she agreed to follow all of these recommendations without questioning purity or safety. Example: One of the health care providers who suggested a home compounded fish oil supplement may have been unknowingly poisoning her with arsenic. In addition, some of her Herxheimer reactions could have been avoided, if only her health care providers had known what we now know. Hopefully, physicians will order TNF-alpha levels before giving patients HBO therapy, Klonopin, or metronidazole, for example, as those treatments can cause terrible reactions in high TNF-alpha patients.

Jill had come to Pocomoke to have me "on call, on site," as she started her CSM therapy. She gradually worked her pioglitazone dose up to therapeutic levels before coming in for her initial CSM visit. At 90 pounds, weakened by her illness and with a history of "crashing" blood sugar, she was nervous about taking the pioglitazone pretreatment but her fears turned out to be just that—fear and not reality. If anyone were going to get "whapped" by CSM, it was Jill.

She did well, surviving the intensification brought on by the

284 Jill: 100 Weeks In

TNF storm. Even now when I think about her case, I see the image of the wind blowing through our ornamental pear trees, creating a blizzard of pear flower petals on the day her intensification reaction began.

The millions of petals, all blown off the tree at once by an outside force, were a clear metaphor for the TNF-alpha storm. Later, when more information about TNF comes from the research labs, I might look at my current model of the mechanism of intensification and the Herxheimer and smile at how "primitive" the idea was, but for now it makes sense.

For anyone who has symptoms like Jill's or who might not have the strength to keep fighting for his health, take heart. At the end of the intensification, there is a soft landing. Never assume the ravages of the terrible illness that is chronic Lyme will be permanent. Find courage from Jill's story.

Never give up!

Update from Diane Stephenson, March 14, 2000

Medina, OH –April, 2000

Oh, I am feeling *so* much better! Today I wanted to kind of reflect on some of the many facets of being ill, and to talk about how wonderful it is to start getting better. Basically, I'm a private person, but I'm willing to talk about these things because I know there are many people who could benefit from hearing about my struggle and about the outcome.

Right now, I'm jubilant. I'm elated. I'm overwhelmingly happy. Why? Because inside, there is only me now. There are no more of the demons, no alien micro-beings, and no invading enemy made of that foreign DNA which I now have come to know as "the neurotoxins." And all of this is because I followed Dr. Shoe-maker's cholestyramine/pioglitazone protocol.

I kind of think of my longstanding illness of 13 years as robbing me of all joy, all happiness, and cruelly and relentlessly kind of dictating every aspect of my life—all of my activities, including my activities of rest, diet, mood, social interactions and yes, even those of intimacy. My chronic neurotoxic disease limited my pleasure, my satisfaction derived from the fulfillment of even the most basic human needs.

Basically, in my mind, I felt like I was on Death Row, in solitary confinement. A place where you're tortured daily. And I had very little hope of escape from the imprisonment of my chronic, neurotoxin-mediated illness. And I was actually frightened to think of my bleak future.

I felt paralyzed. All of my dreams, all of my hopes and aspirations, all of my goals were paralyzed by the icy realization that my plight was to remain trapped and confined to this toxic-diseased body. And basically I thought of my body as my prison and my torturer. Considering all the betrayals and disappointments and heart-breaking disillusionments that can occur in life, basically it was my own state of health that became my biggest heartbreak.

It created a profound sense of loss. Loss of one's self, loss of identity. Since I'd been ill, I was no longer the person I knew, or even recognized. I became someone I really didn't like. Kind of like a shadow, or a hologram. I had no true life, no true emotions. They were all kind of funneled through a grid. I think of it as "The Lyme Disease Grid."

When I was sick, food did not taste the same. It had a metallic taste. And rest was difficult to obtain. I was exhausted after eight hours of sleep, and I awoke in pain, with stiffness and a profound headache. The enemy—the neurotoxins—invaded my mind and controlled my dreams, producing fitful nightmares.

And this next part is difficult to mention, but perhaps other people who have suffered will relate. Sexually, I felt like a robot. I was like that hologram I referred to before, going through the motions. And I could only remember the passions that I once possessed. However, I did not love my husband any less. Indeed, because of my illness and his strength and his encouragement and his help through it, I loved him more.

But I believe the invasion of my body was complete. It was a total overtaking of all functioning. Mentally, physically and sexually. I do remember before my illness, I had a healthy desire for sex. I remember the joy and that wonderful warm feeling of loving and being loved. That sense of oneness with my husband of 33 years. But in my diseased neurotoxic state, I lost touch with my own sexuality. It became somewhat unreal, like I was reading the words in a book. In other words, sex was not the same, and intimacy became synonymous with pain. Pain in my muscles and my joints, and my stomach was terribly sensitive, and I alternated between feeling nauseous and intestinal cramping. I felt like I could not breathe because the muscles between my ribs were so weak.

I felt suffocated, and like every rib in my body was going to break, and that my stomach was actually going to burst up into my chest and squish my heart. My neck was painful and stiff I just could not get comfortable. And my entire concentration was on that pain. I did not feel that I was alone, but I know that the pain and the sickness and the sadness and the lost joy and the burden of hopelessness were all right there with me.

But now I'm well. And I cry tears at times, times of pure excitement and expectation in my life, without that monstrous and cruel tormentor. That neurotoxic disease is gone. And left behind is the real me. I'm a very private person and to tell this story is difficult, but I think the world needs to know that many of us suffer silently with chronic disease robbing us of all joy.

But now, having said that, I'm just beginning to celebrate the fact that I've received a full pardon—one that I desperately sought for 13 years. And right now, I feel like I'm standing in full view of the opening gate of my prison. Very slowly it is opening, and what I see is this bright sunlight. Glorious, healthy sunlight. And I'm traveling this pathway toward a new-found freedom, which I see as releasing the bondage, loosening the chains of paralysis and restoring or illuminating my life's light.

But one man has stepped forward. He stepped out of the long marching-line of tin soldier-doctors that indoctrinated and brainwashed legions of medically trained personnel who are satisfied to practice medicine with a narrow-minded creed. They say: "Accept the status quo; don't make waves. It's business as usual. Just treat the symptoms, and don't go beyond the well-trod path of expectable and usual treatment."

And I felt that my cries for help fell on deaf ears. That same professional group, the doctors of the status quo, called back in unison: "We can't hear you." And they all said, "Here, have an antidepressant. Have a painkiller. Have a mood elevator or a sedative."

And what I really wanted was validation. Not a cover-up, and not a Band Aid. Not a drug to place me in a foggy, semi-comatose mental state, which would then leave me open to hear the ridicule of my sorry state—prescription drug addiction! But that didn't happen in my case; I have never taken these drugs.

But I felt that that was their motive. I just wanted someone to hear me. I was sick. I was in that bottomless pit, like hell on earth, and crying out to God to send me someone. And only one man seemed to hear my cries for help. And what a paradox for me. Because help came in the form of a man in that same professional group that I had come to distrust and yes, even secretly despise. He was a medical doctor, no less, and a man. I'd gone through 30 doctors without success, and here was another one, but I now can experience life in all areas, with joy and with pleasure and without pain, as I did 13 years ago, before this nightmare of chronic illness began.

I've been awakened like Snow White from a terrible, fitful sleep. And to me it's a new dawn of wellness and well-being. And my rescuing prince came in the form of a Family Practice doctor who lives hundreds of miles away from me in Pocomoke, Maryland. I feel that I'll be eternally grateful and I know that the love of my life—my best friend and my husband—is grateful that the woman that he fell in love with 33 years ago and married is back as she once was.

Things are definitely getting back to normal. But illness is a part of life, and we have to talk about it.

I think that recovery from a long-term illlness is very much like the peeling away, layer by layer, of a very large onion. And through the years of untreated disease, these toxins continued to form and circulate and re-circulate. And in my case, the damage caused by the neurotoxins over the years took its toll. For me personally, I had to make a concerted effort every day to exercise, to walk, to eat properly, take vitamins.

This part is really emotional for me. I used to have conversations with my husband quite frequently about retirement. He's going to be 62 this year and it's very strong on his mind. And I would often discuss the idea of remarriage with him, telling him that he should remarry after I was no longer in the picture. He should not be alone for his golden years. And I couldn't guarantee that I would be here in five or ten or fifteen years. And I didn't want him to be lonely or sad, when I didn't make it, or found myself in an extended care facility.

The other thing is that we have a very close relationship with our grandchildren. We're very active with them. And I didn't want them to see their grandfather in any other state than what he normally is. But my husband never gave up on me in all these 13 years. He always told me that we would always be together, no matter what. And in my book, he is truly a saint. I think there should be a chapter dedicated to these spouses and the loved ones who live with a person with a chronic illness.

Sure, the cholestyramine/pioglitazone protocol is the treatment of choice and the right treatment. But I must retrain all of my weak muscles and joints to work again up to par. And I think getting well after a long, devastating neurotoxic disease is a battle. And I must be an active participant.

I think when we are sick, we come to expect that others will take care of us. We expect the medical professionals to do the diagnosing and prescribing, and eventually the healing of our disease state. But having dealt with this illness for 13 years, I have found that I personally needed to become an active participant in my quest for good health. I needed to personally research, and read, join support groups and interact with others fighting this same disease.

I feel like it's a battle. And I think my battle tactics were very much like those employed by our own armed forces. Learn as much as you can about the enemy! And I needed to form an alliance with the people that were on my side—hopefully, medical professionals, fellow-disease sufferers, support groups, my family and my friends. And I needed to reinforce myself with persons who had intelligent game-plans.

I needed to surround myself with positive people. I found that this was a battle I could not fight alone. I felt like I was wounded, weak and frightened. And I was not so different from a young, 19-year-old G.I. going into battle for the first time. But I was greatly comforted by the thought that through my own spiritual meditation, I acquired a sense that God was with me at all times through this battle.

But what I really needed, in a more pragmatic way, I needed a bright, talented and unconventional leader to issue the right orders. Someone of strong, impeccable character, who possessed a sense of fairness and a willingness to take chances—to step out into the line of fire, to exhibit the best judgment during this biological warfare raging within my body.

He fought, though, unconventionally. New tactics! The cholestyramine/pioglitazone protocol. And what he endured for that was ridicule, criticism, mockery from his peers, his fellow-physicians.

What really makes a successful leader? Someone who knows what must be done, and is strong enough to accept that assignment, and with the intelligence to develop a successful plan, along with the courage to implement it. And then the commitment to carry on the fight to the end, to victory.

And at the same time, he must be able to withstand the scorn of those who are either envious, or lack the vision.

I think Dr. Shoemaker came along when I suffered most from battle fatigue. And I felt at that time that I was too weak. I almost felt like God had to carry me through this time. I could no longer trudge along as the foot soldier.

But I believe the battle for me has now ended. And it's been a long, bitter fight. But we have the victory and it is time to celebrate. And I'm going to call it "VL Day"—Victory over Lyme! And now we must spread the news. Victory is at hand for all the battlefronts. The ultimate weapon was not the A-bomb, like in World War Two; it was the cholestyramine/pioglitazone protocol. A few diehards may refuse to believe the outcome and that it's actually over . . . but seeing is believing and the world will come to know the truth, eventually.

You know, I just saw a documentary on Louis Pasteur, and I was struck by the way that most of the other doctors of that era laughed at him. They laughed because he said: "Doctors should wash their hands before surgery!"

Well, who had the last laugh?

But I hope God will inspire more doctors to be like Dr. Shoemaker. I have so much gratitude for him, but I have anger, too. I think my suffering and that of many others continues because narrow-minded and arrogant and ill-informed doctors follow tactics that plainly don't work. We need more doctors who are innovative and willing to step out of that usual rank and file, and committed to treating people, not the symptoms.

They should also be willing to fight for the patient, and to understand that ill person sitting in the office, before they automatically dismiss them or tune them out and abruptly offer them a drug to dull the pain and shut them up, while their disease rages on. Or they shuffle the patient from one so-called "specialist" to another. I went to a neurologist, a cardiologist, a rheumatologist, a psychiatrist and a psychologist. And where does the buck stop?

As a patient, I personally began to feel rejected, abandoned, confused, exhausted. And still the disease raged on. We need patient advocates. We need more education, more practical information. And to tell you the honest truth, that is why I'm talking to you now! But we need more information. We need to have reform in the medical school curriculum. You know, the word "doctor" is almost synonymous with deity. If the doctor says it, it must be gospel.

I think we need to figure out how we can find those few genuine doctors who entered the profession—novel idea here —to actually heal the sick, and to do no harm. And it has been my personal experience that much harm has been done to me and my family by those persons who profess to follow the Hippocratic oath.

Escape from Naushon Island

Naushon Island, MA –1880 to 1970

After more than five years of intense research into the causes of chronic, neurotoxin-mediated illness, I'm still amazed by the way I keep finding clues to the puzzle in my daily life as a practicing family doc.

Take my recent conversation with Steve Merson, for example.

An accomplished writer and a good friend, the talented Mr. Merson was kind enough to show me a draft of his latest screenplay: *Vector.*

Merson hopes that his script will eventually provide the basis for a new television series. Part-sci fi and part character drama, *Vector* tells the compelling story of several characters whose struggle to survive a nuclear catastrophe will ultimately decide the fate of human beings from Alaska to Pocomoke.

In Merson's sample episode, a few gutsy characters manage to survive a massive atomic conflagration triggered by a Middle Eastern terrorist group.

Alone and desperate, the tiny band of *Homo sapiens* seeks to escape the horrors of atomic devastation by hunkering down on an isolated Aleutian island—a remote flyspeck where the prevailing wind patterns won't allow deadly nuclear fallout.

Having gained a foothold on the island, the survivors hang on for dear life. Fortunately, they know they can take advantage of the richness and diversity of the local "food web" that surrounds them. While they feed on island crustaceans and sea mammals, they try to improve their situation by studying the predator-prey ecology to which they now belong. When time permits, they also dream of "repopulating" the world from their own tiny gene pool.

Sounds like a real thriller, doesn't it?

But I did find a minor flaw. "Steve," I told my writer-pal, "that last part sounds a little unrealistic. They can't repopulate the world—the gene pool is too small!

"Before long, their offspring will start coming down with genetic diseases from inbreeding . . . not to mention the mutations that will almost certainly accompany the radiation. And that wind from the West is *sure* to drop fallout on them, sooner or later.

"Besides . . . if they're going to survive, they'll have to live off their food sources without killing them. Of course, if they *could* pull it off, they might gain a significant selective advantage for their descendants!"

Steve nodded, then cheerfully agreed to "think about a few editing changes" in the days ahead. But before we could get down to chewing on the specifics, I found myself thanking him for presenting me with an unexpected gift.

Without knowing it, Merson had just handed me a biological model—a paradigm that would help me understand (and later explain) just how the epidemic of Lyme disease exploded across the United States, starting way back in the 1970s. . . .

Before enjoying Steve's electronic opus, I'd spent a lot of time wrestling with a scholarly review article, "Ecology of *Ixodes dammini-Borne Human Babesiosis and Lyme Disease*" (Annual Review of Entomology, 1985, 30: 439–60.) That provocative and challenging article had been composed as part of a Harvard Public Health and Tropical Medicine team effort led by Dr. Andrew Spielman.

As the Annual Review article pointed out, the Harvard team had identified the white-footed mouse as the preferred host for the immature (larva and nymph stage) *ixodes* tick . . . although the mature ticks seemed to prefer white-tailed deer.

The Spielman team went on to describe how some other species also served as unwilling tick-carriers, and then listed raccoons, opossums, foxes, horses and domesticated dogs (but *not* rabbits) among these species.

Next the Review article argued that the distribution of reported Lyme cases appeared to closely match the expansion of the country's deer population, when millions of Americans migrated from cities to more remote pasture lands and forests in recent decades.

I found the demographics utterly fascinating. As housing tracts increasingly sprouted from farmland, the new residents were creating a marvelous habitat for deer. What happened was that every new housing lot produced a "forest edge" of shrubs, small trees and flower gardens . . . a vegetative cornucopia ("Hey, that doe just ate all the tips off my azaleas!") that soon brought the adult *ixodes* to every backyard in America.

On a recent plane ride from Baltimore to Maryland's rural Eastern Shore, I got an eagle's view of just how these new Lyme demographics actually work. As the sun rose over the gun metal-blue of the Chesapeake, my turbo-prop zoomed above sleeping developments and tract houses adjacent to the urban airport. These new human habitations were honeycombed with sleek cul-de-sacs, from which peeked brand-new houses and the inevitable three-quarter-inch saplings that accompany them. But the housing mix also included more mature plantings and also some older homes separated from the Interstate by mature stands of hardwoods and loblolly pines.

Looking down on all this development from 3,000 feet, I was enthralled by the sight of four separate herds of deer. Each group contained eight to ten animals . . . and all of them were browsing contentedly alongside a ballfield at the edge of a thick forest.

Although very few of these newly transplanted homeowners realized it, the new plantings that supported the white-tailed deer would also be supporting an ever increasing horde of white-footed mice, in which every Mommy Mouse delivered up to ten new litters (eight babies in each) per calendar year.

As Spielman carefully noted, the late 1880s had witnessed a huge decline in the U.S. deer population—to the point that most herds were wiped out. With the advent of the wood-burning locomotive, the great forests of the Northeast nearly vanished as well. Such fashionable neighborhoods as "Millionaires Row" in Williamsport, Pa., featured beautiful Victorian homes built on the money generated by logging primeval hemlock forests. After the trees were gone, however, the town slid into economic decline.

So what happened to the deer and mouse populations that had once thrived in these burgeoning woodlands? Spielman quotes several wildlife experts of that era: "Deer were so scarce that just sighting the tracks of one made headlines in local newspapers."

Nor is he exaggerating. According to several researchers, the entire State of New Jersey hosted fewer than 200 deer by the turn of the century. Similar losses had occurred in Massachusetts, New Hampshire and Vermont . . . while the threatened animals actually became extinct in Indiana, until repopulation finally began there in the mid-1930s. (By 1983, Indiana's deer population had soared to more than 100,000.)

For reasons that I'll explain in a moment, however, the tiny enclave of Naushon Island remained well populated with deer (and ticks) throughout the period of national decline. Spielman documents the fact convincingly: "The only site in which *I. dammini* was known to be abundant before 1960 was Naushon Island."

In order to understand the dynamics at work in this isolated ecosystem, we must picture a small island—one of several that flank Cape Cod—teeming with deer, mice, ticks and Lyme spirochetes, along with the latter's near-cousins, the Babesia parasites, or "piroplasms."

Such an ecosystem works very well—as long as the disease producers don't kill the ticks, and the ticks don't kill the mice or deer. Under those conditions, the limited gene pool cycle can proceed without disruption. Except for the appearance of an occasionally different blood-meal source for the ticks (in the form of a human hunter), the biological balance of power on Naushon remained remarkably stable. The deer converted their antibody status, but didn't seem to be affected by Lyme (unlike people, horses, and dogs).

Do deer contract illness from Babesia the way people do? Apparently not!

Next question: How would the disease be transported off the island? Answer: The transmission would have to occur via birds, or perhaps with deer swimming to the mainland. And what about the hunter with his tick-infested trophy buck stretched out in the back of the Chevy pickup?

A mystery! But logic suggests that there were probably similar pockets of deer—and Lyme—scattered throughout the country. Perhaps one of them was located near Lyme, Conn., back in 1975, when Dr. Allan Steere first described the disease as a clinical entity. By then, of course, the characteristic Lyme rash—*erythema chronicum migrans*—had already been formally identified in Wisconsin (1970) and anecdotally reported in Butte County, Calif.

But perhaps Lyme had *also* affected the deer on Naushon Island, killing off those which contracted the disease? Any deer from this limited gene pool would be resistant to the spirochete . . . so that when the Naushon deer eventually repopulated the Northeast, the stage was set for the modern epidemic of Lyme disease, with non-resident deer as hosts.

Babesia was spreading from its relic population on Naushon, though more slowly. Remembering Theobald Smith's landmark research on cattle, I couldn't help wondering: was the reduced rate of spread of Babesia partly due to the harm that it caused its host?

After all, killing a host (or a food source, for that matter) amounted to nothing less than a biological dead end . . . whereas, impairing a host while still keeping it alive usually served as an effective evolutionary survival tool.

As I looked back on all of these insights about the etiology of Lyme and other chronic, neurotoxin-linked illnesses, I found myself breaking into a round of spontaneous applause for *Vector* and its creator.

My Maryland buddy had given me the model for understanding a whole new family of diseases! Still, I do wonder how —and why—he chose that particular epidemiological term as the title for his new show. Are *people*, themselves, perhaps vectors for some unknown illness?

And here's one last question, while I'm at it.

Why has my own life become so full of puzzles involving people, ticks and Lyme disease that even the simple act of reading a pal's screenplay brings me right back to working on the enigma that is chronic, neurotoxin-mediated illness?

Famous Falsehoods

Salisbury, MD –April, 1999

- The River is Safe
- Lyme Disease Gets Better in Three Weeks
- No One Gets Sick from the Land
- This Building Isn't Sick

*SICK BUILDING, SICK BUREAUCRACY
LEAVE WORKERS FEELING QUITE ILL*

Office Staffers Victimized by "Appearance of Good Science"

It's a proven fact that all fungi—including those which make toxins—need a favorable habitat.

If a *penicillium* species or a *cladosporium* species or a *stachybotrys* fungus is given a bit of cellulose to digest, along with enough darkness, heat and moisture, it will grow successfully.

And if the creature's habitat is located behind a sheet of plywood paneling, or maybe behind some ceiling tiles under a leaky roof, the people on the other side of the paneling or ceiling tiles (or maybe above a moisture-soaked carpet) are at risk. These unfortunates are going to be breathing fungal spores and toxins every time a door opens or the AC comes on. That's because the HVAC return exerts a "negative pressure," sucking fungal toxins out through cracks, splits and gaps into the building's air.

It's also true that some fungi are quite capable of growing on sheet metal in building ductwork, just like those extraordinary epiphyte plants that grow in the Amazon Rain Forest. Why not? Everything the toxin-forming fungus needs in order to survive and thrive is brought to it by the wind! Just turn on the AC on a hot day, and prepare for the worst. Remember that fungus doesn't need much water or organic matter to get caught by the fungal colony that disrupts the flow of air in the duct. Like a small snag on a river that catches and holds mini-flotsam fast, the fungus can count on having its nutrition and water delivered continuously.

The Sheriff's Office in Wicomico County provides a dramatic example of how to construct a sick building. When the sheriff's employees started complaining that they were getting sick on the job back in 1998, the county bureaucracy immediately resorted to the "politics of denial." The result was a depressingly familiar scenario . . . a series of false statements and bureaucratic evasions in which the ruling strategy, the Appearance of Good Science, allowed public officials to avoid admitting that this building was a house of poison.

As it turned out, however, the father of one of my pediatric patients is a deputy sheriff. I saw him frequently. Fortunately, he didn't present with any neurotoxic symptoms, himself, and his FACT was normal. But he knew all about the problem with the building, and he told me that many of his co-workers were frequently sick. My patient's father didn't have to enter the building often, but he'd spent enough time with the sheriff's staffers to be able to paint a convincing picture of windows that leaked, carpets that stayed wet and ceiling tiles that sometimes dripped for days after a rain.

"You should go see the place, Doc. Some of my friends are real sick, and nobody's paying attention."

Where had I heard those words before? *Ah, yes: Pfiesteria!* I hadn't gone looking for that battle, either. It had found me, soon after I began diagnosing patients who were sick from the toxins produced by the one-celled dinoflagellate that had invaded our coastal waters back in 1997.

The *Pfiesteria* controversy had taught me a great deal about the ways in which government bureaucracies deliberately distort public health issues in order to avoid "upsetting" powerful business figures and powerful politicians. But the struggle to sound the public health alert over *Pfiesteria* had also taught me the importance of "staying the course" in the face of attempts to discredit my accurate diagnosis.

And now I had no intention of "blowing off" the threat from Sick Building Syndrome at the local sheriff's office.

After reading the headline in that day's Salisbury Daily Times ("SHERIFF OPENS INVESTIGATION OF SICK BUILDING"), I telephoned our top law enforcement officer, but caught him in a meeting.

"But it's important!" I told the receptionist who was answering the phones that day. "I'm calling about Sick Building Syndrome. My test can diagnose it and a medicine can treat it."

"I'll put you through, sir."

I told Sheriff Hunter Nelms about FACT, Contrast Sensitivity (CS) and neurotoxin symptoms, then warned him: "Sensitivity to bright light is one of the most common symptoms." The sheriff excused himself for a moment in order to poll his staffers. Were they sensitive to bright light? Five of eight raised their hands.

"Certainly, Sheriff. I'd be glad to make a site visit, no charge."

The Sheriff's Office is a concrete-block building that houses the Wicomico County Communication Center, an investigations unit, a secretarial staff, administrative offices and a processing center. The building is situated at the bottom of a hill, with paved parking areas on three sides. The fourth side adjoins a wetland drained by a broad, slow-moving creek. Because it's full of debris, fallen trees and invasive *phragmites* grasses, there's no way that this overloaded stream can act as reasonable water control structure.

The small entryway into the building features a window that opens onto an enclosed information desk, two steel doors and two chairs. The rug is perpetually wet from water seeping under the main door. Paneling covers the cinder-block walls, and the gaps in the plywood are plainly visible. A hot air duct rattles and groans directly above the information desk and communications center.

"Hello, doc!" Sheriff Nelms greets me cheerfully and takes me to a conference room, where I set up my CS test. One by one, officers and staff members drift in to take it. I don't notice my headache and chest tightness at first . . . but after three hours, my own body is signaling the obvious: this building is contaminated. Incredibly, the employees are all well aware of the wet entry, the leaking windows and the wet carpet. One officer even volunteers to show me the ceiling-side of a ceiling tile. It's black from obvious fungal growth.

In the end, more than 25 employees appear for testing, and 14 of them display the classic CS Deficit from SBS. The symptoms vary from person to person, but all of the abnormal CS patients meet my case definition, which means they're presenting in four of eight neurotoxin symptom categories without other explanation.

Later I review my findings with the sheriff and his two top aides. I point out that a proper building diagnosis must include fungal identification, mycotoxin analysis and negative pressure assays with the HVAC running. Identified patients must be treated, with documentation of clinical cure followed by observation for reacquisition of illness symptoms and CS Deficit upon return to the workplace. Susceptible individuals should be informed of the risks of chronic illness from exposure to the building, even though sick buildings usually do not affect all of their inhabitants. It's also important to explain the benefits of CSM as a preventive therapy to everyone involved.

Finally, good disease management in this scenario means that affected patients should be given the option of transfer. The building itself will require extensive and expensive retrofitting.

Sounds like a pretty good plan, right? Too bad it never went into effect. And what happened instead was painfully predictable. Although the sheriff had done his best to confront the problem directly by discussing it openly with the news media, calling on me for preliminary testing and then updating his supervisors, his recommendations were soon overruled by the county commissioners.

While ignoring my report, which would have required some major fixes, the commissioners agreed to hire a firm to perform a "building analysis." That probe was accomplished in less than four hours—and with the HVAC unit turned off. Abnormal numbers of fungi were found, but not an incredibly high number. No negative pressure assay was attempted. No workers were interviewed, and no inspection of the "backside" of ceiling tiles, paneling or carpet took place. No mycotoxin analysis was ordered.

The report confirmed the evidence of water damage, and that was about it. And the bottom line conclusion? You guessed it. "This building isn't sick!"

Soon after the release of this ersatz analysis, six officers came privately to my office for repeat testing and treatment. All improved with therapy, and all got sick upon returning to the workplace. Each offered a similar, derogatory quote from an administrator about "that meddling Dr. Shoemaker." It's not the first time I've been hit with "hyena attacks" on my credibility. But the officers were fearful for their jobs and they dared not speak out publicly.

The one officer who did break the departmental code of silence was sent to a physician hired by the county. The diagnosis was "depression," of course, and the officer soon found himself undergoing anti-depressant therapy. Then, because of his "mood disorder," this dissident staffer was relieved of his active duty status and forced to turn in his badge and gun.

Depression is one of the best damage-control strategies of all. When in doubt, discredit the patient!

The final tactic in the arsenal of The Appearance of Good Science—burial by endless testing—hasn't been used yet.

All of this struck me as rather pathetic. In other parts of the U.S., affected patients demand that their right to a safe workplace be honored. In those situations, employers must answer to liability lawyers. But not here in Maryland. Not yet.

For the moment, the issue of Sick Building Syndrome at the Sheriff's Office has simply been buried. I've had no further contact with employees or employers. I feel sad that many of the nice people I spoke to will go on believing that they just have allergies or asthma or irritable bowel disease . . . or that they're "just getting older." Still, I wonder what might happen when some of the most affected patients (those who work in the communications unit under that rumbling heating duct) are required to think quickly and clearly in a life-and-death situation.

I just hope the chronic cognitive deficits those patients "don't have" won't injure someone else.

chapter 20

Event

Getting behind
"Sick Building Syndrome"

Wayne, NJ –January, 2000
Snow Hill, MD –May, 2000

Got your pencil? Great. It's time for a ten-second Environmental Health quiz!

To find out how much you know about how ordinary buildings (whether home or office) can make you deathly ill, simply answer the following question.

QUESTION: What do such unusual-sounding names as *Cladosporium, Trichoderma, Chaetominium, Fusarium, Aspergillus, Penicillium* and *Stachybotrys* all have in common?

If you answered "They're all toxin-forming fungi, and right now they're infecting more than 1.3 million American office buildings," go immediately to the head of the Sick Building Syndrome (SBS) class . . . where you'll soon discover that this rapidly accelerating human illness has reached epidemic proportions in recent years.

It's an alarming fact: according to the latest data from the U.S. Occupational Health and Safety Administration (OSHA), more than 20 million American workers—nearly 15 percent of Uncle Sam's entire work force, in fact—may now be affected by toxins from SBS fungi.

Add in the 10 million U.S. school kids (out of a total of about 70 million) who are also exposed daily to building-related fungal toxins, and it's easy to see why the word "epidemic" isn't an exaggeration, when it comes to describing the recent surge in SBS.

One of the most troubling aspects of the SBS phenomenon, of course, is that millions of its victims actually blame their illnesses on something else. Like David Jasinski, whom you're about to meet, many of these sufferers live hellish lives but somehow manage to drag themselves to work each day.

In many ways, the loss of their good health amounts to a tax they pay in order to continue enjoying the so-called "benefits" of employment.

Their determination to hang onto their jobs seems commendable . . . but how did we ever get to the place where *it's okay for the workplace to make you sick?*

All too often, the tragedy of SBS hinges not on the disease —but on the widespread ignorance about its true source. So many of these patients never realize that they've come down with a major illness! Sure, they've been through the required check-ups, and many have spent hours describing their vague, toxin-related symptoms to frowning, and often doubting physicians.

But the answers these patients usually receive (as documented in many chapters of this book) soon begin to sound discouragingly familiar. *You're depressed; I'm going to write you a prescription for Prozac!* (See Chapter 12: "Fad Medicines" For America's "Fad Diseases.") Meanwhile, the few health researchers who have been active in this field can't help wondering: How many cases of SBS are being mis-diagnosed as something else, as these "Chemical Era" diseases become more and more pervasive?

Like depression, which often seems to take the blame for any illness that can't be easily identified, such vague medical conditions as reflux, anxiety, stress, irritable bowel syndrome, chronic sinus congestion and asthma are all on the rise today, even as physicians rarely understand that the symptoms often are actually caused by dozens of different fungal toxins. How many patients with these unproven diagnoses actually have Sick Building Syndrome?

In order to understand the SBS invasion in 2000 America, we must first recognize that the dynamics of this particular group of illnesses (they're all allergic, irritative or toxin-based) were first identified during this author's researches into the human-illness effects of *Pfiesteria* and *cylindrospermopsis*.

While studying these painful ailments in recent years, I gradually assembled some general principles about the relationship between habitat and toxic disease agent. All of these explanatory criteria apply accurately to SBS, as follows:

• Introduce toxins into a poorly flushed area and you can be sure they will *remain* there.

• Insert additional toxins, and the increase will soon be noticeable throughout the habitat.

• Add residential, recreational and occupational exposure to the ever increasing toxin load and you'll eventually witness the emergence of an environmentally acquired, chronic, neurotoxin-mediated illness (especially if the environmental niche —or the organism—is a new one).

Welcome readers, to the ugly and often heartbreaking indoor world of *Desperation Medicine*. The health effects of poorly flushed air in buildings aren't much different from those produced by poorly flushed *water* in estuaries!

Before we take a quick look at the effects of SBS on people, however, we need to remember that the allergic and irritative effects triggered by toxic fungi also occur whenever humans are exposed to certain chemicals. These substances, which you can find listed in any standard toxicology textbook or review article, provide powerful evidence for the fact that we are all now living in the Chemical Era mentioned above—in a world increasingly dominated by high-tech-engineered substances that are altering our environment at an ever accelerating rate.

The following table, courtesy of OSHA, shows how toxic chemicals contribute to some of the major respiratory diseases found in the American workplace, including rhinitis, laryngitis, upper airway congestion and bronchitis.

Chemical Causes

Ethylenediamine in adhesives

Acidic or alkaline cleaning solutions and powders

Ammonia

Hypochlorous acid (bleach)

Volatile organic compounds (ubiquitous, especially in paints, thinners, solvents and industrial cleaning solutions)

Certain pesticides (carbaryl, malathion, parathion, mevinphos, pyrethrum)

Rock and mineral dusts (used in road construction and digging or foundations)

Cement dust

Phosgene (used in chemical manufacturing; notorious history as a WWI warfare agent, "On Flanders Fields")

Acid anhydrides (used in epoxy adhesives and paints, coatings, circuit boards, polymers, polyesters and plasticizers)

Aldehydes

Acrylates (used in paints and adhesives)

Dusts from wood finishes (furniture making and cabinetry)

Ethylenediamine, monoethanolamine, and other amines

Formaldehyde and glutaraldehyde (used in sterilizing medical instruments)

Isocyanates (used in polyurethane paint and in the manufacture of foam for roofing materials)

• • •

Household Chemicals: The Inside Story

Although the effects of industrial and occupational chemicals on human health have been exhaustively studied, only a few investigators have explored the subtler, more insidious impact of household compounds on human health (See Chapter 21: "How Sick Is Your Building?").

Take rugs, for example. These days, most rugs are pre-treated with special coatings designed to help in the removal of stains. But few people realize that small particles of these noxious chemicals are continuously released from rug fibers. Nor are these toxins removed by such traditional housekeeping tools as the vacuum cleaner. Remember: a "clean-looking" carpet can still make you and your loved ones very ill!

As a family practice physician, I treat this kind of environmentally acquired health problem almost daily. And whenever I find myself treating a family which has experienced a sudden onset of wheezing and nasal congestion, one of my first questions is: "When did you get that easy-to-clean carpet?"

All too often, I learn that the new living room centerpiece "was installed only three months ago!"

It's amazing how often patients fail to think about their environment as a possible source of symptoms. Example: I often talk to parents about the need to eliminate dust mites from the bedroom of a child with asthma. Yet I rarely hear those same parents thinking out loud about the possibility of removing the carpet. Don't they realize that bare floors are beautiful and much safer when it comes to protecting indoor air quality?

It's also important to remember that treated wall coverings can also release their isocyanates. Other harmful substances include toxic chemicals from air fresheners (among the worst offenders) added to "climate control" systems, insecticides contained in floor-cleaning solutions and volatile organic compounds (VOCs), used in everything from copy paper and fax machines to spray-on cleaning compounds. (Fumes released from humming computers and plastic phone elements also add to the VOC air-count from hour to hour.)

Another helpful suggestion: it pays to look carefully at the labels of products containing "triclosans." These antibacterial preservatives are often targeted by SBS activists who see them as the major culprits in spreading the disease. Astonishing, isn't it, how these Chemical True Believers are able to pin the blame for an entire health condition on a single malefactor? But don't assume they *aren't* right.

The triclosans *do* rank high on the list of possible triggers for an unusual form of building-related, chronic, neurotoxin-mediated illness known as "Multiple Chemical Sensitivity Syndrome." (More on this subject later.)

Before we blame chemicals and toxins from fungi for all of these problems, don't forget that the "human component" in SBS also looms large. Many buildings today feature elevated levels of carbon dioxide, volatile fatty acids (including the butyric and proprionic versions), along with plenty of methane and hydrogen sulfide. Let's face it: these deleterious substances are generated by human activity and nothing else. Add to the toxin load from these ingredients the toxic chemicals that emerge recycled from sweat, saliva, sputum and vomit, and it's easy to imagine the result.

Ask yourself: How many times have *you* wanted to violate political correctness by telling a co-worker that he or she "makes you sick" because of body odor, stale perfume, bad breath or bowel disturbances? Based on the latest research findings about SBS, your accusatory comment is probably *literally* true!

Another key factor in the misery of SBS is simply money. That's right: the Good Old Buck. There's no getting around the fact that in most situations, the buildings where people work or live are owned by someone else—and frequently by Corporation XYZ. If that building makes somebody sick, who pays? But if the building can't be shown to be unsafe, then there is no illness and no liability. Some of the most outrageous "Appearance of Good Science" statements I've ever heard were directly related to egregious cases of SBS. And indeed, a quick look at the CDC internet website on (See Chapter 25: "Getting Behind The CDC") is enough to illustrate my point!

There's no denying the fact that allegations of "Building-Related Illness" (the very *name* sounds like a whitewash!) are usually—and instantly—met with categorical denials by those liable for the health-effects of the building. In most cases, the cry goes up immediately: "But no one *else* is sick!" to be followed by the choral reply: "Actually, *all* of us are sick!"

In the classic power struggle that follows, workers who don't have much choice other than "Love it or leave it!" usually cave in and wind up paying their debts for their jobs at the "company store" with months or even years of cough, fatigue, headache, abdominal pain, confusion and brain fog. Indeed, the situation in some workplaces has gotten so bad that companies with identified Sick Buildings are simply shutting them down, boarding them up—and moving the entire operation lock-stock-and-barrel to new quarters, for fear of losing their sick employees to healthier competitors!

As an aside, it should also be pointed out that the conversion of agricultural lands to office space frequently puts a different spin on the SBS problem. In that scenario, the government regulators and the corporate bosses attempt to cudgel the farmers into selling off their land for development . . . by blaming them publicly for "ruining the watershed with their crop-related nutrients!" (Later, the new building that the company needs will probably be located on abandoned farmland.)

After years of watching the struggles that explode around Sick Buildings, I can almost predict the wearying course of events. First the affected workers will demand action. Soon thereafter, area building-owners will generate a "consensus statement" that talks solemnly about the "health-safety of the structure in question."

Next the owners will attack the complainers by suggesting that the "building-related" health effects are actually disguised versions of symptoms generated out of the private lives of the employees. "A number of these employees are longtime cigarette smokers—doesn't *that* explain the high rate of bronchitis we're seeing at the Amalgamated Widget Building these days?"

These declarations are invariably followed by such misleading (and usually empty) announcements as: "We've hired a highly regarded indoor air quality engineering firm to study the problem. Let the chips fall where they may!"

(You can be sure that "the chips" will fall just inside the door marked "Corporate Public Relations"—first time and every time.)

What to Do When SBS Strikes?

At first glance, you might think that the simplest and easiest medical strategy for battling SBS would be to require all employees to take the Contrast Sensitivity (CS) test in order to diagnose the illness, and then to treat it with cholestyramine (CSM) where appropriate. But that approach doesn't work in situations—fairly frequent, actually—where patients are developing Multiple Chemical Sensitivity (MCS) from chronic exposure to fungal toxins—and possibly triclosans—in a building that features re-circulated air. By the time that MCS appears in SBS patients, the damage can be irreversible. Diagnose SBS early, don't be put off by the personnel officer or the phony indoor air quality report or the direct attack on you as the cause of your illness.

It's extraordinary, really, how many people think nothing of adding noxious chemicals to our shared environment. Example: I have a sign in my office that reads: "The doctor is allergic to perfume and cologne. Please go home and wash off what you put on this morning." I can usually tell in a flash when a patient has been drenched in Fake Gardenia—because my stomach immediately knots, my head starts aching and my chest feels anvil-heavy. The right to wear perfume in my office stops at my nose.

Although these aromas easily offend me, I don't actually have MCS. True MCS produces far more severe symptoms of much longer duration. Expose a veteran SBS patient with MCS to an air freshener, and she may become violently ill for a week or more. Is it simply out-of-control emotion? Is she neurotic? Psychotic? No . . . because this situation is *real*.

The good news here is that pioglitazone has worked wonders for some MCS patients. They soon discover that the side effects of the medication can be minimized by eating small, frequent meals . . . and by scrupulously avoiding the artificial sweeteners, preservatives and food dyes that form a large part of the typical diet.

After treating them for several years, I can tell you that most MCS patients lead miserable lives. I recall one classic situation, for example, in which a female patient moved deep into the Maine woods in order to get as far away as possible from the chemical-laced urban pollution that had been tormenting her for a decade. Her strategy appeared to work well during the winter, when she occupied a log house with bare floors, curtain-less windows and a vented woodstove.

But spring brought a burst of growth in the nearby balsam firs—and the turpenes released from the trees nearly killed her.

Extraordinarily challenging, research on MCS is still in its infancy. Still, a few courageous individuals agreed to take pioglitazone on an uncontrolled basis in a small clinical trial last winter. Those patients did very well. But will their improved condition last? I have to wonder, since pioglitazone helped, is TNF involved in the biochemistry of MCS? Also: what CS changes are associated with MCS in SBS patients—but not with SBS patients unaffected by MCS? These questions will only be answered by further research.

At this point, I don't have a medical opinion on why MCS is found much more commonly in my patients with SBS than those with other chronic, neurotoxin-mediated illnesses. Still, a few of my Lyme patients did present with MCS, along with a ciguatera patient and two others suffering from *Pfiesteria*. Did they have SBS also? (The problem, of course, is that no conclusions can be drawn, given this small number of patients.)

So much for the MCS component. For the many SBS patients who *don't* come down with that ailment, the conventional wisdom up until now has been that their illness is linked closely to indoor air quality. As a result, terms such as "asthma" and "allergy" have dominated recent review articles about SBS. For the most part, the literature contains no discussion of the impact of multiple *simultaneous* chemical exposures on workers. Clearly, we need to begin applying the "systems approach" to this epidemic!

The systems (or "landscape") approach to understanding ecosystems requires the observer to assess multiple factors simultaneously—whether the ecosystem consists of the attack zones of *Pfiesteria* or the muck farms of Central Florida . . . or even the allegedly SBS-riddled Greenwood Trust Building in Delaware. When buildings are involved, the landscape approach should always include identification of toxic fungi by an accredited mycology lab and also identification of mycotoxins. Nor is such testing very expensive, when compared to the cost of treating illnesses caused by the resident toxin forming fungi.

The landscape approach does raise one troubling question, however. How reliable are these tests—especially if the investigator feels compelled to assay for a broad spectrum of potential toxic agents? Remember that such species as *Stachybotrys* come armed with at least 24 different toxins. Sophisticated testing —such as chromatography—will obviously be required in order to begin building a "library" of chromatographic toxin-patterns . . . and such a library could quickly prove invaluable in pinpointing the presence of suspected fungal toxins. Remembering that the fungicides added to paint might cause mutations, how will the lab boys be able to pick up a new toxin made by a new fungus growing on the new paint?

Routine CS testing will also assist investigators in determining which areas of a building should be targeted for extended analysis. Such tools will help administrators decide when and where to spend money for mycotoxin analysis. Example: If all of the workers in a headquarters building show both physical symptoms of SBS and a CS deficit, it probably won't be necessary to engage in costly assays in order to learn if the offending organism lives in standing water (a toxic algae, for example). Look instead at what's living inside the HVAC—the typical hiding place for toxin-forming fungi.

In situations where the investigator finds a cluster of sick patients, the landscape approach would probably suggest that the best strategy is to earmark time and money for seeking local causes such as leaky ventilation ducts or dripping pipe junctions hidden behind walls.

Always begin your landscape-assessment of a suspected SBS site with the one solid, reliable biomarker that physicians everywhere can trust: the Contrast Sensitivity test. Remember that the "medical detective work" required to sniff out Sick Buildings must always begin with the clear identification of individual sick patients! Sick patients with CS deficits, not smelly basements, remain the marker for Sick Building Syndrome.

David Jasinski:
To Hell and Back at American Cyanamid

David Jasinski, now 51, has never forgotten the moment when his hand stopped working.

It happened two years ago, at a McDonald's restaurant in suburban New Jersey.

Jasinski was eating a cheeseburger and a cardboard container full of piping-hot french fries. But he was eating slowly, without much interest, because he felt so lousy.

In recent months, the International Sales Manager for American Cyanamid had felt increasingly ill. Thin and hollow-eyed, he'd lost more than 30 pounds, while struggling with "a case of killer-flu that just didn't want to give up."

As a top executive at the $3 billion-a-year international manufacturing conglomerate, Jasinski lived with ferocious pressure. While working a "basic 12-hour day" for weeks at a time, he had been told again and again that the company was depending on him to make sure that "the factory lines" were kept busy. His task: sell as much product as humanly possible, to clients scattered all around the globe.

Jasinski spent half his life on the road, it seemed. For more than a decade, he'd been hustling non-stop from Taipei to Jakarta to Beijing in a never-ending quest to unload more and more of the fiber, fertilizers and pesticides and chemical solvents that were the heart of Cyanamid's product line.

After so many years of living out of a suitcase and eating on the run, Jasinski had grown accustomed to "putting up with a bad stomach." Was it his irritable bowel syndrome or his gastroenteritis which caused the brutal gut-cramps that so frequently tortured him? And what about those monster headaches he'd been enduring for the past year or so—those agonizing blasters in which he felt sure that the top of his skull was about explode into a thousand twitching fragments?

Having been diagnosed as suffering from depression, Jasinski was living a miserable life. By 1999, his diet consisted primarily of "Maalox and tranquilizers." Like millions of other Americans in the stressed-out 1990s, he lived in terror of the next "stomach attack" . . . and actually refused to leave the house without a bottle of Maalox at the ready, in case "the acid" decided to launch a sudden assault.

It was "hell on earth," he says.

And then it all got worse . . . on that mild, September afternoon in Wayne, New Jersey, when he tried to pick up a McDonald's French fry and discovered that his hand didn't work. "I looked down and I realized that I couldn't feel what was in my hand," he recalls today. "As a matter of fact, *both* of my hands and arms were numb, all the way up to the elbows.

"I had to look at my hand in order to see if it was holding a french fry, because I certainly couldn't feel it!"

Up to this point in his increasingly tortured life, the long-suffering Jasinski had assumed that that his illness was simply the result of "stress piled on top of more stress." As he would later explain, it had never occurred to him that the buildings in which he worked might be making him sick.

Several months after the McDonald's incident, I put David through my standard Contrast Sensitivity test and determined beyond any reasonable doubt that bio-toxins were actually responsible for his chronic illness. Thoroughly puzzled, he sat down to reflect on his work history, and on the series of "damp and moldy buildings" in which he'd spent most of his career.

"I started to work for American Cyanamid in 1974," he pointed out, "and I worked for them in various functions for 22 years. I spent most of my time in three buildings, and all three of them were sealed.

"They had windows, but the windows didn't open. So we were all subject to the re-circulated air, and who really knows what-year-air we were breathing"

Jasinski first noticed a pattern of continuing illness while working in the second building, back in the late 1980s. "Interestingly enough, that building had its intake for the heating and air conditioning right next to the loading dock for trucks.

"There were times when you could actually smell the exhaust in the building. The diesel. That's good for headaches and nausea, among other things. I did some investigating on my own—and I was the one who uncovered the fact that it was an engineering flaw."

Already poisoned by his steady diet of diesel fumes, Jasinski was moved to yet another contaminated building in early 1993. This time the offending office complex was located in West Paterson, N.J.

"That building had a number of problems with its heating and air conditioning," the sales manager recalls today. "And there were many times that the place was actually flooded in different areas. And by flooded, I don't mean ankle- or knee-deep water, but enough water to wet the carpets. In retrospect, looking back, it must have been something in the mold spore type of contamination.

"The stuff growing in the heating and air conditioning systems, that was one problem. But also, if there were heavy rains or snow melting, it would leak through the roof. It wasn't widespread so that the entire building was like a sieve, but certain areas were prone to it. They fixed the roof while I was there, but the heating, air conditioning and sprinkler system problems really existed right up until the day I left there."

Looking back, Jasinski realized that the computer-operated system for "controlling the climate" in the West Paterson building had been designed without the slightest regard for the people who worked there. "The interesting thing was that this system was entirely controlled by computers. And the computers said that if it's December 22nd, then it's usually 22 degrees—and the system was going to turn the heat on, regardless.

"And the override to that took many days. So if it was just a quirky situation where you had a couple of mild days in the winter, you would go to work and perspire like you wouldn't believe. There was just no way to turn the heat down. The computers wouldn't let them do it!"

Does this sound like technology run amuck?

But Jasinski says that the absurdity of the "computer climate-control" was fully equaled by his company's bizarre failure to prevent water from running down the walls and then continually soaking the carpets. "I really can't explain it," he says today. "I guess at that point, nobody really believed that if mold and fungus grew around these wet spots, it could really make you sick.

"I learned it the hard way. I really think the headache and the insomnia I was experiencing, along with the muscle aches and joint aches and depression, was caused by the buildings. It may have started with the original building, but the more I think about it, that West Paterson building, with all that dampness and contamination: I think that's what contributed mostly to it."

By the time David Jasinski visited my Maryland office in late 1999, his health was almost completely shot. Beleaguered by endless headaches, sore muscles, chronic stomach pain and short-term memory problems, he was in danger of becoming completely disabled by Sick Building Syndrome.

I took one look at him, and went straight to work.

After making certain (via the CS Test) that his symptoms were part of a bio-toxin-mediated illness and eliminating confounding variables, I immediately placed him on a four-doses-a-day regimen of cholestyramine. I have a high regard for David, and I was quite pleased when he began to show signs of improvement after only a few days of CSM therapy.

"I started to feel better within 48 hours of my first dose of cholestyramine," he will tell you today. "The numbness in my hands has completely vanished now. My stomach is normal, too. I can eat anything, and I don't have to be worried about onions or Chinese food or any of the other things that used to instantly trigger problems.

"I don't think I've had one headache since I started this treatment. I've been so 'up' during the past few weeks that I need to get off my medication for the depression. I truly don't believe that I need it anymore."

He pauses for a moment, reflecting on his good fortune, then floods you with a brilliant smile. "My energy level is much improved, and I sleep like a baby. I've started to conk off about ten o'clock [at night] now. In the past, when I was sick, I had absolutely no desire to sleep. I'd find any excuse at all to stay awake."

Although David doesn't use multi-syllabic "science words" when talking about human physiology, his description of the process in which CSM filters harmful bio-toxins from fatty tissues is perfectly accurate. "The cholestyramine has the ability to attach itself to the toxins that have been absorbed into my body [from the contaminated office buildings].

"In the past, those toxins just kept circulating, brain to stomach to nerves, and that's how these different symptoms would be continually present. This CSM is a cholesterol medication, and much like it does with the cholesterol, it has the ability to attach itself to the toxins, and then they are expelled in your waste.

"Like I say, I've been so excited about it. It's so nice to feel good, to feel upbeat, to enjoy my job for the first time in many years. To really enjoy life! I don't look my age and I don't feel my age anymore."

David Jasinski was fortunate. Unlike millions of other SBS victims, he was able to find a cure for his illness—a cure based on a clear understanding of what bio-toxins really are, and how they "hide" in fatty tissues scattered throughout the major organs of the body, in order to continue wreaking their havoc year after year.

What the Pediatricians Haven't Talked about: The Monster under the Bed

Although many people don't realize it, Sick Building Syndrome isn't limited to offices, schools (See Chapter Chapter 26: "Why Johnny Can't Read") and airplanes (later).

The fungi that manufacture mycotoxins share some selective habitat requirements, but there's absolutely no biological reason why a wet basement at your local bank wouldn't harbor the same species of fungus that you'd find growing in a home-owner's wet basement in Snow Hill, Maryland . . . or anywhere in the flood zone of the Tar River in North Carolina.

And once that fungus starts to grow, watch out: If left unchecked, a few spores of *Stachybotrys* or one of its nasty cousins can morph quickly into the kind of toxin-spewing monster that you might expect to encounter in the pages of a Stephen King bestseller.

As a kid, I used to worry about what might be underneath my bed when the lights went out. Forty years later, I realize that if that same bed had been located in a Sick Building, I'd have had a good *reason* to worry! Something was lurking beneath the bed-springs, all right, even if I couldn't see it or smell it. Remember that by the time a room smells musty or you can actually spot the mildew, it's too late to take preventive measures. But if the fungus is a toxin-former and you *do* smell something "moldy," look out—because you're likely to be breathing toxin at that moment.

In other chapters of this book, I've outlined a great deal of information about residential and recreational acquisition of chronic, neurotoxin-mediated illnesses. But it's also true that the term "SBS" (as applied by OSHA, at any rate) usually refers to occupational exposure. Still, I'm concerned that large numbers of patients with mycotoxin-induced illness aren't being diagnosed properly. For this group, the source of the exposure wasn't the office or factory floor . . . it was located inside their very own homes.

And why wouldn't it be? Aren't the contractors who build residential housing just as dollar-conscious as the developers of large office complexes? Don't the home builders fret over heating and cooling costs as much as the billion-dollar shopping center and highrise apartment builders?

These days, our climate-controlled, perfectly engineered indoor environments certainly don't include drafty windows and doors that leak air whenever the wind blows. Add a "plant room" (the old, bad days of the window-leaking "conservatory" are gone forever!), spritz the bird's nest ferns a few extra times and *presto!*, you've got yourself an indoor ecosystem, complete with fungi of all species.

An even bigger problem is the new fad of building fancy rooflines and elaborate entranceways for all those spiffy new housing units. But every break in a roof line is a gold-plated invitation for water entry. And when the proud new homeowners try to *save* a few bucks by purchasing a "pre-fab" building, the eco-results are often worse. Why? For starters, if the junctions between sections of the pre-fab haven't been cut perfectly, the fungi will move into your Sick Building even before you do!

A family in nearby Snow Hill came to me recently with just such a case. As it turned out, their pre-fab assembly had been held up by several days of heavy rains. Soon they noticed a black mold growing around the entryway and under the paneling. The kiln-dried wood that had been used in construction changed its shape after getting soaked . . . and the front door never fit properly after that.

First the mother got sick. Then the children quickly followed suit. As you might expect, the pre-fabbers insisted they were not at fault; their $80,000 mold factory had been *sold*, and it was time to move on. (No charge for the chronic illness, I guess.)

As usually happens in America, an attorney was quickly hired. The company responded by sending in consultants who found the construction to have been impeccable. Meanwhile, the family's 12-year-old son was beginning to have problems at school. The psychologist examined him, then suggested that the combination of a new school, a new home and some unresolved peer interactions were contributing to an attention deficit disorder. The primary care physician at the family's HMO didn't miss a beat, and instantly prescribed Ritalin (without bothering to examine the child, however). The prescription was actually phoned in to the pharmacy . . . although Mom *was* required to drop by the physician's office for a hard copy.

Ghastly? You bet. But this family's misery had only begun. Within a few weeks, the child began to attend counseling sessions, at $115 per. He seemed moody and confused and continued to lag at school. The psychologist wanted to bump him up to a stronger medication, but Mom didn't like the idea of powerhouse stimulant meds being poured into 12-year-olds.

Then the school's guidance counselor read an article in the *American Academy of Pediatrics Journal* suggesting that "individual isolation" in children was often accentuated by violent computer games (usually a solitary experience). Suddenly, Mom found herself confronting yet *another* possible explanation for her child's increasingly dysfunctional behavior. Were the kid's problems actually the result of severe adolescent turbulence, combined with a steady diet of shoot-em-up video games?

Eventually, the mother dropped by my office for a new patient consult. As she outlined her family's situation, I began thinking about CS testing. And sure enough: within a matter of minutes, her FACT showed a significant deficit. I listened to her description of her neurotoxin-linked symptoms and immediately recommended CSM therapy.

It took her two weeks to get better with CSM, but her home was still full of mycotoxins. If she stops the CSM, she knows the symptoms will return immediately. Incredibly stressed, she now worries incessantly about her court case . . . and about the way her strange-acting son recently trashed a neighbor's garage.

Why such violent behavior? The boy says he can't remember. Look out: here come the juvenile authorities and Social Services, all at once . . . not to mention the family pastor, who also has an opinion. Next thing you know, the kid is suspended from school for throwing textbooks in the library.

Pretty grim, no? And yet it keeps getting worse. In recent days, the counselors have decided that the father's occasional beer is a "drinking problem," and he's now required to attend substance abuse sessions twice a week. The boy continues to take numerous medications—including a blood pressure pill, clonidine—which supposedly helps in "bad ADHD cases."

After nearly a year of sleeping in a moldy-smelling room beside a leaking window, the child has become tired and phlegmatic. Mom keeps thinking about home schooling, but who has the time (or the strength)?

So how does this story end?

Does the boy end up smoking dope, getting into more trouble, maybe stealing a car and wrecking it or getting arrested for a felony?

No.

His CS test was positive . . . which meant that I could start him on CSM therapy immediately. He improved slowly but steadily. The family eventually settled the dispute with the builders and moved out of the tainted house. The child is 14 now and doesn't take mood-altering drugs. Instead he's active in the youth group at his church and his grades have gone back up where they should be, since his IQ is 119.

It's remarkable to think about . . . but our society actually functioned quite normally, in the case of this troubled family. Every intervention that took place was "by the book"—and perfectly useless. Each public bureaucracy that became involved did its best to help—and accomplished nothing. Every professional who joined the case practiced according to the established standard for best care.

And yet they all missed it.

They hadn't learned: *toxins hurt children's brains.*

But don't *you* forget that lesson. If you aren't sure about your home or work environment—if you're experiencing symptoms that might be signaling neurotoxin-linked illness, or seeing them in other family members—don't put off your CS test, or theirs.

Go ahead: let the doctor make the right diagnosis . . . and then prescribe the proper therapy!

Toxins at 30,000 Feet

I'll admit it: I always get a little nervous when the spouse of an attorney signs on as a new patient.

I don't know why it happens, exactly . . . I guess there's just something about the interaction that gnaws away at my "Be careful" button.

So when Ms. Rita dropped by my office recently for a neurotoxin-illness consult (she suspected Lyme disease), I made sure I was on time and on my toes.

Ms. Rita had no history of a tick bite, no ECM rash, no pain in her small joints or wrists or feet. She was a marathon runner, in fact! Nor did she complain of memory impairment, confusion, or a reduced ability to assimilate new knowledge.

Surely this was *not* a chronic Lyme case? Still, Ms. Rita was sick, and she knew it. She described herself as feeling "incredibly exhausted" at the end of each of her shifts as an airline attendant, and she said she now needed huge amounts of time to recover from an ordinary workout at the gym. She also suffered from chronic sinus congestion (*"All* the flight attendants seem to have it!") . . . although it wasn't accompanied by shortness of breath or wheezing.

Occasionally afflicted with night blindness and daytime glare-sensitivity—along with a bit of blurred vision, especially after working four consecutive days away from home—she felt sure that something had gone wrong with her health.

"It just isn't *like* me to ache like this, Dr. Shoemaker! My taste is off, too, and everything tastes like cardboard or aluminum foil!"

Then she rushed on to point out that she was *also* struggling with headaches, some intermittent abdominal pain and some funny tingling in her feet.

So what's the diagnosis, doc?

It didn't take me long to realize that this patient displayed enough symptom categories (including fatigue, muscle, sinus, neuropathic headache and prolonged recovery) to warrant a CS test. Bingo! It was positive.

This woman was clearly suffering from Sick Building Syndrome . . . but she didn't work in an office, and her home had been carefully inspected for fungal toxins. So where was she getting sick?

When I finally stumbled upon the answer, it nearly floored me. Ms. Rita's exposure was in the airplanes her company flew . . . and *most of them were just a variation of what a sick building can be.*

Amazed, I began to ask her some questions about the ecosystem aboard all these 747s. What chemicals did they use to clean the aircraft? Answer: the same ones any building maintenance supervisor would use. What kind of chemicals were contained in the fabrics and carpets, in order to permit rapid cleaning between flights? (You know the answer.) And what about that powerful blue toilet chemical that had to withstand at least 100 flushes between each takeoff and landing?

Pesticides? You bet. With more than 500 people a day riding the airplane, how else were they going to prevent lice and fleas from being served with the peanuts and the breath mints?

"They clean the air conditioning units every six months or so," explained Ms. Rita. "And you should *see* the mold that builds up on the wet side of the airflow device!"

As you might imagine, all of this was quite unnerving for me. I spend a lot of time in (not on!) airplanes as a physician who frequently attends conferences and consults around the country. Maybe my headaches, sinus congestion and "jet lag" are just another form of illness related to indoor air quality.

The story of Ms. Rita and her adventures while flying the friendly (and apparently toxic) skies over America does serve to make a crucially important point about SBS and other chronic, toxin-mediated illnesses.

Our understanding of these rapidly escalating illnesses has barely scratched the surface.

Up to now, science has answered almost none of the questions about the etiology, the symptoms and the treatment of SBS. Can any researcher anywhere in the world tell us how many times a patient must be exposed to these fungal poisons, before the first negative health effects begin to be felt? Is the pathological impact of fungal toxins cumulative in some ways we don't understand?

When it comes to SBS, how much is enough? Does a patient need to work in the same contaminated building for six months or a year or *three* years, before life-changing pathology sets in? And why do some patients work for years at a time in environments highly contaminated by fungi . . . without ever developing so much as a light cough?

More than anything else, we need to begin developing a set of data-based guidelines that might bring some uniformity (to say nothing of clarity) to the diagnosis and treatment of this increasingly threatening, environmental illness.

chapter 21

Reflection

How Sick Is Your Building . . . And What Can You Do about It?

Princess Anne, MD –October 15, 1986

My daughter Sally is too young to remember the gasoline shortages of the 1970s, when OPEC flexed its supply-muscles bigtime, and the lines at the gas station often stretched to the distant horizon. Everywhere you turned in that frantic Jimmy Carter-era, government economists and oil industry experts were giving speeches on the need to "make sure that we never allow ourselves to become vulnerable to 'petroleum blackmail' again!"

Question: does that scenario sound a bit . . . *familiar?*

Of course it does. If you're like most Americans of middle age, you probably also recall how the gas crunch inspired a lot of automakers to get out there and design cars that "sipped" fuel, rather than gulping it by the gallon. Remember those "waves of imports" (mostly Japanese, of course) that boasted of "getting 40 miles to the gallon on the open highway?"

Suddenly, all those tail-finned highway monsters of the 1960s were "out," replaced by needle-nosed, supremely fuel-efficient cars like my 1972 Subaru, which racked up 42 miles to the gallon and never looked back.

Ah, the good old days. Was it Yogi Berra (or Lao-Tze?) who once described the world of ever changing and ever returning fashion by pointing out: "It's *deja vu* all over again?" Welcome to the brave new world of the New Millennium, in which more and more folks seem to be driving $28,000 Sport Utility Vehicles (but without the tailfins), and in which the Arab Emirates are once again leveling their petroleum-gun at our heads.

Why can't we learn? Twenty-five years ago, the experts in the environmental think tanks talked endlessly of solar energy, ethanol-based gasoline, wind power, geothermal power, hydro-electric power, methane recycling and a dozen other "alternative energy" sources that were going to "free us" from dependence on fossil fuels. Back then, the conventional wisdom said: "Diversify your supply; don't get into a place where you must depend for your energy needs on a single source!"

But it didn't happen. For reasons that remain crystal-clear, the great energy corporations continued to put all their eggs in the basket marked "internal combusion engine," and the rest of us continued to empty our wallets every time we pulled into a gas station. Ask yourself: do you really think the Shells and the Texacos of the world would have continued sitting on their hands in the research labs, if there had been enough Big Dollars available from these new energy sources to offset the loss of making capital improvements to the petroleum infrastructure?

Unlike the oil moguls, however, the nation's building industry *did* respond aggressively to the 1970s demand for increased fuel efficiency. They probably didn't do it out of civic high-mindedness, though. Most of the developers simply realized early on that designing and constructing airtight buildings was in their own best financial interests.

Enter the era of the "sealed" office building or shopping emporium, in which the sweet promise of "climate control" seemed to offer *homo sapiens* an endless, balmy springtime—along with clean, crisp "recirculated" air that would remain forever untainted by contact with the outside world. How magical it all seemed . . . the idea that we could solve such problems as smog, high humidity, cigarette smoke—and even the energy shortage —by simply manipulating the HVAC system!

It was a pleasant enough daydream. But then reality showed up, in the form of various nasty fungal species that seemed to thrive in the moist, warm air being wafted their way by computer-operated heating and air conditioning systems guaranteeing a steady 73 degrees, as well as changeless humidity.

There's no doubt that these new building designs and climate-controlled HVAC systems have saved America some energy dollars in recent years. Almost overnight, millions of homeowners and office workers were gazing at the outside world through "double-paned, fixed windows," secure in the knowledge that the Breath of Winter would never gain entry.

And so what if these hermetically sealed fortresses never allowed their occupants a single lungful of fresh air? (Nor is the problem limited to office buildings, by the way, in a world where climate-controlled homes are rapidly becoming the norm.)

The same philosophy—"Lower Costs, At All Cost!"—also helped to shape new construction methods aimed at reducing the need for maintenance by owners. Just look at the vinyl siding on all those new tract houses springing up across the land. Or take a few minutes to read the fine print on the can of indoor paint, along with the chemically treated wall coverings and rugs, in a typical new home. Supposedly, these treated materials will make life much more difficult for the kind of bacteria and fungi that used to gnaw happily away at floors, walls and baseboards, in the bad old days before we found a "chemical fix" for virtually all of life's problems.

Ask yourself: what role do the built-in fungicides really play, in that can of latex paint that just went on the wall? What are the unexpected human health effects that can be triggered by a wall-covering treated with chemicals engineered to kill bacteria and fungi? Sure, these nifty contrivances serve to "reduce maintenance" . . . but what *other* unintended consequences may flow from such high-tech devices, without our even knowing it?

These days, the computers purr contentedly inside the sealed buildings, and we tell ourselves that we've finally managed to engineer the various "risk-factors" completely out of our new office buildings and increasingly popular "smart houses."

Too bad it isn't true. Like every other weapon in the struggle for space among living organisms, our nifty engineering designs and our toxin-sprayed wallpaper and chemically treated throw rugs all have a "downside"—a price that must be paid for relying on this particular strategy of self-defense.

Take that "climate-controlled" heating and air conditioning system I mentioned a minute ago, for example. Sure, it's "energy-efficient." But what happens when you trap the same stale air inside a system for weeks and months at a time? Answer: It becomes a *habitat*—a world in which one or more biological species can "feed and breed." And that's the key theme of *Desperation Medicine*, really: the recognition that changing the habitat frequently opens the door to new organisms that can threaten human health. If we are going to live safely in our spiffy new homes, we must not ignore the eco-niches we are creating with all of our wondrous new technology.

One of the key problems in any interior environment is that we humans need some airborne moisture (I recommend 40-percent humidity in the home at all times, by the way), in order to prevent our mucous membranes from drying out and then triggering attacks of ear, sinus or lung infection.

Some moisture is good, then. But when the humidity climbs too high in a home or office—or when "standing water" is allowed to remain on the premises for more than a few hours—we soon find ourselves confronting a host of pathogens designed by nature to thrive in this more tropical environment, with potentially serious consequences for our own good health.

In order to understand why water is the real "enemy" in the enclosed human habitat, let's step back for a moment and imagine that we're about to buy a new home. In this imaginary scenario, I'll use a few useful tips gleaned from the "Historic Remodelers of the Eastern Shore," an extraordinarily savvy group of home-design and engineering experts. (I'll also assume that you aren't putting too many toxic chemicals into your house and that your windows open!)

The first important thing we need to remember, says Historic Remodelers, is that the lower you go in a building that contains a water problem, the more likely you are to encounter health-threatening toxins (aka "mycotoxins") spawned by various fungal species. Example: *Stachybotrys*, a particularly versatile toxin-former (at least 24 different toxins identified so far) grows better in sub-basements than basements and better in basements than on ground floors. (But don't forget that upper level-entry of water can contaminate a home from top to bottom with numerous other toxin-spewing fungi, in addition to *stachybotrys*.)

So how can you quickly determine if your new home is fungi-free or not? The quickest approach, of course, would be to conduct a Contrast Sensitivity (CS) Test on the former owners . . . while also examining the school records of the children who lived there before you, in order to make certain that they weren't learning-disabled due to neurotoxins caused by fungi. (See Chapter 26: "Why Johnny Can't Read.") But since that kind of interrogation probably won't happen ("You want to do *what?*"), you'll probably prefer to follow the steps described below.

First: start with the simple things. Remember that a "wind barrier" placed 80 feet from the north and west sides of your new home will lower heating costs dramatically. At the same time, it will blunt the wind's ability to drive water into your home. Make sure the barrier includes both deciduous trees (for pleasing summer shade) and conifers (their evergreen limbs provide an efficient, year-round windbreak). If possible, plant shrubs that taper in height to improve the aerodynamics of the break. This foliage will provide cover and food sources for the new species that will soon be arriving to enjoy your new eco-system. Just make sure the vegetation isn't quickly gobbled up by deer!

The south and east sides of the house should be outfitted with a variety of deciduous shade trees. Plant your best "ornamentals" here, and you'll enjoy an earlier spring and a later fall season of blooms. The shade will help in summer, and the early morning winter sun will provide almost as much radiant heat as you'd get from a wood stove. And who can forget the thrill of watching a flock of cedar waxwings flutter through an ornamental crabapple tree at dawn, outlined in the burnt gold luminescence flooding from the just risen sun?

Remember, too, that planting your windbreak too close to your foundation will defeat the purpose. That's because thick plantings retain moisture at the foundation line. Their roots tend to wick surface water beneath the house or into the basement. For best results, plan exactly how you're going to move water that gets dumped on your house quickly away from it.

Other key moisture-problems include interior leaks from overflowing washing machines, shower faucets that drip water and condensation that occurs beneath the house. You should also take a careful look at your roof. Has the flashing been properly installed at the junction with the masonry? (Look for stains on the brick and watermarks on the joists, underneath.)

Make sure, also, that at least 18 inches of flashing protects every junction where a roof line joins the side of another wall. Look for algae growing on the northwest side of a roof joining a wall . . . a likely sign that you've got too much water (or two little airflow) in that section of the roof.

As for the windows: don't forget that they let in a lot more than just sun and air. Install flashing atop each, with double caulking on the sides and bottom. The window stool should feature enough angle and lip to drain water off at the top and not behind the siding.

Next step: make certain that your attic has adequate ventilation. Soffit and ridge pole treatments usually work well together. Remember, too, that attic heat on a summer day can make any air conditioner's duct-joints sweat up a storm. But not to worry: you can easily find a flexible glue that will prevent water entry from this source.

Now it's time to inspect your outside walls. Remember that any vapor barriers you install should go on the outside of your plywood, but under your siding. That's because moisture infiltration is greater during warm, humid days. You don't want a lot of wet, outside air penetrating through your house sheathing to a vapor barrier beneath your drywall . . . or to an impermeable wall covering. So build your barrier while remembering that a stiff interior wall covering (such as luan plywood or paneling) may wind up giving the indoor toxin-forming fungi the habitat they love most: cellulose from your drywall, moisture from the inside of the house that's retained by the outside vapor barrier, heat and darkness.

So far, so good. But now it's time to step into the watery world of the bathroom. Here I enthusiastically recommend that you spend a few extra dollars for a cement backer for your tiled shower—and especially for your pre-fab insert shower stall. Don't settle for a "water-resistant" drywall! The cement is heaver, and takes more time to install and seal. But remember: Every tile treatment will eventually leak (along with the factory-made, plastic enclosure).

Another bathroom tip: make sure you have a good exhaust system from your bathroom to the outside, and that you aren't venting all that moisture into a closet. You do *not* want to open the door to your winter coats and get a summer's worth of spores, toxins, and enzymes in your lungs. Remember, also that you should never vent exhaust into your attic or crawl space.

Be sure to vent your dryer with a downslope and a short run to the outside. To show you why, let me describe one of the worst examples of "bad dryer venting" I ever witnessed. It occurred in the for-sale home of a nearby prominent builder, whose dryer exhaust inexplicably ran uphill, then through a cold closet and a heated room en route to the outside. As you might expect, the lint collected at the junction of cold and warm pipes, where it soaked up moisture and contributed to a leaky pipe in a wall cavity behind a child's headboard. Even worse, every time the dryer door opened, outside air whirled fungi toxins into the device . . . and into the bathroom. Remember that "out of sight is definitely not out of mind" (or lung, for that matter).

If you happen to live at the bottom of a slope, don't make your basement or crawl space the local "birdbath." In this situation, you'll have to build terraces, swales, or dry wells . . . or maybe even install lawn pipes to direct the water away from your living spaces. Do it! The effort will be rewarded, each time you realize that you can breathe freely at night. Besides, your interesting water-control structures will attract an incredible diversity of species, including amphibians and birds. Beautify your yard, even as you save your basement! Water really does run downhill, and you can't change that. Use it to your advantage, instead.

Another suggestion: build a ventilated shed for your firewood. Do you really want the water from three cords of green wood evaporating into your basement?

Now here's a warning: if you're looking at a dirt floor in your crawlspace, you're also looking at a moisture factory. I've heard many pros and cons about crawlspaces, and I'll tell you flat-out: I don't like them. But if you're forced to live with one, remember a key rule: If you close off your ventilation grates in summer (reducing the flow of hot, humid air), be sure to open them in the winter to let in the cold—so that the fungi population doesn't increase over the winter. And never put a vapor barrier on the house-side of your sub-floor. (Try and tell that to a contractor who insists on putting his sub-flooring on the moment his floor joists are in place.) The construction will go a bit more slowly, but you'll keep moisture out of your living space.

To solve the crawlspace problem, cover your dirt floor with a 20-mil sheet of plastic, then secure it with a thin layer of ballast stone. An exhaust fan can help keep the moisture level lower . . . but don't mount it on the wood-joists for your floors, because you'll feel and hear it constantly after that, no matter how quiet it's supposed to be.

It helps to remember that basements are always the worst offenders, when it comes to home-acquired fungal illnesses. To defend against them, study your basement water inputs first. Example: a hot water heater can easily trigger condensation and create pools of standing water. Insulate that heater. And don't forget that if you have a humidifier attached to your central heat, it should not become a fungus hatchery. Keep it dry and clean by applying a five percent solution of chlorine bleach (no more) regularly.

Never forget that the key to protecting your basement is to keep water out. Downspouts shouldn't stop at the foundation line, for example. If you can't waterproof the basement concrete walls, the best solution is to excavate the outside of the foundations so that you can then apply waterproof paint to the exterior of basement walls. Better yet, in new construction, apply the wall treatment at the start of the process, not the finish.

Think it through! One mycotoxin patient of mine back-filled the outside of his basement walls with 20 inches of pea gravel enclosing perforated drainpipes that were covered with red resin paper on the uphill sides of his basement. The pipes ran around the house on the downslope side. He then built eight-by-12-foot fish ponds under each of the screened exhaust ends of the pipes. Now he enjoys a clear waterfall year-round, and it doesn't freeze up, even in the dead of winter. His neighbors still don't quite understand why his ponds don't freeze. This gentleman's basement remains quite dry, thank you—because he knew how much water pressure was being exerted on his basement walls. Make water a friend and not an enemy!

I think it's quite helpful to know that you can be creative with your "water solutions." Like ag chemicals, water is safe in the right amounts, and at the right times, and in the right places. Otherwise, that unruly H_2O can provide the necessary habitat for toxin-formers that will grow fast if you let them.

And one final recommendation: If you do fall prey to fungal toxins in your home, don't panic. You can easily obtain quick, inexpensive and effective treatment by consulting your physician and launching a regimen of cholestyramine therapy.

Take heart, but don't forget that fungal organisms don't stop growing just because we don't see them. To be effective, any "building remediation plan" you come up with (after water entry is controlled) should include liberal use of dilute bleach, or a quaternary ammonium cleaning compound. Anything else is a standing invitation for continued illness.

I also recommend that you contact an approved indoor environmental engineering firm before launching renovations aimed at restoring healthy air quality. Ask about their expertise in mycotoxin analysis, however. Remember that the new growth-industry of indoor engineering has attracted plenty of "experts" outfitted with plenty of get-rich-quick schemes.

Don't let them get rich at your expense!

A New FACT for
Occupational Medicine

Pocomoke, MD –April, 2000

After 20 years as a primary care practice physician, I've learned not to be surprised when I find a strange car with an unknown driver waiting outside my office at 7:30 in the morning.

Good morning, Early bird!

Like many physicians, I'm often amused by the way my schedule has changed over the years. In the early going, I'd arrive at 8:30 to prepare for my first patients at 9. But my practice grew quickly, and within a few years I was showing up at 8 each day to get ready for an 8:30 start.

Of course it wasn't long before the office hours got bumped back to 8—and my arrival on the parking lot to 7:30. Which was fine with me. Getting started that early allows me a bit of real privacy in which to prepare for outpatient medicine. Like an eager high school wrestler getting ready for a match, I love to "prepare mentally" for the day ahead. And why not? In primary care practice, after all, everything turns on the small details in patient history and physical exam. Getting sharply focused on those details requires a different mind set than working in the yard on Saturday afternoon (an activity I *also* cherish, by the way).

Anyway, here I am: another 7:30 on the parking lot.

But the police car parked over there on the asphalt *is* a surprise. And the middle-aged officer behind the wheel looks worried.

"Are you Dr. Shoemaker? I just want to know if I'm gonna be okay."

He's anxious, but he doesn't look sick.

"Of course, come right on in. What's your name?"

●   ●   ●

John is a new recruit. He's been given the graveyard shift, and he's spent a lot of nights patrolling the quiet streets of Pocomoke this cold winter. But the job is exacting a price, apparently; every time he goes to work, he develops a headache, a cough and nausea. Yet his symptoms always clear up after he's been home for a few hours.

Interestingly enough, those same unpleasant symptoms only show up when he drives one particular police cruiser. Has he reported his troubles to the Chief? No, John explains haltingly; this job was hard to get!

"I just thought my health problem was like a tax I had to pay to stay on the job," says John. "You see, most departments are only hiring young academy graduates now. My wife has a bad back and we've got two kids in the middle school. I get home in time to pack them off to school. Then I pick them up after I wake up in the afternoon."

He gives me a cheerful smile. "Somehow, it all works out. But I can't afford to make waves with the chief. I'm still on probation, you know? And if I lose this job, I'll lose the health insurance along with it. My wife gets these back treatments three times a week, and that costs about $1,000 a month. The treatments seem to help her for a few days—but then she always needs another adjustment."

John is telling me this story in a jumbled fashion. He stops and starts and often repeats himself. He's acutely confused. His eyes are red but his skin isn't. If his police car is poisoning him, is it odorless carbon monoxide, maybe mixed with something in the heating system? Fungi sometimes grow in car air conditioners, and they can cause the symptoms he's described. Still, a fungal toxin wouldn't trigger a brief illness that's cured by exiting the car.

Next he tells how he went to see the "HMO doctor" down the street. The doc didn't have much time for him, but he did manage to prescribe antibiotics for a sinus infection—along with stomach acid blockers for indigestion and a mild anti-anxiety pill for his job stress. Maybe they even helped a little bit.

"I just want to know if this is going to harm me permanently," says John, and I can see the fear lurking in his eyes. "I don't like taking pills. I'll do it if I have to . . . but I don't seem to be getting any better."

John has the typical chronic neurotoxin symptoms. He's sensitive to bright lights (hence the dark sunglasses at 7:30 on a cloudy morning). He feels short of breath all the time, and he suffers from nagging muscle aches and nasty headaches. And his "mental confusion" is real, no doubt about that.

"John, sit down in this chair. Hold this device, the FACT, up to your cheekbones. Lean forward, but watch out—don't bump your knees on my desk like everybody else does." (BUMP! He grimaces as his knee bangs the desk.)

"Now, John, I want you to notice that there are five rows of nine columns each on the FACT card. Each box contains lines that do one of three things. Some of the lines lean to the left, some lean to the right, and some stand staight up and down, or perpendicular.

"Taking this test is quite easy. You simply read the card by covering one eye with your hand. Start in row A and read from left to right. Then call out the position of the lines, by saying 'Left,' or 'Straight,' or 'Right.' Remember, the lines will get fainter as you go from left to right. When you reach the place where you can't tell the direction of the lines, you'll receive a test-score which tells us exactly where your brain loses the ability to distinguish between white, gray and black.

"And here's another key point: If your brain is carrying a biological toxin, the loss of your sensitivity to contrast will form a distinctive data-pattern. This is a great diagnostic tool, John, and I've been using it a lot lately for people with different kinds of problems.

"All set? Okay, you can start. Which eye will you cover first? Good. Now, just read Row A. No, don't go down column 1! No . . . just say 'Left, Straight or Right.' You don't need to say stuff like, 'A tiny little bit!' or 'Maybe up?'"

It's amazing, but I've been through this drill so often that I can almost tell who has a neurotoxin illness by how well they follow my simple instructions!

John's test turns out to be strikingly positive. Quickly, I send him in the poisoned police car (but with the windows open) toward the local hospital for a carboxyhemoglobin level. Then he sits inside the closed car, heater on, for 30 minutes for a repeat carboxyhemoglobin level.

The ER staff nurse, Shelley Byrd, agrees to monitor him so that this provocative test won't result in a death sentence from carbon monoxide.

Both of his carboxyhemoglobin levels check in at 2, a normal finding in a non-smoker. But Shelley also confirms one of John's earlier observations: There's definitely an "unusual smell" in that car.

Two days later, off work after the weekend, John feels fine.

"There it is, Doc: we proved that it's the car! But I still want to know if it will hurt me permanently." He isn't confused anymore. He picks up the FACT and reads it perfectly. "Whatever you do, don't tell the chief anything. I'm not going to ride in that cruiser anymore, that's for sure."

Ken Hudnell came up with the answer. We'd talked about this case after John first came in. I'd actually expected John's Contrast Sensitivity to remain impaired, since I'd thought the problem was related to combustion of gasoline. We see improvement in 36 hours with CSM treatment of biological toxin-mediated illnesses . . . but chemicals, and especially those related to internal combustion engines, create a permanent deficit. With the rest of his work up to normal, what was the problem?

"Glycol ether," said Ken. He thought there probably was a small leak in the antifreeze line that emitted fumes when the heater was on. (No, not ethylene glycol; it was a glycol ether.)

Now, how can I tell the Chief to look at the antifreeze line without breaking confidentiality? An interesting problem of medical ethics! Do I have a legal duty to safeguard the next policeman driving that poisoned car?

But before I could make a move, John was assigned to a narcotics sting operation out of town. There was no way I could contact him. Yet I didn't stop worrying about the situation, or asking myself: is glycol ether-poisoning a dose-related event? How long will it be before someone else got sick?

Pocomoke is a small town with a small-town approach to grocery shopping. People stop and talk. In Checkout Lane No. 2, I bumped into Bill Thomas, the DARE officer. I hadn't seen him in a while.

"Bill, are you feeling all right? Your eyes look a little red [not good for the officer who teaches kids to stay away from drugs!]."

"Doc, I don't know what to tell you. I had to drive that old cruiser last night. I was filling in for an officer who made such a big stink about that car that they transferred him! Maybe he's right, though. Something smells funny in that car. I tell ya, I'm really beat; working that double gave me a real headache."

"Sick to your stomach, too, Bill? Sounds like glycol ether poisoning to me. Before you let somebody else drive that car, check the antifreeze line. I'll bet it has a small leak when the heat's turned on."

"You got it, Doc. I'll call the chief right now."

John's been doing fine lately, I'm told. No more "flu symptoms" on the job. *Hang in there, Early Bird!*

chapter 23

Event

Surviving
Chronic Fatigue Syndrome

Pocomoke, MD –August, 1999

"The road to Heaven leads through the heart of Hell."
—William Blake, "Songs of Innocence"

Dawn.

A mild summer morning in August of 1989. Six o'clock.

White curtains fluttering gently in the bedroom window of the house on West Sycamore Lane.

Sally Barkley, 37 years old, opens one eye. Blinks it slowly. Something isn't right. She doesn't feel so hot. She feels . . . *sick.* Her heart is racing, and her raw tongue burns as if slicked with liquid fire.

Her heart sinks. She can't miss work again! But already, she feels the familiar exhaustion creeping over her. The heaviness in her bones and muscles . . . as if her body were a black hole collapsing in on itself. What the hell is the matter with her?

The doctors don't know. They can't tell her a thing. One specialist says it's nothing more than "depression"—a "chemical imbalance in the brain, no problem, we'll get you started on Prozac right away."

Prozac for aching muscles? For fierce attacks of unremitting diarrhea? For blurred vision and sensitivity to light and sudden attacks of devastating exhaustion so terrible that they leave her crawling along the bedroom floor, begging her husband Henry to carry her into the bathroom?

What the hell is the matter with me?

Nobody knows.

Another specialist—a veteran endocrinologist from Johns Hopkins—says the culprit isn't really depression. It's "fibromyalgia," compounded by Sally's hiatal hernia, and her peptic ulcer, and her ever increasing hypertension.

They can't *both* be right.

Is it lupus? Multiple sclerosis? Some other auto-immune disease, in which Sally's body has somehow rebelled against itself —throwing her body chemistry into chaos and triggering these brutal daily headaches, this "icy burning" sensation along the skin of her arms and legs?

Don't cry. Don't think about it. Get up and function, before you lose your goddam job!

With superhuman effort, she drags herself to a sitting position. She groans once, and Henry stirs beside her. He coughs, yawns and begins to stretch.

"Oh, my God!"

Startled, Henry sits bolt-upright. "What is it, Sally? What's wrong?"

"Oh, my *God!*"

She turns to him, her face a mask of frozen terror.

"Look at my hands, Henry. Look at my feet!"

He looks. And gasps. His wife's hands and feet are completely covered with yellow, leaking blisters.

The white curtains flutter gently in the window. . . .

The patient had all the symptoms of a neurotoxin-mediated illness, and she responded to cholestyramine—but she didn't have any exposures. Was she making the toxin herself?

• • •

It began in Nevada, in a tiny community on Lake Tahoe known as "Incline Village." It was here, starting back in 1985, that two observant physicians began to notice a strange pattern of symptoms in patients who complained of blurred vision, faltering short-term memory and debilitating exhaustion.

During the months and years that followed, this mysterious ailment (was it caused by a virus?) would evolve through a series of ever-changing names: Lake Tahoe Disease, Chronic Epstein-Barr Virus Syndrome, Yuppie Flu.

And finally: Chronic Fatigue Syndrome, or CFS.

During this same period, the two physicians who had made the initial diagnosis—internists Dan Peterson and Paul Cheney —would be thoroughly discussed, chewed up, and then completely ignored by the influential scientists who run both the National Institutes of Health (NIH) and the U.S. Centers for Disease Control (CDC).

The story of what happened to Drs. Peterson and Cheney deserves a book in itself. Although their basic theory that Chronic Fatigue Syndrome is caused by a "mono"-like virus perhaps related to herpes simplex would never be dis-proven, the powerful administrators at the great medical think-tanks continually insisted otherwise. For more than a decade, the scientific intellectuals in Atlanta and Bethesda issued a never-ending series of contradictory —and often just plain wrong—medical advisories that ascribed the disorder to half a dozen different factors, none of which turned out to be involved in the pathogenesis of this disease.

The U.S. Congress also joined the debate in the late 1980s, and eventually allocated millions of dollars for CFS research at the CDC. But that money somehow disappeared, apparently after being re-routed to "more important" projects. According to one knowledgeable insider, the money was transferred to encephalitis research at a top-secret research facility (Plum Island) located near New York City.

That scenario sounded a little far-fetched to me. And yet nothing seems too bizarre, these days, especially for a physician who has spent a few years watching how this country's public health system reacts to the accelerating spread of chronic, diagnosis-defying illnesses. And it's also true that, as of this writing, nobody has yet accounted for the millions of dollars that vanished from the CDC's Chronic Fatigue Syndrome budget.

Neurotoxins and Chronic Fatigue: The Strange Case of "Cathy P."

So how does CFS actually work? Perhaps the best way to understand the physiological dynamics of Chronic Fatigue Syndrome is to examine the 20-year history of one of my most challenging patients—a struggling retail employee whom I'll refer to as "Cathy P." for purposes of this discussion.

Now 47 years old, Cathy P. is a white female whose complaints perfectly fit the classical description of Chronic Fatigue Syndrome as an illness that "primarily attacks middle-aged and middle-class women, with symptoms that often remain vague and difficult to categorize."

When Cathy first visited my offices in Maryland nearly two decades ago, she complained of "continuing, overwhelming fatigue" that made even the simplest tasks difficult to complete. After taking her history, I conducted a physical exam and ordered all of the standard lab tests, hoping to find something . . . a clear cause for her fatigue such as a blood sugar problem or an allergy or some type of hormonal imbalance.

After those tests all came up negative, I re-examined her and ordered additional laboratory probes . . . one of which paid off handsomely when I discovered that she was suffering from a low-level anemia that was *not* related to iron deficiency, but probably related to a deficiency in a membrane-associated enzyme, pyruvate kinase.

I also picked up convincing evidence of a low-thyroid condition. I treated both of these conditions aggressively, but the patient obtained no relief from the grinding fatigue that had brought her to me in the first place.

During one of Cathy's office visits, I detected some wheezing. Her pulmonary-function tests were slightly low. Was she exposed to molds at work or at home? Were her sudden bouts of weakness the result of a so-far-undiagnosed allergy?

Once again, I treated what I'd found in her, only to discover that her fatigue persisted. Increasingly frustrated, I turned to the disease models provided by Peterson and Cheney. Cathy clearly displayed the blood-clues that linked her to chronic mono, in addition to her other symptoms.

Responding, I treated her for chronic mono with an appropriate mono virus-killing medication that is also employed against herpes infections. What if she really did have what Peterson and Cheney had diagnosed in their patients—namely, a mono virus that had somehow integrated itself into her own DNA? And what if that DNA was manufacturing some substance that left her perpetually ill?

Logic told me that I had to kill the virus.

Before taking this step, however, I decided to put in a call to one of the leading U.S. authorities on such viruses—Dr. Steven Strauss at the NIH. Strauss was a top world expert on chronic mono, and the first thing he told me was: "Only half of my patients improve, when I prescribe medication aimed at killing their viruses."

Unfortunately, Cathy P. did not improve, either.

Two years after I treated her for the virus, she returned to my office, this time suffering from a clear case of clinical depression. "I just can't take it anymore," she told me. "I'm not like I used to be, doctor. Yesterday, I wanted to drive my car off the road and into a tree, but I didn't.

"I came here, instead."

I immediately started her on antidepressants, which helped to correct her sleep disorder and her suicidal ideation. But the fatigue continued. Looking back on my original diagnosis and treatment a few years later, I kept wondering, knowing what I now know, how I had missed the obvious clues that should have told me Cathy P. was struggling with a chronic, neurotoxin-mediated illness. This patient had been telling me what was wrong with her, but I not been able to hear it!

Cathy P. returned to my office a few months after I began treating her, however, in order to hand over the last of her anti-depressant pills. "You can keep these," she said glumly. "I've accepted the fact that I just need to learn how to live with this condition. I don't need these pills, because my problem isn't really depression, and I know it."

Nearly twenty years after Cathy P. first presented with her symptoms, she visited my office in November of 1999 to complain about a particularly painful condition—a new, searing "pain in the neck, and it's just plain driving me crazy!

"For the last five years, I've been doing fine," Cathy explained. "I've learned to live with my fatigue. But this neck pain is really terrible. You've got to help me!"

This time I listened as hard as I could. Because her description did not seem to point toward a pinched nerve or herniated disk, I asked her to describe the pain in more detail. She immediately started talking about two other problems that were causing her increasing concern: a growing, painful sensitivity to bright light, and an unsettling state of mental confusion that she had come to call "brain fog."

These were symptoms that I'd often heard about before, while examining other neurotoxin patients.

"It's terrible, Dr. Shoemaker," she told me at one point. "This total confusion creeps over me, and I can't remember a thing. I have to write everything down, or I'll forget it for sure."

I was in the middle of writing these observations down, when a sudden thought broke through my own mental fog: *Neck pain, light sensitivity, memory impairment—my God, those were the clues I needed!*

The key to the puzzle had been right there in front of me. Cathy P.'s neck pain was the same symptom I'd encountered dozens of times in patients suffering from the neurotoxin-mediated

Sick-Building Syndrome and chronic Lyme disease!

Her fatigue and her light-sensitivity were also the same.

For several years now, I'd been seeing these same symptoms recur endlessly in my neurotoxic patients.

What were the medical implications, if Cathy P.'s chronic fatigue turned out to be no *different* in its essentials from the chronic Lyme, the Sick-Building Syndrome and the *Pfiesteria*-related illness I'd already been treating for three years . . . even though this patient had *never reported any toxic exposures?*

What if her body somehow manufactured its own toxins?

With increasing anticipation, I asked Cathy P. to take the Contrast Sensitivity test.

This simple test of visual sensitivity showed the neurotoxic basis for her symptoms in less than three minutes. Overwhelmingly positive for visual contrast deficit, she clearly displayed the "Hudnell Sign"—a key indicator of the presence of neurotoxins.

Her chronic fatigue was just one of the many toxic-effects that were wiping out her ability to think and making her neck sore!

I was jubilant, but also troubled. How was I going to be able to distinguish between such well-documented toxin-illnesses as sick-building and chronic Lyme, for which identifiable microbes were demonstrably the source, and these bizarre illnesses, in which no pathogen had yet been discovered?

Fortunately, I had spent a great deal of time reading about Chronic Fatigue Syndrome before Cathy P. arrived with her sore neck. Again and again, during my literature search, I'd noticed that Chronic Fatigue usually involved one symptom that almost never appeared in other types of neurotoxin-linked illness.

That symptom was "postural hypotension"—a condition which causes dizziness in patients who stand up quickly after they had been lying down.

"Cathy," I quickly asked the patient, "do you get dizzy when you stand up?"

"I sure do, Dr. Shoemaker. For the last two or three years, I've had to make sure that I get up slowly. Otherwise, I get so dizzy that I'm afraid I'll pass out!"

With that comment, the light dawned fully: Cathy P. was suffering from postural hypotension, and her Chronic Fatigue Syndrome was just another form of neurotoxin-mediated illness . . . except that her particular ailment *could have been caused by endogenous neurotoxins!*

In order to test this promising hypothesis, I carefully documented Cathy P.'s progress, during the first two weeks of her cholestyramine treatment. The results were quite positive: her vision continued to improve, even as her symptoms (including the postural hypotension) abated.

At the end of the first two weeks, I said to the patient: "If my theory is correct, stopping the medicine will result in your symptoms slowly coming back. I don't know if that is certain—or how long the process might take."

At that point, Cathy P. agreed to stop taking the medication.

The suspense lasted only three weeks. Each day she became more fatigued. At the end of her trial time off medication, she complained of being "right back where I was," as the fatigue, the mental confusion and the distracting neck pain once again began to degrade her quality of life. Her CS again showed the diagnostic deficit—and once again I prescribed cholestyramine . . . and was pleased to see her vision return to normal within two weeks. Once again, the debilitating symptoms dissipated, not to return.

Research shows that when *Pfiesteria* patients improve and are then re-exposed, they *abruptly* deteriorate. So do cylindrospermopsis, sick building and Lyme patients. In the absence of exogenous acquisition, there is no recurrent illness. But when the acquisition is endogenous, the neurotoxins will be produced within the body. These endogenously manufactured toxin molecules accumulate day by day, until they reach concentrations sufficient to trigger the chronic syndrome.

But what toxin, exactly, causes the symptoms that we know as CFS? Is the syndrome actually the result of an unwanted functioning of a viral segment incorporated into human DNA? Or is the syndrome caused by something else. At this point, the only honest answer is: "I don't know."

I'm sure about *one* thing, however—which is that every time Cathy stopped taking CSM, her symptoms returned at the same rate as before. Given that re-exposure was not the cause in her case, could there be any doubt that her body was causing her fatigue . . . or that her illness was controlled by CSM?

Cathy's clinical course has since been repeated by many other patients. Yet the source of their chronic fatigue remains a mystery. According to my model of chronic, neurotoxin-mediated illness, the toxins impair the operations of the sympathetic nervous system in addition to all the other nervous system elements, as well as the usual organ systems. Do the endogenous neurotoxins attack receptors for adrenaline (epinephrine) . . . and is *that* why patients with this illness have difficulty maintaining their blood pressure while standing upright?

Experience shows that patients with postural hypotension usually benefit from sympathetic nervous system stimulating medication, midodrine. When this substance is given in small doses, steep blood pressure drops are averted . . . but the other neurotoxin symptoms persist. Blood pressure and other symptoms improve, however, when midodrine is given with CSM. (Only occasionally does CSM alone correct postural hypotension.)

I remain grateful to a prominent CFS patient (Dr. Allan Bickling), who suggested I give midodrine a try. His medical prescience was greatly appreciated. Believe me, when dealing with new approaches to old illnesses, I'm happy to use all the help I can get!

For Chronic Fatigue Syndrome patients like Cathy P., the proven effectiveness of the VCS Test and cholestyramine is very good news, indeed. What it tells us is that the CFS folks are no different from any other victims of neurotoxin-mediated illnesses—and that their symptoms can be managed successfully, so that their good health can be quickly restored.

Like Tommy East, a local waterman who has learned to prevent reacquisition of his *Pfiesteria* symptoms by taking cholestyramine daily so that he can earn a living on the river each day, Cathy P. has proven that she can maintain good health simply by using CSM on a preventive basis. In the same way, anyone suffering from a disorder that produces bodily toxins can gain quick relief from the debilitating system impact of the poisons by first taking the diagnostic test and then ingesting carefully monitored doses of this safe, inexpensive substance.

The long campaign to cure Cathy P.'s Chronic Fatigue Syndrome resulted in two key insights that have informed my clinical and research work ever since, as follows:

1) Whenever patients present with a constellation of symptoms involving postural hypotension, blurred vision, nagging fatigue and short-term memory loss, the physician should look first for the presence of neurotoxins. The best approach is the use of the CS Test, which demonstrates these toxin mediated effects clearly;

2) While doing his or her level best to uncover the etiology of the toxin-linked pathogen at work in the patient, the physician should *proceed to treat the symptoms and obtain relief from them, regardless of the prevailing medical opinion about the cause of the disorder.*

Cathy P.'s healthy outcome provides a beacon of hope for patients like her. (How many are there? Millions?) Thriving today, she has gone back to work full-time. Her symptoms have diminished to the point that she's usually not even aware of them. Better yet, she no longer even complains about "how bad the cholestyramine tastes!"

For me, Cathy P.'s case provided a compelling example of why responsible physicians must do their best to ignore the "conventional wisdom"—especially when that wisdom is incorrect! Again and again during the past twenty years since the first diagnoses of this painful illness were made at Incline Village . . . CFS has left millions of sufferers without the help they needed and deserved.

Deductive Vs. Inductive
Reasoning: The Gospel According to Kuhn

In order to understand why American medicine has so far failed to perceive the growing threat from neurotoxin-mediated illnesses, we need to step back for a moment and talk about how—and why—scientific research in this country now finds itself in the crushing grip of a "paradigm" fueled by deductive and analytical thinking that is for the most part rigidly controlled by "Medical Establishment."

What is a "scientific paradigm?"

According to one of the great scientific historians of modern times, Thomas S. Kuhn, a "paradigm" is simply a structured, logically consistent way of "framing scientific reality" in order to analyze and define it.

As most contemporary thinkers will readily admit, the Modern Scientific Paradigm is based almost entirely on so-called "objective reasoning," in which investigators conduct endless observations of phenomena, then analyze those observations carefully in order to look for similarities in structure and outcomes that can be used to logically "prove" a given hypothesis. This approach relies on "deductive reasoning," a mode of thought in which general principles are deduced from repetitively predictable patterns of information.

Ruthlessly logical, the deductive approach allows scientists to document "complete objectivity" in their approach to scientific questions—even as they insist that their quantifiable results must be "reproducible." In addition, any new medical procedure must be duplicated by other researchers who carefully follow the protocols of the experiment.

Question: What's wrong with this "deductive paradigm," which at first glance appears to produce findings that are thoroughly objective and untainted by "subjectivity" on the part of the investigator? Believe it or not, only rarely is the "objective" clinical study actually objective. The taboo truth here is that bias actually *rules* science. Some of that bias may be intentional (especially when it comes to Lyme disease). But even in cases where investigators aren't "proving" an already agreed upon conclusion, achieving absence of bias in patient selection and interpretation of results is usually impossible.

You don't have to be a Ph.D. physicist to understand that the 20th Century phenomenon known as "quantum physics" has by now completely invalidated most of our traditional attitudes about "scientific objectivity" on the part of the observer.

Even a brief look at such epochal advances as Heisenberg's Uncertainty Principle, or Schrodinger's theories about the unpredictable movement of atomic particles is enough to shatter forever the myth about "objective observations freed from the taint of subjectivity." But such paradigms die hard . . . and while they live, they tend to control the shape of the scientific dialogue that unfolds around them—to say nothing of the millions of research dollars that flow to those scientists who remain safely within the "conventional wisdom" offered by the paradigm.

Thomas Kuhn seemed to be saying as much, in *The Structure of Scientific Revolutions*, when he pointed out:

> Philosophers of science have repeatedly demonstrated that more than one theoretical construction can always be placed upon a given collection of data. History of science indicates that, particularly in the early developmental stages of a new paradigm, it is not even very difficult to invent such alternates.

> But that invention of alternates is just what scientists seldom undertake except during the pre-paradigm stage of their science's development and at very special occasions during its subsequent evolution. So long as the tools a paradigm supplies continue to prove capable of solving the problems it defines, science moves faster and penetrates more deeply through confident employment of these tools.

The reason is clear. As in manufacture so in science —retooling is an extravagance to be reserved for the occasion that demands it. The significance of crises is the indication they provide that an occasion for retooling has arrived.

Bulletin: The "crisis" that Kuhn describes as the key to achieving a "major paradigm shift" in science is now upon us. Its effects are already being felt, and they are devastating. And they will only get worse, in the months and years immediately up ahead.

And the name of the crisis?

Chronic, neurotoxin-mediated illness.

Narrative of a
Journey through Hell
Sally Barkley's Story: Part II

After awakening on that terrible summer morning to find her hands and feet completely covered with grotesque blisters, Sally Barkley realized that her situation had become truly desperate.

As a trained laboratory scientist with a special gift for running tests that were remarkably accurate, Barkley had gained an outstanding reputation at both Harvard and Johns Hopkins, where she frequently conducted toxicology studies that surveyed minute quantities of exotic poisons.

"That was my claim to fame," she would tell me in 1999, "the fact that I was just so accurate. I love repetitive things! I love the things that other people find too mundane—like drawing up blood and getting it exactly the same every time, and adding all the reagents. And then with inhalation toxicology, always exposing the animals to the correct and exact and constant conditions all the time. It's my forte."

Given this background, it's easy to imagine Sally's frustration, when doctor after doctor explained that there was simply no way to account for her astonishing symptoms.

"It was torture," she said to me at one point. "How I wish someone had been able to tell me what was wrong with me! I was never sure . . . but I guess it started with the blisters. And yet, before the blisters even came up, I'd been complaining of some fatigue and an icy burning sensation on my skin.

"When I think back on it, I had also been complaining about fatigue and the inability to sleep at night. I went through a huge series of tests, and it got down to where they just couldn't figure out what was going on.

"They were accusing me of imagining things! And it got so bad that at one point, I even went to a psychiatrist. I think I had three sessions with him, and he finally said, 'There's nothing wrong with you, mentally.'"

Physically, however, Sally Barkley was falling apart. Here's her description of what it was like, year after year, to live in the "Hell" that is Chronic Fatigue.

I was tested for lupus and multiple sclerosis, along with Lyme disease and brucellosis. I can't even name them all. They went through all the exotic diseases. But the blistering, I think, is when it truly came to a head and everything started to go downhill for me.

I started having respiratory problems that were likened to pneumonia, but it wasn't pneumonia. I developed skin problems that looked like fungal diseases, but never came out in the culture. I had an inability to sleep, diarrhea, incontinence, chest pain, headaches, a ringing in my ears. It just went on, and the muscle pain was just excruciating, absolutely.

I also had temper tantrums and changes in mood. I had an inability to concentrate. I couldn't read and I couldn't add. That was probably the most devastating thing to me. The day I realized that I couldn't add. I couldn't add two and two. Awful, awful, awful.

Then I started having car accidents. Little ones, running over curbs. Hitting fences. Getting startled easily, and sensitive to light. Just on and on. And I was diagnosed in 1992. And I suppose this

had a lot to do with the fact that they couldn't come up with any
better name. They called it "fibromyalgia." And by that point, I
had been getting routine and regular shots of cortisone, I believe.
And my skin was changing colors.

Well, I'm a redhead and redheads don't truly tan. We burn
and then we might get a little bit of a light tan, but not something
that someone with dark skin would get. And I was as brown as the
dirt! I was swollen. My face and my hands . . . everything was
swollen. And I'd go on ten-day prednisone treatments that would
bring it down, just temporarily, and then it would go up again.

I couldn't sit still because I hurt so badly. My husband would
have to pick me up out of bed to help me get to the bathroom. Or
just to get off the bed. If he wasn't around because he was off at
work or something, I could roll out of bed, but I'd be on my hands
and knees and I'd be lucky to make it to the bathroom.

•   •   •

While the Search
For a Cure Goes Forward . . .
Let's Get Busy Treating the Patients!

After more than a decade of physcial and emotional misery, a
desperate Sally Barkley finally rang my office telephone in the
fall of 1998.

"Can you help me, Dr. Shoemaker? I'm sick and tired of being offered antidepressants . . . and I'm sick and tired of being
told that I need a psychiatrist. I've heard that you've got a new
approach to chronic fatigue. Is that true?"

"Yes, ma'am. I'm convinced that CFS is a neurotoxin-illness,
even if the toxins are produced internally. I also suspect that
we're confronting a new kind of illness with this disease—maybe
a virus with the uncanny ability to actually become part of human
DNA. Or maybe a chemical that we ourselves make is causing
the illness. Whether that chemical is programmed genetically or
not, I don't know.

"But those are only theories. I'm much more interested in results. You need to take a test for Contrast Sensitivity. If it shows a deficit, I think my treatment protocol can help you."

When she took the CS test and her results came up highly positive, Sally didn't waste any time. She began taking the standard cholestyramine regimen, starting right away.

The first two weeks were difficult. "Everything ached," she grimly recalls. "I was so weak that I could hardly get out of bed, and my tongue felt like it was on fire. But I was absolutely determined to stay the course, and in the end, that decision paid off."

Two weeks after she began taking this simple medication, Barkley's energy started to return. The debilitating "brain fog" began to lift. Suddenly she found that she could enjoy a long walk—even go horseback riding—without being "wiped out for the next three days."

"I can walk again!" she told me during a recent follow-up call. "I can go to the mall with my daughter, without being in excruciating pain. I've gone horseback riding twice recently, and not been incapacitated for two weeks, as I know I would have been, had I tried to do that prior to taking this medication.

"Why, I can even drive an automobile again! I drove 300 miles today, doing inspections on my job. I'm really feeling good now. I do not hurt. Oh, I know I'm still sick. I still have trigger-point pain, for example, and some other nagging symptoms. But these are minor.

"The really important thing is that I sleep well at night now. My life is normal, and I couldn't wish for much more."

A couple of months later, Sally called me about comments her daughter shared. She described how—as a four- and five-year-old—she had often jogged with her energetic mother to a nearby country store.

"Those were special times for me," Sally quoted her daughter, "and I've felt pretty sad, because my mother hasn't been able to run with me like that for the past ten years. She was always too sick. But do you know what?

"We did it yesterday! Thank you very much!"

First, Treat the Patient. . . .

Whenever I picture Sally Barkley on horseback, galloping across some verdant meadow near her home in Tampa, Fla., I find myself more convinced than ever about the vital role that clinicians can play in diagnosing—and then effectively treating —illnesses that have so far defied medical definition.

Unlike most of the "scientific heavyweights" in the academic research centers, the all-important Family Practitioner is perfectly positioned to take the knowledge gained directly from patients in the consulting room and run with it.

By *listening hard to patients* (always the key to a successful diagnosis), the clinician can often pinpoint the kinds of telling details—such as Cathy P.'s "sore neck"—that will lead to new breakthroughs in treatment.

For too many years, medical research in this country has been relegated to the big university think tanks and the government labs. Fueled by the big dollars of Big Science, and controlled by well-connected careerists eager to cozy up to political power, American medical research has lost its true focus: that suffering patient out there in the waiting room.

Instead of asking "why" a patient's illness doesn't seem to fit our preconceived categories, which is precisely what has happened with Chronic Fatigue Syndrome, we need to treat the patient now, and worry about the medical mysteries later.

After treating more than a thousand victims of Chronic Fatigue, Chronic Lyme Disease, Sick-Building Syndrome and several other forms of neurotoxin-mediated illness, I'm convinced as never before that the CS Test is a superbly effective diagnostic tool for pinpointing the presence of destructive bio-toxins in brain tissue.

I'm also convinced—along with Cathy P., Sally Barkley and all the others—that cholestyramine is the best way to begin relieving symptoms and thus allowing these stressed-out, long-suffering patients to get on with their lives.

Relieving suffering and healing the sick . . . how's *that* for a revolutionary medical concept, here in the America of the 21st Century?

Toxins, Chronic Soft Tissue Injury And Fibromyalgia

Pocomoke, MD –June, 1999 / September, 2000

It's one of the murkiest, most difficult to define conditions in all of medicine.

And maybe that's why the medical name for it keeps changing.

Once known as "non-articular rheumatism," the chronic muscle pain experienced by millions of Americans became "trigger-point pain" back in the 1980s, after physicians noticed that applying pressure to a tender point would leave many patients hurting for hours. Within a few years, however, this trigger-point condition had metamorphosed into "myofasciitis." But that nomenclature didn't last long, either—because "itis" means "inflammation," and it turned out that most victims of this disorder didn't have that.

Enter "fibromyalgia," which by the early 1990s had become the latest buzzword for a condition that seemed to be permanent. During endless symposia and continuing education meetings, physicians were coached to tell their patients that the disorder could not be cured, and that their trigger-point pain was some-thing they would have to "learn how to live with." Is it any won-der that for most patients, this excruciating condition gradually came to dominate their waking hours?

In the end, of course, "fibromyalgia" became nothing less than a medical industry. The rheumatologists spent many hours trying to discover an "autoimmune" cause for the illness, while the anesthesiologists were busy injecting trigger points with steroids and Novocaine. The neurologists reached for their prescription pads, since regular doses of amitriptyline and other antidepressants (not to mention Neurontin) helped to provide patients with lots of restorative "Stage IV" sleep, a major factor in reducing chronic bodily pain.

Oh, sure, these antidepressant medications *do* seem to help a few patients. And a few other sufferers undoubtedly gain a measure of relief from peripheral therapies such as exercise, massage, vitamins and bee-venom treatment—along with dietary and other lifestyle alterations aimed at combating the effects of this strange malady on the human body.

What the drug-prescribers and the lecturers at the crowded symposia failed to grasp, however, was fibromyalgia's true identity—as a neurotoxin-mediated syndrome.

Meanwhile, the lawyers were also helping to complicate the picture by introducing yet another name for the misery the doctors couldn't fix. They called it "chronic soft tissue injury," or CSTI, and they argued persuasively that it often follows a high-speed auto accident.

All too often, they also used CSTI to justify expensive, unnecessary tests—along with endless physical therapy and chiropractic bills at which the insurance companies understandably blanched, but then eventually paid. Question: Why does chronic pain so often become "disability," when someone else is paying the bills?

Because my own continuing interest in sports medicine had given me a chance to provide "expert witness" testimony in numerous chronic muscle pain cases, the Maryland Automobile Insurance Fund had routinely tapped my services over the years. Again and again, I'd found myself gazing at a photo of a barely scratched fender, before reading a report in which a rear-ended driver was claiming "permanent severe injuries requiring surgery, along with continuing therapies and medicine."

Ludicrous or not, the cases often wound up in front of a judge and jury, with the plaintiff's attorney solemnly intoning: "Your Honor, my client clearly had mild degenerative arthritis before the accident, but she rarely experienced any pain. Since the accident, however, her life has been sheer misery! She can't work, and she needs psychiatric help. And as for her marriage . . . well, I can assure you that any kind of physical intimacy is simply out of the question!"

As you might expect, the chiropractors testifying for the plaintiffs had a field day. While their "surface EMGs" and related machinery buzzed and clattered, the "deep-muscle therapists" were giving "soothing massages" that lasted at least an hour. All things considered, however, these opportunists still offered better dollar-value to their clients than the physicians—most of whom quickly grew weary of listening to patient complaints about "excruciating pain," especially when nothing abnormal turned up on x-rays. Their lack of empathy was easy to understand, though, since the tests were always "inconclusive," and most patients had a possible hidden agenda (and a not-so-hidden attorney who would be "calling soon").

But now and then, the patient's symptoms were easier to identify. Some patients displayed clear-cut muscle atrophy, for example, and others could point to trigger-point sites that were almost palpable. Frequently, even a gentle push on a tiny piriformis muscle (located inside the gluteus muscle, on the outside of the buttock) could set off an attack of classic sciatic pain.

If the piriformis had gone into spasm, so that it pinched the sciatic nerve where the latter left the pelvis, the pain would radiate down the patient's leg. Sciatica? No doubt from the accident! Toss in a "bulging disk" (spotted during a $1,500 MRI), and bingo!, you could easily claim a terrible "exacerbation of a pre-existing condition."

Now add "PT sessions" (or more chiropractors) three times a week at $125 a pop, featuring those exciting new machines that throw sparks and even an occasional convincing blue flame, and some practitioners could ride this therapeutic pony for months on end . . . instead of merely showing the patient how to stretch the affected muscle a bit and driving off the "sciatica" without further fuss.

Another type of chronic misery involved so-called "chest pain from trigger points," which usually occurred at costochondral junctions, or rib-sternum joints. All too often, this symptom led to an expensive "look-see" heart catheterization, as the front-line practitioner asked himself: "How else can we be . . . *sure?*" But the list of impossible-to-define ailments certainly doesn't stop here. What about all those shoulder and neck pains? Surely they require MRI scans, carpal tunnel evaluations, EMGs and frequent "multiple consultations!" And if the "injury" occurred on the job, why so much the better: Now Workmen's Comp is involved!

Long experience shows clearly that when "back pain" won't go away, the vocational counselors (hired by the payor insurance companies) will appear as if by magic . . . and the private investigators with their long lenses will soon be on the scene to snap revealing photos of back-injured patients hefting 50-pound sacks of dog food along the driveway.

The bottom line here is that physicians simply don't *like* dealing with chronic soft injury patients. The paperwork is endless, and the questions from patients impossibly lengthy and complicated. Lots of forms to fill out and lots of referrals—who needs them? And besides, isn't it a truism that once the lawsuit (aka, the "green poultice") is settled, many of these afflictions seem to be cured overnight?

There's no doubt that working with these patients can be difficult at times. But you can also learn a great deal from them— which is precisely what happened in the case of Carlane Burns. She's a hard-working technician at the local waste water treatment facility, and it was her bad luck to get highway broad-sided in 1993. On the other hand, she was lucky in another way: she *did* survive a 55-mile-an-hour automobile crash . . . even if she wound up with knee pain, shoulder pain, back pain, neck pain and lots of trigger-point pain as a result.

My regular treatment regimen helped to ease Carlane's piriformis and chest-wall pain, but she still hurt. And it was interesting to discover—given what finally happened in her case—that I had written the phrase "chronic soft tissue injury" on her chart soon after I began treating her.

Before Carlane, another high-velocity accident victim had already taught me that some patients of this kind tend to develop a chronic, neurotoxin-like illness after being injured in auto accidents. I found that bizarre. What was the neurotoxin, I wondered. Wouldn't it have to be an internally produced, or "endogenous" neurotoxin?

From the beginning, Carlane's symptoms were familiar. They included fatigue, muscle aches, cramps, non-anatomic distribution of tingling, headache, memory loss, blurred vision and sensitivity to bright light. "It's really terrible," she told me, describing that last symptom. "Most of the time, I feel like I'm living in a cave."

Intrigued by her list of symptoms, I asked Carlane to take a Contrast Sensitivity test, and I wasn't terribly surprised when the results turned out positive. She was suffering from a neurotoxin-mediated illness! Moving quickly, I started her on the CSM regime, and sure enough, her symptoms evaporated after three weeks. At the same time, her FACT scores returned to normal.

Next step: I stopped the CSM. And why? It was simple. I knew that if Carlane's toxins had been exogenously acquired, then the cholestyramine would have cured her. But if the acquisition was endogenous, the toxins would begin to build up in her system again, as soon as I halted the administration of CSM.

Sure enough, she returned to my office after three weeks instead of the scheduled four.

"I couldn't wait any longer, Dr. Shoemaker! Everything is getting worse. The headache and the neck ache came back first, followed by the cough and the abdominal pain. It was just like when I had my gallbladder taken out. Then a few days ago, I got lost in the grocery store. That's when I knew for sure 'it' had come back.

"I hate that [CSM] powder—but I hate hurting all the time worse!"

I quickly discovered that her FACT scores had dipped again, almost to their pre-treatment level. There could be no other reasonable explanation for the falloff in her Contrast Sensitivity. During the next few months, Carlane was able to regain her health and maintain her improvement by taking two scoops of CSM one day and three scoops the next. And the cost? About $1 daily. Affordable and easy on the body, CSM is a therapy that will *work* . . . at least until something better comes along!

I was pleased with Carlane's progress, but the question remained: what was going on here? Intent on answering that question, I turned again to one of the country's best medical librarians—my friend Russell Kujan at the Maryland Med-Chi Library. He did his usual superlative job during a wide-ranging literature search for "endogenous toxins." But he came up with nothing. What to do? Was I being far-fetched, to speculate that CSM might somehow be helping auto accident victims? It seemed too unbelievable to believe . . . and yet the results spoke for themselves.

But then came a breakthrough. Once again, I managed to find a key clue to a neurotoxin puzzle by studying the medical literature on obesity.

The article was entitled: "Ciliary neurotrophic factor and weight loss." And what was a "neurotrophic factor," exactly? Interestingly enough, this chemical—when infused via special catheter into the brains of patients with Alzheimer's and Huntington's chorea—somehow stimulated the growth of neural tissue at the site of damaged brain cells.

Even more surprising was the fact that patients who received these infusions also developed "trigger-point pain" and "diffuse aching." And when the infusion was stopped, the pain went away. Start it up again, but at a lower rate, and the pain returned

. . . *also* at a lower rate. This was too much! Somehow, I was getting a "dose response curve" for a trophic factor associated with fibromyalgia pain.

On second thought, the biochemical sequence made sense. Was this phenomenon any different, really, from the way in which a maple tree sends up "watersprouts" after its trunk is cut? Wasn't this the same kind of process in which small growths of nerves (neuromas) form at the site of damaged nerves? Why *wouldn't* a nerve that had been damaged in an auto accident of sufficient velocity release a healing compound? Was TNF involved, perhaps? Probably not, since there was no Herxheimer. . . .

As I thought about the problem, I took a look at the scars on my own hands, where saws and beams and falling glass had sliced up more than a few nerves over the years. I had cut through lots of neurons, yet I had no trigger points or chronic pain or fibromyalgia to show for it.

All I could do was assume that the velocity of these auto accidents had something to do with the systemic nature of the problem . . . and that trauma-killed nerves didn't release neurotrophic factors in the same way that merely damaged nerves did.

Is cutting a neuron in half a different event, biochemically speaking, than severely bruising it to the point where repairs become impossible?

My friend Ken Hudnell remained more than a little skeptical about my hypothesis. He told me that I'd need a lot more data than just a few cases, if I hoped to convince a skeptical scientist about the reality of "endogenous neurotoxins." I agreed . . . and took immediate steps to have the office staff call in about 20 patients who'd been diagnosed with fibromyalgia. Sure enough, all displayed neurotoxin symptoms. They also carried the FACT deficit.

A trial lawyer of my acquaintance seemed especially excited by my findings.

"Are you telling me that my insurance company won't be paying hundreds of thousands of dollars for fibromyalgia claims any more?"

These days, I perform FACT testing on auto accident victims on the first day they present for evaluation. I ask the same questions about neurotoxin symptoms at the two-week follow-up and at one month, as well. Routinely, the symptoms appear, the FACT scores come up as "Failed," and I offer CSM therapy. What a shame that eight of my first ten "plaintiff patients" refused the treatment!

"Dr. Shoemaker, if my lawyer says I'm cured of my pain, I don't have a case. He told me that CSM wasn't an 'established treatment' yet. Can I have a referral for my orthopedist, please?"

(None of the "defendant patients" refused treatment, by the way.)

So what do we have here?

Answer: Chronic soft tissue injury is simply another example of how "habitat-change leads to chronic neurotoxin-mediated illness." Only this time, the "habitat destruction" is internal, and not visible until the damage has been done.

Startled by this discovery, I began to wonder: How many *more* examples of complex chemistry gone awry would I be able to find and prove?

As my researches continued, I was greatly encouraged by a high-profile case that provided credibility for my "Endogenous Neurotoxin Theory" of chronic soft tissue injury. The case involved one of Maryland's top defense attorneys—and it demonstrated how finding the right *subject* for a treatment regimen can be almost as important as the effectiveness of the treatment, itself. (Think of Androcles pulling the thorn from the lion's paw, or the shaman relieving the pain of an opposing chief with willow bark—the *salix* species—and you can see how curing a VIP brings instant credibility to the healer!)

This particular treatment began when Attorney Russell Dashiell sent me a case to review. The patient had been through a low-velocity accident that should not have left her with significant injuries. Yet she presented with the clearly defined symptoms of a neurotoxin-mediated illness—and that condition was in fact later proved by Mr. Dashiell to have been caused by a second, unreported accident.

As I prepared to testify, my interest in the case grew quickly: this would be the first time my theories about chronic soft tissue injury would be presented in court.

But then the unexpected happened, when Russell's paralegal professional—Irene Aubain—read my summary in preparation for the trial.

"Russell . . . he's describing *me!*"

Ms. Aubain was about to become the medical VIP who would be the right subject for my CSTI theory.

Irene had been seriously injured, after being struck from behind during a 1998 accident. In the months that followed, however, she began to develop the same symptoms as all my *other* neurotoxin-afflicted patients. No medical treatment seemed to help. She knew a great deal about the treatment of automobile accident-inflicted injuries, yet could find no relief from the after-affects of her own. And she seemed to be getting worse by the day.

One of the things I like most about Russell is that he's a history buff. He often participates in Civil War reenactments, for example, and he loves to apply the lessons of history to contemporary problems.

"Irene," he told his suffering paralegal at one point, "you have to remember that many advances in medicine must have sounded quite bizarre to the practitioners of their day. Imagine how many soldiers in the Civil War might have survived—if only the surgeons had washed their hands or changed their blood-soaked coats. Imagine how many *wouldn't* have died of dysentery (by far the most efficient killer of those who survived combat) if water supplies had been kept clean, or food had been refrigerated.

"Think about all those brave pioneer women who survived the trek to California—only to die in childbirth from an infectious disease caused by the lack of basic hygiene. Remember Louis Pasteur, Irene—and give this man's treatment a chance to work for you. I've known Ritchie Shoemaker for years, and he doesn't propose any medical theory that he can't back up with hard facts!"

To her credit, Irene listened. She was nervous when she arrived at my office, but she *got* there. And her CS score quickly told me what I needed to know: she displayed a typical deficit associated with neurotoxins. She was struggling with all of the other symptoms of chronic toxin illness, as well. Yet her only exposure had been the accident!

This was the most clearly defined case of soft tissue injury that I'd ever seen, and I was delighted when she quickly agreed to get started on CSM.

Irene's improvement was startling, to say the least. Her CS deficit improved within five days, and her 15 different symptoms began to melt away.

Will Irene achieve full recovery with CSM? Only time will tell. At this point, she's content simply to know that her health has been restored, and she's continuing to take cholestyramine for maintenance.

Another interesting aspect of this case was the way that Irene began to gain a new perspective on her illness, as one practitioner after another failed to provide her with the relief she sought. Baffled and endlessly frustrated, she nonetheless managed to keep battling. Like Diane Stephenson, Irene is a woman of character, and she somehow managed to endure both the ravaging effects of her illness *and* the ineffective, frequently indifferent medical treatment she received. Irene had suffered through a public silence—although the depth of her loss of quality of life haunted her during every waking hour.

Like diabetes and heart failure, chronic soft tissue injury never takes a day off. Knowing that, Irene is doubly grateful for the fact that she can now spend Saturday afternoons working in her garden and doing what "normal" people do, without suffering the endless fatigue and muscle aches that used to accompany such efforts. She's also pleased that her mental faculties have been restored. Imagine wandering through the supermarket, struggling to remember the ingredients you need for supper!

Irene's day-to-day aching and the expensive therapies required to blunt her unbearable chronic pain (along with brain fog and enveloping fatigue) had been caused by someone else smashing into her automobile. How could the legal system compensate anyone adequately for the loss of years of normal life?

Irene's medical future remains uncertain, and I'm convinced that she'll need to take CSM daily for an indefinite length of time—or at least until another, more effective therapy arrives on the scene. Meanwhile, she continues to demonstrate her courage in the face of an unremitting and progressive illness. At the same time, CSM has restored the vitality and love of life she had enjoyed before her accident.

As you might expect, I'm deeply grateful that Irene has now joined the ranks of hundreds of my patients who've gained life-enhancing benefits from CSM therapy.

I'm also pleased that Russell Dashiell never doubted my work. I suspect that he will be among the vanguard of attorneys who are already beginning to revolutionize the way in which chronic soft tissue injury is treated in the courtroom. Just imagine, as an attorney, being able to identify physiologic correlates of chronic pain with CS testing . . . and then *confirming* those findings with the Heidelberg laser-doppler device.

For the first time in the history of American litigation, we won't have to argue about whether or not a patient's chronic pain is the result of an accident! Nor will we need to quibble over alleged "injury exaggerations" by the plaintiff. How much money will the American insurance industry be able to save on unnecessary physical therapy, on chiropractics, on massages and acupuncture and vitamin therapy and cortisone shots from anesthesiologists and chronic pain therapists?

How many millions of dollars lost annually to "employment disability" will be recovered . . . and how large will the savings be to the ordinary consumer, who no longer has to pay those sky-high insurance rates?

A word to the wise, then: If you or your loved ones have the symptoms and find out that you display the CS deficit, find a doctor who will prescribe CSM and start treatment! Find a friend with "fibromyalgia" and gently ask about other neurotoxic symptoms. Then insist—gently, gently—that they take a FACT and also pay a visit to "chronicneurotoxins.com" on the World Wide Web.

Don't be surprised if skeptical friends shake their heads. So what? The key thing to remember here is that you've got a real chance to enjoy your life again.

For chronic soft tissue injury-sufferers everywhere, the news today is very good.

Your pain doesn't have to last forever.

You didn't ask for this misery—so why put up with it any longer?

chapter 25

Reflection

Lenny Wein. A Survivor—Thanks to Daily Cholestyramine—Was He a Victim Of Genetic, Endogenous Neurotoxins?

Stuart, FL –June, 1998
Pocomoke, MD –August, 2000

How effective is cholestyramine at cleansing the human body of debilitating toxins?

Ask that question of 54-year-old Florida retiree Lenny Wein, and he'll tell you that without regular daily doses of this common, therapeutic substance, he probably wouldn't be able to function —let alone enjoy his "early retirement" on the surf-lapped beaches of tropical Florida.

He called me from Stuart, Florida following my research effort there in June, 1998. The reference to CSM, in treatment of patients exposed to toxic forming dinoflagellates in the St. Lucie River, caught his eye.

"I was diagnosed 20 years ago with an obscure disease known as Charcot-Marie-Tooth Syndrome [CMT]," says the former print shop operator from New York City. "This is the most common form of an inherited neuropathy. It results from a mutation in a gene that produces a neurotoxin that eats away at the protective sheath [myelin] around nerves that run to muscles and joints. When the nerves die, the muscles connected to them will soon expire as well.

"When the doctors explained how my illness slowly atrophies your muscles, they told me I'd soon be confined to a wheelchair.

But I'm still walking 20 years later, even though I do use a cane.

"I never would have believed that developing a *cholesterol* problem would lead to stopping the progression of my CMT. But that's what happened. Amazingly, when I started taking cholestyramine for my high cholesterol, it began filtering the CMT-related toxins right out of my body.

"As a result, I'm not confined to a chair, and I'm very grateful for that. I've been taking the cholestyramine—in the form of Questran—for more than a decade. Along with removing the cholesterol in my body, I'm convinced that it also removes the neurotoxins produced by my disease. I feel sure there is more than just a genetic defect involved in my illness . . . and I'm astonished daily by the way that I seem to be defying the natural history of this disease.

"Believe me, I've consulted with many of the country's top CMT experts—and they're just as amazed as I am."

Like most patients who suffer from neurotoxin-mediated illnesses, Lenny spent several frustrating years listening to doctors tell him that he had "arthritis"—or that the symptoms he began discovering at around age 30 were "all in his head."

"When I started losing feeling in my hands, I went to the doctors," he recalls today. "They told me I had bilaterally compressed nerves, and they said that was the reason my hands were getting somewhat deformed. They were also telling me I had arthritis. It was kind of bizarre, but that sort of diagnosis is not uncommon with this disease.

"A lot of people have to go through numerous physicians, including neurologists, who will misdiagnose this kind of illness. But once I was [accurately] diagnosed, I felt happier. Before that, I'd been told that it was all in my head, and that I should go see a psychiatrist!"

Cheerful and easygoing, Lenny Wein says he doesn't resent the fact that he got stuck with a chronic illness, even though the disorder is slowly destroying the muscles in his hands, feet and legs.

"Naw, I don't think I got screwed!" he told me with a booming laugh. "This kind of rare disease is just one of things that can happen in life. And you have to take care of it. I can tell you without exaggeration that if I go two days without any [CSM] powder, I can feel it. I can actually *feel* my muscles getting weaker and weaker. And soon my feet will begin to tingle. Hey, I'm probably the most compliant CSM-taker you'll ever meet, doc!"

"It could be a lot worse, and I feel very fortunate that this isn't one of the fatal neuromuscular diseases. I'm going to die from something else, not this!

"I have a very good outlook toward things. I continue to do whatever I can, and even probably what I *shouldn't* be doing!"

Although Lenny is convinced that his nerves are being attacked daily by toxins released from his Charcot-Marie-Tooth, his doctors haven't been able to pinpoint the biochemistry involved. Nor is there a cure for his illness. But these theoretical questions about "why" don't seem very important, at his stage of life. Today he says he's simply grateful for the fact that he can stroll down the beach at Palm City and watch the seagulls skim along the Atlantic wave tops.

"I give the credit to cholestyramine," he says candidly. "The stuff *works*, and that's all I care about!"

Struggling to Reach a Patient

For a medical doctor, there's no satisfaction on earth quite like the feeling that comes from helping patients cope with illnesses and then to have them thrive. Such had been the case with the always upbeat and affable Lenny Wein.

But what happens when the patient refuses to accept the "doc's" advice—and chooses instead to go right on suffering needlessly?

Believe me, that's a recipe for enormous frustration.

Let me tell you about a recent treatment scenario that was fraught with legal and ethical complications. It happened a year or so ago, when a college junior—escorted by her worried mom —arrived at my Pocomoke office for a consult. Was this young woman suffering from chronic Lyme? That diagnosis seemed more and more likely as I listened to the unhappy catalogue of her complaints, which included fatigue, muscle ache, shortness of breath, sensitivity to bright light, cough and much more.

Interestingly, this patient's family history included a father, an aunt, a grandfather and a great-grandfather who at various times in their lives had labored with the same symptoms. Question: Was the college kid before me suffering from chronic Lyme . . . or from a classic case of genetically based CMT? How could I be sure? No, she didn't seem to have the highly arched foot or the other physical features that usually signaled the presence of CMT in older patients. . . .

Still, my troubled patient *did* display some of the other signs of CMT, including a "tingling" in her toes and hands and a weak hand-grip. But it was also true that she'd triggered two bands on her Western Blot blood test for Lyme!

Her CS test was far from ambiguous, however, and as soon as she saw her deficit-score, she agreed to begin taking CSM. Within two days, her improvement in strength had become obvious . . . although her muscles still ached. Her reaction to the CSM suggested a Herx-like event, so I started her on pioglitazone at once, even as I asked myself the unanswerable question: *Okay, has she got CMT or Lyme?*

There was only one way to find out: by giving her a special blood test (costing more than $1,000) for CMT. But she didn't want to take it. She simply couldn't bear to face the truth of her condition, whatever it might be.

She continued to get better during the next couple of days. Ironically, however, her improvement only served to alarm her: did this huge gain for her health *also* mean that she had CMT, and would she be condemned to that painful condition for life? Obviously intent on remaining "normal" in her own mind, she balked at the blood test—not at the cost but at the implications: "Doctor . . . I don't want to *know* if I have CMT!"

Two more days passed—and then she refused any further medication.

"No, I won't take any more of that powder."

She knew that her grip-strength had improved from 18 to 28 in her dominant hand in less than a week. Her non-dominant hand had also gained power, surging from 16 to 26. Her CS scores were improving . . . even as the tingling faded away and her light-sensitivity receded. "You're getting better!" I told the distraught young woman. "You aren't as fatigued as you were. Your muscles ache less. The headaches are easing . . . how about staying with the treatment until you feel like your old self?"

She hesitated, and I could see the pain in her eyes. Then: "Sorry, doctor . . . but I won't take this. If I get worse, maybe I'll come back."

Was it Lyme? I don't think so. Does CMT cause a Herx? Since she hasn't taken the repeat test, I don't have the standard drop-off in Contrast Sensitivity to prove that assertion.

Deeply frustrated with the outcome of this case, I later grew more philosophical about a patient's right to know (or *not* to know) her genetically programmed destiny.

As I reflected on her decision, I recalled several studies that had been conducted soon after the development of a blood test for Huntington's chorea, a fatal disease. The studies showed that most of the patients at risk for that illness had chosen not to take the new test. It's also interesting to remember that medical science recently put the finishing touches on a new blood test for Alzheimer's. That test isn't 100 percent accurate, of course. Still, I wonder how many of us would be willing to take it?

Question for Lenny Wein: Got any suggestions on how I can reach this kid? How can I convince her that even if she's been sentenced to an inexorable, genetic wasting disease, CSM will put the brakes on most of her misery and allow her to live a healthy, virtually pain-free life . . . the same life that *you've* been enjoying all these years!

Getting behind the CDC

Atlanta, GA –1997 to 2000

> Q. *What's Wrong with Medical Research in America?*
> A. *All Too Often, It's Controlled by the Bureaucrats*
> *Who Run the "Centers for Discussion Crushing!"*

It's one of the most revered scientific acronyms in all of American life, CDC.

What are the U.S. Centers for Disease Control and Prevention, if not the citadel of American medical research . . . as well as the headquarters for the mightiest array of disease-fighters on Planet Earth?

Hoping to test those attitudes among the lay public, I recently asked 30 of my family practice patients in small-town Maryland to take a brief quiz designed to test the credibility of the Atlanta-based science monolith, which now receives more than 300 million federal tax dollars each year.

I wanted to see what would happen if I added the phrase "according to the CDC" to a series of obviously inaccurate statements, such as:

• New research confirms that contrails from high-flying jetliners are causing increased incidence of skin cancer in the United States;

- Children who are taught math by having flash cards rapidly shown to them tend to choose careers in science, rather than in liberal arts;
- Dietary cutbacks in fatty foods predispose patients to osteoporosis.

Even a quick glance at these "scientific observations" is enough to show that they're logically absurd, right?

But guess what happened when I added the single phrase "according to the CDC" to these off-the-wall conjectures?

You got it: once the CDC "seal of authority" had been attached, most of my quiz-takers assumed that these ludicrous statements were 100-percent accurate!

Although I readily admit that my study wasn't "controlled," or "double-blinded," or "randomized," or "age-sex-matched" (or "worthy of peer review," for that matter!), the results were nonetheless quite revealing about current attitudes toward the Big Science Bureaucracy in America.

The results showed that my patients were willing to believe just about *anything*, if it carried the all-important label marked "certified by the CDC." When our most hallowed institution proclaims a finding as "good science," it *is* good science. And why not? Aren't the people who conduct the experiments for the CDC among the nation's most qualified physicians and researchers?

Well, maybe some of them are . . . but what about the youthful interns who *also* work in these hallowed halls? For most lay people, they wear the same mantle of impeccable scientific authority . . . even though they haven't "earned their stripes" yet. Should they be treated with the same breathless reverence usually accorded their supervisors in Atlanta? *Of course not.*

Absurd or not, this same attitude of worshipful awe can also be seen in federal and state legislators who interact daily with CDC officials. Example: I won't soon forget a 1997 interview with U.S. Senator Barbara Mikulski (D-Md.) on the subject of *Pfiesteria*-related human illness in the mid-Atlantic region. After announcing that she would work to obtain funding for research on the predatory dinoflagellate, Senator Mikulski declared: "This issue is bigger than the individual states involved. We need to bring in the CDC—they're the best investigators in the world!"

As it turns out, however, ordinary individuals cannot actually "call in" the CDC—a lesson I learned the hard way in Florida, during efforts to help residents of that state cope with outbreaks of an unusual illness perhaps caused by mutant fungi near the Casteen Roads nursery site owned by Frank Fuzzell. (See Chapter Nine: "Chronicles From A Poisoned Landscape.") In fact, the official request must come from a state or federal agency . . . and preferably, from an agency involved in public health.

But when the Georgia-based brass decide to respond to these requests, they often ignore the most likely sources of information about health threats and epidemics. In the case of *Pfiesteria*, for example, those of us who were working on the front lines with patients expected that we'd soon be receiving phone calls from the Center.

It didn't happen. Of course, we also expected that the calls would be followed up by a door-to-door study of patterns of illness compared to patterns of exposure.

But that didn't happen, either. No outreach for "case identification" was ever performed. Still, the CDC did maintain a presence of sorts . . . but primarily as a mechanism aimed at funneling research monies toward selected academic practitioners! Trying to report a case of an acute *Pfiesteria* illness (*not* a mandatory reportable disease, by the way) often seemed to resemble a kind of bureaucratic gymnastic routine. Do I phone the Maryland DNR hotline? (Yes. But the reporting goes no further.) Do I call the Maryland Department of Health? (Yes . . . but no one answers the phone there.) Do I call the CDC directly, while bypassing Maryland and Virginia? No. Do I let myself become involved in bureaucratic in-fighting? (No.) And guess what happens?

"No new cases of *Pfiesteria* were reported to the CDC," that's what!

In the end, the CDC's case definition statements were invented by health officials who had never seen any *Pfiesteria* patients. As a result, "asthma-like conditions" were not included in the original case definition, because "no patients with wheezing were in the group reported to the Centers." Light sensitivity? They forgot.

The recent *Pfiesteria* epidemic in the mid-Atlantic region provides yet another compelling example of the negative consequences that can flow from the failure to communicate with the country's practicing physicians. After treating several patients who were suffering from this brand-new malady in 1997, I had written the first medical articles in the world's literature on *Pfiesteria* illness in humans acquired in the wild (not in a science laboratory, that is). I was also the first in the world to publish on successful treatment of chronic illness from *Pfiesteria*, in 1998.

But no one from Atlanta ever called . . . even though I could have shown them plenty of patients who stopped wheezing only after taking cholestyramine.

How could the nation's major "disease prevention" agency have chosen to ignore this key evidence of a new disease outbreak along our coastal waterways?

You can be sure that these esteemed national scientists—whose ranks do, indeed, include some of the best scientific minds in America—made very little, if any effort to gather information from practicing physicians who were actually treating patients.

As far as I'm concerned, that's a tragic oversight. Why not take advantage of the huge fund of experience accumulated by the nation's 450,000 practicing physicians . . . the highly trained health care providers who are out there practicing "bedside science" day in and day out? Why deprive the "bench scientists" of this important source of knowledge? Maybe both types of scientists could share skills. Researchers could access more data and physicians obtain more insight by working together.

In order to understand how the CDC's refusal to consult physicians on medical issues can distort public health policy, consider the recent flap over Dr. Jeffrey Koplan's recent and widely quoted article in the *Journal of the American Medical Association* (JAMA), an essay in which he came to some remarkably dubious conclusions about the "epidemic of obesity" in America. That study, of course, was widely quoted because —according to the CDC—our society is becoming too fat. Yet the Koplan study failed to control for amylose (a key carbohydrate that is partially metabolized by enzymes in human saliva), or for insulin, the hormone most responsible for making fat.

As most weight-loss experts will readily point out, the CDC approach to obesity in recent years has been based on measurements of body mass and weight (the Body-Mass Index, or BMI) that are entirely unreliable. At the same time, it ignores the confounding variables that come into play among the millions of citizens who follow "low-fat diets"—ineffective weight-loss programs that take the fat out of your cream cheese (for example) and then substitute corn syrup in order to make the spread palatable.

The CDC approach to this important public health issue also ignores the impact on weight-gain from cessation of smoking. What if they had subtracted out those patients in their analysis who had quit smoking? (Interestingly enough, the CDC's home state of Georgia ends up as the state in Koplan's paper with the greatest per-capita increase in obesity during recent years!)

My point is simply that such epidemics as obesity cannot be studied exclusively in the laboratory, merely by examining statistics. Health trends are analyzed best when practicing physicians provide reports to collaborating scientists like Dr. Ken Hudnell, who can focus solid clinical facts into well controlled studies.

This same kind of misleading science has also contributed to public perceptions of the "surging epidemic" of diabetes in our society. Sure, the numbers of adult onset diabetic patients are going up—and by 33 percent, according to the latest statistics. Yet the blame for that is inevitably placed not on the types of food we now emphasize in our diets, but on mere caloric intake. But what happens when a borderline diabetic is placed on a diet full of pasta, whole-wheat bread and low-fat foods? All at once, the patient is eating foods that instantly turn into sugar.

In reality, the major factor behind the recent "explosion" in diabetes is the fact that the medical *definition* of the disease has changed.

Almost overnight, a fasting-glucose score of 110 has become the marker for diabetes, compared to 125 in past years. (How many Americans would end up as "speeders," if the speed limit were lowered overnight? And how many geniuses would instantly materialize, if the definition of "genius" shrank from an IQ of 150 to 110?)

Let's stop saying, "Diabetes is surging"—and start admitting that our definitions are changing.

There's no doubt that the science bureaucrats at the CDC are significantly hampered by their failure to listen to the nation's physicians on public health matters. But the record also shows that this huge public health agency has been enormously effective, when it comes to investigating and then fighting infectious disease epidemics.

Take the recent, threatening epidemic of *ehrlichia*, for example. During that complicated scientific investigation, the CDC labs quite properly performed the elegant PCR research, and then published compelling scientific papers. The scientists who worked on that project were outstanding, and they did a terrific job.

In the same fashion, the agency earned high marks in recent years for its ground-breaking research on the epidemiology of hantavirus and the West Nile-like "Virus 2." In those investigations, the bench scientists were well-equipped to analyze the physiology of the pathogen and the process through which it was spread by disease vectors.

When the scientists at the CDC exit their laboratories and enter the realm of public health policy, however, they often stumble badly as a result of the distortions caused by their own bureaucratic and political identity.

The problem here is that American citizens in recent years have made the predictable mistake of placing their faith in scientific organizations based not on science but on politics. As many observers have noted, the government science bureaucracies have strayed from their original research-base and are no longer in touch with the kinds of public health issues confronted daily by the nation's primary care physicians.

Nor is there anything to suggest that this basic trend will soon be reversed. The cornerstone of the CDC initially was epidemiology, the study of patterns of illness that occur in populations of people. As for old-fashioned, door-to-door "shoe leather research"—well, the agency researchers simply won't investigate issues related to this aspect of medicine anymore. (These days they delegate that job to the states.) Besides, there simply isn't the *time*, these days, to do the road work that originally defined "epidemiology!"

Make no mistake: whenever "availability of funds" becomes the limiting factor in public health decision-making, you can be sure that medical and scientific judgments will soon begin to "follow the money." And since the CDC relies on public dollars —just like any other government agency—there's little doubt that the decisions made in Atlanta will factor in plans to keep those taxpayer-dollars flowing, regardless of the health issues involved.

Because the politicians who hold the CDC on this short string of grant money are primarily interested in pleasing the political lobbyists and the voters, primary physicians remain nearly voiceless on national health issues. Sure, the CDC publishes a weekly summary of reported diseases (MMWR). But we all know that the reporting forms on which these summaries are based demand significant amounts of time from physicians. In today's high-speed, HMO-dominated world of health care, how many doctors can afford to interrupt their labors in order to alert the agency to possible new illnesses? Forget it!

Let's face it: If a busy physician must choose between spending an hour filling out six Lyme disease reports or spending it on "quality time" with his family, chances are that the illness will wind up in the "underreported" category!

This continuing exclusion of practicing physicians from CDC decision-making is nothing less than a national outrage. Imagine the outcry, if some rural county in Maryland (Worcester County, let's say) unveiled a 20-year development plan that didn't include minorities, landowners or the medical profession. Obviously, any planning body that takes itself seriously must allow everyone a voice. The CDC deliberately excludes the "outliers" from having such a voice.

The record shows that the CDC is a highly conservative organization. Yet science depends on healthy skepticism—and on the willingness to constantly challenge the "conventional wisdom" as new information becomes available. If a new idea (such as the use of cholestyramine to treat *Pfiesteria*-related human illness syndrome) emerges from the daily practice of medicine, it should be evaluated on the basis of its merits. Instead, the CDC often regards a breakthrough of this kind as "outside the mainstream." All too often, in such situations, the Atlanta administrators end up telling reporters: "This idea is premature!"

That's precisely what took place in November of 1998, when the CDC declined to evaluate my protocols for the treatment of *Pfiesteria*. Without even bothering to investigate the matter, the agency brass chose to ignore this highly effective treatment method . . . a decision which left hundreds of U.S. *Pfiesteria* patients deprived of vital information that could have helped them in their struggle to win back their health. "Premature," indeed!

Of course, this was hardly the first time that the CDC had failed to respond effectively to a new disease outbreak. For more than a decade, in fact, physicians all across the South had been reporting Lyme cases in which the vector was the Lone Star (dog) tick, and not the more familiar and smaller deer tick. But the Atlanta experts had ignored this powerful evidence, while always insisting: "There is no such disease!"

If only the CDC had asked the Army what it knew in 1992 about Southern Lyme (Struggling to the Light, Chap 29).

Finally, after more than ten years of diligent research by physicians at the Medical College of Georgia, the CDC admitted the obvious: Lyme disease has a southern cousin, now known everywhere as "Southern Tick-Associated Erythema Migrans-Like Illness." (Wow! Is that a mouthful, or what?) That "newly discovered" disease is found today in South Carolina, Georgia, Alabama, Louisiana and Texas.

And what about Florida? These days, there's increasing evidence to show that the Sunshine State has the biggest Lyme population of all. A key factor in the Florida epidemic has been the presence of slow-burning fires in the Apalachicola swamps along the Florida-Georgia border, which has been driving disease-infected ticks out of the undergrowth for several years now.

But the hardest-fought bureaucratic battle over Lyme disease has taken place in the Northeast, and it happened because the CDC insisted on such rigid clinical definitions of the disease (including a five-band specific antibody response to the *Borrelia burgdorferi* bacterium, when only one band was needed) that it became impossible to give a CDC-authorized diagnosis to many clearly infected patients.

While the medical power figures in Atlanta continued to insist on the "Western Blot IGG" test as the most reliable indicator of the presence of *Borrelia,* primary care practitioners all across the country were shaking their heads. Hadn't many researchers, including a CDC-linked researcher in this field, Dr. Alan Steere, demonstrated again and again that blood-antibody tests simply weren't reliable as a diagnostic tool? In fact, the only really effective means of pinpointing the true presence of Lyme is based on a *clinical* diagnosis.

Like Dr. Steere, most practitioners long ago concluded that treatment with antibiotics must not be withheld, pending a blood test result. The record shows clearly that some patients don't get better when treated with antibiotics—and some with defined clinical criteria don't even show a positive blood test. (Contrast Sensitivity wasn't being used then.)

Recognizing these facts, a few doctors who were pioneers in

their own right began to treat Chronic Lyme patients with intravenous antibiotics for prolonged periods. Suddenly, insurance companies were facing claims of up to $10,000 a month for therapy. Is it any wonder that the big insurers soon began to demand "medical proof" of Lyme . . . or that the clinical definition of the illness was turned over to the academic scientists, including those affiliated with the CDC, rather than to the clinicians out in the field?

There's no doubt that the CDC's Lyme panels were stacked with scientists from the academic community—or that many of them had well-established reputations for being "anti-chronic Lyme." Meanwhile, the primary care docs may have well been told that they "need not apply." (Don't forget that first defensive-layer of the Appearance of Good Science: "Consensus!")

Suddenly, the order of the day was: "Publish, or your dominance will perish!" And the results were entirely predictable: The health insurance carriers soon wound up relying on "position papers" by influential academic scientists (according to the CDC?), especially when they made their "eligibiity" decisions on Lyme patients . . . rather than relying on the diagnoses of the doctors on the firing line of primary care medicine.

In the end, the perfect defense for denying a Lyme disease HMO-claim became: "This is not a Lyme case, according to the CDC definition." End of discussion, and quote-unquote. "The expert medical witness may leave the stand!"

In part because the CDC position plays such a major role in determining how health insurance claims are paid, this federal agency has gained enormous influence in U.S. public health policy. And why not? How can any investigator with new information hope to gain ground in the politics of science—when it's crystal clear that the Atlanta monolith will always respond by announcing: "If we say it isn't science, it isn't science!"

That attitude has transformed the CDC into the Centers for Discussion Crushing and Prevention (of new insights from ever taking hold, that is!).

And the CDC's failure to investigate Sick Building Syndrome has been equally egregious. In spite of clear and unequivocal data that show the neurotoxic effects of fungal toxins on millions of sick Americans, the government researchers have chosen to do nothing about this problem.

Did the feds ever convene a panel of scientists and practitioners who have actually treated this pathology? No. Did they consider the pioneering work of Dr. Eckhardt Johanning—the editor of two textbooks and many scientific papers—who has reported that fully 20 percent of the Sick Building patients he treated conventionally failed to improve . . . an outcome which clearly suggests a "chronic" effect?

And what about those persistent, documented reports of severe illness (and even death) from the toxins produced by the *stachybotrys*? After confronting this indisputable evidence, the CDC bureaucrats announced that "the causal link from the toxin mold to the illness has not been proven," and that "the hazards presented by molds that may contain mycotoxins should be considered the same as other common molds."

There's no need for alarm, either, because the same federal health experts have assured us that "large mold infestations can usually be seen or smelled." (Here's an analogy that will illustrate the logic of that last statement: "All snakes that are poisonous will rattle their tails before they strike—and any bites from those that *don't* are statistically insignificant!")

According to the CDC, no test can confirm an association between stachybotrys and health symptoms. The Atlanta bosses have spoken; what further need for discussion? Is there any doubt that the CDC Division of Bacterial and Mycotic Diseases would reject the Contrast Sensitivity data taken from our small cohort of stachy patients, as well? (See Chapter 20: "Getting Behind Sick Building Syndrome.") Look as the CDC position on Lyme, Pfiesteria, Stachybotrys, Sick Building Syndrome and Fuzzell's land-association illness; does anyone *not* see the pattern?

It's all rather frustrating and discouraging, but I'm convinced that the situation will begin to improve soon. Stay tuned . . . and watch for the coming changes in the "medical power pyramid," as a broad-based group of primary care physicians begins to make itself heard, even at the sharply pointed head of the pyramid! Increasingly, the demand for Contrast Sensitivity testing is going to be heard, as patients struggling with the painful symptoms of neurotoxin illness demand relief from their misery.

Eventually, the joined voices of patients cured by CSM therapy will trigger huge political demand. And that process will change research-funding methods, as well as attitudes. A new day is coming in American science, if only the "bedside scientists" can hang on a little while longer.

And please make a note: You heard it here first!

●   ●   ●

**Bulletin . . . This Just in from
The "Miracles Do Happen" Department . . .**

The CDC heard us. Amazing!

Is there actually a reason to hope that the Centers for Discussion Crushing might be willing to listen to reason and logic . . . even if the message happens to come from outside their own Atlanta-based headquarters?

Maybe. I still want to believe that the CDC listens dispassionately to scientific data, presented credibly.

That was my first reaction, anyway, when I discovered in June of 2000 that the Center's management team had back-tracked on several earlier decisions . . . in order to officially recognize the importance of Contrast Sensitivity in the neurotoxic history and diagnosis of *Pfiesteria*-related human illness syndrome.

Not surprisingly—given the number of patients I'd already treated and the amount of research I'd already done—*Pfiesteria* turned out to be the first chronic, neurotoxin-mediated illness to ever be accepted by the CDC. After years of disrespect and indifference from Atlanta and numerous public health departments up and down the East Coast, things suddenly began to change.

The great CDC flip-flop got started after the Morbidity and Mortality Weekly Report, or MMWR (a time-honored publication that specializes in infectious disease patterns in the U.S.) devoted a special section on May 5, 2000 to *Pfiesteria*. The bottom line: the agency had found "no cases" in 1998–99!

Was this some kind of zany joke? The report seemed laughable . . . yet it carried the agency's authoritative imprimatur, right there on the cover: "According to the CDC . . ."

Some of my veteran *Pfiesteria* patients enjoyed a hearty laugh as they skimmed the report and read about the non-existence of the illness that had brought them to my office in the first place.

Amazing, but true! Apparently, the *Pfiesteria* coverup was firmly in place—both at the state and the national level.

Back in March, you may remember, the State of Maryland had convened a special *Pfiesteria* conference at St. John's College in Annapolis. The purpose: to review all the latest findings (as of early 2000) on the increasing threat of human illness caused by *Pfiesteria*.

When I learned about the approaching conference in early March, I immediately called Ken Hudnell. "Can you believe this, Ken? They don't want anybody to know about human illness. They refuse to confirm the fish kills that are taking place all around us, and they won't tell the public about the high *Pfiesteria* counts in known attack-zones.

"Ken, you need to attend that meeting. They won't invite me to speak, that is for sure, so you've got to speak out."

Ken agreed, and then got busy on the telephone. Suddenly, Dr. Rob Magnien was inviting him to give one of the lectures on the final day (once the reporters were safely out of town, that is). Fortunately, Dr. Ramsdell and Dr. Burkholder had already made it clear to Dr. Magnien that Ken should be allowed to present our *Pfiesteria* data to the conference.

Like Marc Antony addressing the citizens of Rome, Ken took the podium as the last speaker of the conference. He didn't waste any time. After the attendees had all been assured again and again that "no one was sick from Pfiesteria," Ken rocked the proceedings by announcing just the opposite.

In a flash, Dr. Hudnell was presenting his dwindling audience with my documented case histories of 54 *Pfiesteria* patients and the clear data analysis of those cases that showed just how much of a problem *Pfiesteria* was, even without big fish kills.

Yes, said Ken, there was also a double-blinded, placebo-controlled, crossover clinical trial . . . and it showed the indisputable benefits of CSM therapy in patients who shared exposure, symptoms and Contrast Sensitivity deficits. It took Dr. Hudnell only a few minutes to demonstrate that the CDC case definition was inadequate, incomplete and for the purposes of practicing physicians, unusable. Then he pointed out that an expanded definition of this ailment would include patients of all ages, independent of exposure to fish kills. Ken also noted that many of my 54 sufferers had been misdiagnosed by other health care providers in the past.

In the year 2000, patients—not fish kills—are the marker for *Pfiesteria* activity.

Ken's presentation made it quite evident that the illness clears up promptly with CSM therapy, followed by careful monitoring via CS testing.

Confronted by both Ken Hudnell's impeccable scientific credentials and the undeniable significance of his data, the Maryland's officials and the CDC, too, were forced to back-pedal, and quickly.

But the battle wasn't over yet. During a conference call in May that followed the MMWR, Ken asked the CDC executive in charge if she wished to see our data. No, she did *not*. The numbers hadn't been assembled by her agency, after all, so why waste valuable time looking at them?

In what was almost a single voice, however, the 20 other participants in the conference call announced: "Well, we *do* want to look at his data!"

Soon thereafter, Dr. Robert Venezia, the Maryland Department of Health liaison to the CDC, phoned me to discuss the possibility of a meeting in which he could share data and learn more about what I was doing.

What *chutzpah*! After I'd spent four years working on this problem—while enduring countless put-downs from Maryland's scientific establishment—Venezia & Co. wanted me to give them data my patients had insisted remain confidential!

Nonetheless, the turning point in this strange scientific odyssey had finally been reached. It had actually arrived a few days earlier, during a Harmful Algal Blooms meeting sponsored by Ken's lab, the U.S. EPA National Health and Environmental Effects Research Laboratory. Entitled "Human Health and Environmental Indicators," that conference brought together some of the heaviest hitters in the world of Environmental Health . . . including Dr. Wayne Carmichael, one of the world's top blue-green algae experts. (We had talked in detail about his work and mine regarding *cylindrospermopsis* in Florida during one of the breaks in the conference.)

Dr. Burkholder also attended the Environmental conference, along with Dr. Glasgow and Dr. Ramsdell. This was the varsity team, no doubt about it. And the ranks of the experts also included several key experts on Sick Building Syndrome—along with several leaders of the North Carolina *Pfiesteria* contingent, such as Kathleen Buckheit and Paul Webb. Suddenly, all of these neurotoxin-illness titans were listening to Ken as they had never listened before!

"We want to be part of the solution," Buckheit and Webb told Ken Hudnell earnestly, "not part of the problem that we all had several years ago." A few days after the conference ended, on June 22, the CDC-affiliated team—including Venezia, Webb and Buckheit—along with Amy Chapin of the State of Maryland, came to Pocomoke to begin reviewing my data and touring the region in a new spirit of cooperation.

"I'll work with you," I told them, "but you have to *understand* what I know about estuaries. Come on down . . . but only if you're willing to feel what toxin-water is really like. Take off your shoes and feel the difference between silty loam sediments in areas of palustrine emergent vegetation and the sandy silts elsewhere. Look at the deposition sides of the river, and learn the ecology of *Pfiesteria* firsthand.

"Get your toes in the mud and learn what life in the attack-zones really involves."

Believe it or not, they actually showed up!

And suddenly, CDC *Pfiesteria* coordinator Luke Nahearn was sending out welcoming e-mails. "Sure, you can present a poster at our international *Pfiesteria* conference! And Dr. Hudnell and you can make a presentation of your collaborative study."

Was I exhilarated by this sudden shift in direction? You bet. Still, every one of my colleagues who heard about this 360-degree turnabout by the CDC advised me to be "real careful."

"Look," said a few of my savvier friends in the Maryland medical community, "they aren't suddenly acting nice to you for no reason. They're either scared to death that you're going to make them look like back-bench bureaucrats . . . or they're looking for some way to trap you. Watch your back!"

What will happen next? Right now, our two recent *Pfiesteria* papers have been submitted for publication, one through the CDC, along with two articles on Lyme. Those papers will be followed by articles on ciguatera, lionfish, sick building syndrome and *cylindrospermopsis*.

Question: Is there a realistic chance that the CDC will respond to the hard facts and solid data in those papers . . . when the same data will instantly expose the many mistakes made in the past by the medical administrators who actually *run* the Centers?

Answer: The science will carry the day. The CDC listens to scientific facts; we have bushel baskets of truth to present.

chapter 27

Reflection

Why Johnny Can't Read

Pocomoke, MD –June, 1999

It happened among the roaring cataracts and jagged cliffs of the Snake River Recreation Area, and it wasn't pretty.

It happened during a "wilderness expedition" of "outward-bound" professionals . . . all of whom got the surprise of their lives after they encountered some *real* wilderness in the form of a snarling Momma Grizzly intent on protecting her two cavorting cubs.

The fun began when two male guides who were leading the human group of adventurers made the tactical error of walking between a peevish, seven-foot Grizzly and her gamboling young. She was not amused. In a flash, the guides were beating a hasty and undignified retreat—and then vaulting high into the branches of nearby trees.

They left behind two human females and *their* children, and both women instantly made it clear that they would brook no interference from this ursine invader, with one of the ferocious moms angrily bellowing: "You better leave my kids alone!"

What followed was a Gary Cooper-style "Mexican standoff," as humans and bears stood rooted in place, glaring at each other. (The men folk remained perched on their distant branches, silent as mice.) At last the bear growled a command in the direction of the cubs, who quickly scattered into the underbrush. Ms. Griz then rose to her full height and pawed the air for emphasis— before stepping off the trail and vanishing into the scrub.

• • •

Wouldn't it be wonderful, if the rapidly emerging threats to our children's literacy skills from organic neurotoxins were as clear and starkly defined as the danger presented by that muttering grizzly? And wouldn't it *also* be wonderful if parents would stand up to the seemingly insurmountable forces that are always telling them: "Nothing is wrong with your child, or her ability to learn!"

No such luck. Unfortunately, the toxin-based dangers facing our kids aren't so easy to discern. As a matter of fact, children are markedly under-represented in all of my cohorts of toxin-sickened patients . . . a disturbing fact which makes me wonder: are they partially protected from symptoms by their youthful energy and resilience?

Or am I missing something in many of the kids I routinely examine and interview, day in and day out?

Is it possible that children could be immune to toxins, through some mechanism we don't yet understand? According to my disease model, the fat-soluble toxins circulate perpetually, while binding for short periods to specific receptors. And wherever they go, cell damage is the result . . . whether that damage takes place in nerve tissue, muscle, lung or brain or bile storage areas.

Here's another question: Since we know there's been an explosion of asthma cases in toxin-exposed areas of the United States, should we start investigating the possibility that many asthma attacks in children are triggered by toxin assaults on cell receptors in airways?

That's a tough one. Let's face it: I don't know enough about biological toxins in children to be sure. So what am I missing?

Already difficult, the problem of accurately diagnosing toxin-mediated illness in children has been enormously compounded by today's grotesque over-emphasis on pharmaceutical chemicals to control behavior problems. And that particular distortion seemed especially glaring to me a few months ago, when I treated a 10-year-old named "Adam" for his so-called "hyperactivity" problem.

Adam had been referred to me by his long-gone pediatric psychiatrist, who could no longer make a living in our town . . . since children everywhere are now being diagnosed as having "hyperactivity" or "impulse disorder" or almost any other behavioral ailment that can be used to justify a prescription for Ritalin.

After a careful examination, it became obvious that Adam's problems weren't linked to "hyperactivity" at all. In fact, the child had been attending a school with a badly leaking roof. And when the school authorities finally got around to investigating this problem, they discovered that some of their students were being attacked by a *stachybotrys* fungus growing in the area of the leak. The school system responded by calling in a group of environmental hazard experts who fixed the roof and then assured the teachers that the fungus might cause an occasional cough or headache, but that it would soon go away.

Adam failed to improve, however—until he took a Contrast Sensitivity test that showed a deficit, then corrected it with CSM. His good health restored, he began tackling his schoolwork in earnest . . . and finished his middle school with academic honors.

All too often, as in the case of Adam, childhood illnesses caused by toxin-forming organisms are being blamed on such "behavioral" culprits as hyperactivity and attention deficit. What can you say about a society in which Time Magazine devotes a cover to "The Menace of ADHD"—but never mentions the insidious effects of mycotoxins on learning?

Is this increasingly diagnosed behavioral malady a real illness, or just the latest pediatric fad?

Everywhere you look, these days, the experts are lining up at the talk-show microphones, eager to wax eloquent on the "new era of stress, of high-speed Internet communications and global competition for knowledge . . ." all of which are supposedly wiping out our children's emotions and triggering "attention deficits" across the board.

Break out the Ritalin!

Or maybe we should conclude that Johnny can't read because he's watching too much violent TV? Playing too many "shoot-'em-up" video games, while sitting alone and isolated in front of a computer screen all afternoon? Better head for the medicine cabinet . . . grab that bottle of Ritalin!

But wait a minute: maybe Johnny's problem is *actually* caused by the huge amounts of sugar in his daily diet?

Or perhaps our daycare and school systems are trying to teach him to read too early (starting at age 4, in many areas), when he should be out there playing happily with the other kids in the neighborhood? (You guessed it: *it's Ritalin time!*)

Sorry, but I'm not buying any of that stuff.

After several years of research on the problem, it seems crystal-clear to me that many of these troubled "Johnny's" can't read because they're carrying deficits in their neural function shown by CS . . . which means that other nerves are undoubtedly affected as well. A recent California study suggests that one-third of all learning disorders are actually "biological" in origin—and that impaired brain-perception of auditory inputs (hearing) can be demonstrated easily in any clinical lab.

For example, a child might be able to recognize the sound of the letter "R" when it is pronounced as a single sound, while remaining unable to identify the same letter as occurring in a word such as "storm."

The key point here: neurotoxic illnesses hurt brains.

All too often, Johnny can't separate "e" from "a," or "g" from "p," or "b" from "d."

Failure of edge detection (contrast sensitivity), gets called dyslexia if Johnny can't recognize where one letter stops and the next starts. Letter reversal is just a symptom of the illness. Toxins? Hudnell, in 1996, documented a large CS deficit in learning disabled children in Czechoslovakia. Sure, learning disability is multi-factorial, but before Johnny gets on the bus to special ed classes, lets try to identify the cause.

And here's the most challenging question of all: is Johnny perhaps suffering the effects of an environmentally acquired toxin? Is the neurotoxin the true culprit here—rather than "learning disability" or "attention deficit" or "amotivational syndrome?"

For many patients today, the answer to that key question is actually quite simple.

All too often, these kids have been exposed to micro-organic toxins that impair nerve function, learning ability and numerous other executive cognitive functions. Almost overnight, it seems, they find themselves unable to concentrate adequately in order to complete a task or associate a concrete construct with an abstract thought. Moody and withdrawn, these affected kids often begin to experience distracting abdominal and muscular pains, along with their other problems.

Suddenly, the reason behind Johnny's inability to do his homework comes clear. He's a slow learner not because of some vague "syndrome" . . . but because environmental toxins have prevented him from concentrating adequately to complete a task or associate a hands-on learning experience with an abstract thought.

What would Johnny's parents think, if they knew the real story behind his inability to perform in school? If they understood that the kid's "attention deficit" was actually due to *Pfiesteria* toxins in the slowly flushing estuaries of New Bern, North Carolina, would they be as quick to "drug him up" as they are now? Or would they stand their ground and fight the politicians and the big pesticide manufacturers, like that Old Momma Grizzly Bear at Snake River?

I think you know the answer to that one.

To illustrate my point even more, let me tell you about little "Jimmy, Jr.," a troubled third-grader I've gotten to know pretty well in recent months.

Jimmy showed up in my office one morning, accompanied by his mom, who was in search of treatment for the child's pneumonia. Jimmy had been sick off and on for more than a year, and his regular doctor had grown accustomed to prescribing antibiotics.

Meanwhile, the allergist was recommending "desensitization" shots, and the ear-nose-and-throat surgeon kept suggesting "ear tubes"—followed by speedy removal of the little boy's tonsils and adenoids.

It didn't take long to figure out that Jimmy was having a tough time in school. His standardized Maryland State test scores were running far below the predictions from his teachers, most of whom had already decided that the kid was saddled with ADD. But the physical exam I gave this troubled child showed that he was suffering from a lot more than just enlarged turbinates, middle-ear fluid and chest-wheezing.

Jimmy was moody; in fact he was downright depressed. Definitely labile, he smiled one minute and glared with rage the next. His teachers reported that they'd "tried to encourage him in class," but that he just didn't care.

He also went to the nurse frequently—in a futile quest for relief from "aches and pains" that kept changing all the time.

Interestingly enough, however, the school psychologist had detected the fact that Jimmy was quite bright—his aptitude tests were ranked in the 90th percentile, or better.

How was it that this smart kid, who had done quite well in school before his previous summer vacation (at Williams Point on the nearby Pocomoke River), couldn't seem to pay attention in class without regular doses of Ritalin?

I'd already treated several cases of neurotoxin-mediated illness in people who'd spent time at Williams Point, so I couldn't help wondering: Could Jimmy have picked up an environmentally acquired impairment of his ability to learn? It was time to find out. Without hesitation, I gave him the standard Contrast Sensitivity Test that same day and was confirmed in my suspicions when it reproducibly displayed the key "Hudnell Sign" of impaired visual ability.

Next step: CSM to the rescue! At pediatric dosages, cholestyramine binds toxins but doesn't seem to cause the unpleasant side effects that adults so frequently report.

Jimmy got better fast. It wasn't long before his delighted mother called to tell me how nice it was to have her son back, after a year-long absence: "Thanks for rescuing Jimmy from those nasty toxins!" Within a matter of days, the allergy shots had been suspended and the ENT surgeries were canceled. The Ritalin prescription flew straight into the trash. Jimmy didn't seem to need the school psychologist anymore, and his grades and in-school test scores soared.

Thrilled by his success, I fired off a passionate letter to the President of the School Board and received the response I expected: total silence.

But the word was beginning to get out in the neighborhood. Jimmy's dad told Sammy's dad about the changes in Jimmy. And soon the word reached Josh's dad, who liked to drive the kids around on his big fishing boat. All of these children were frequent swimmers in the Pocomoke . . . and all of them had been seeing the same psychologist, who had diagnosed ADD in every one of them!

So I went right to work. Within the space of a few days, I pinpointed their CS deficits and started them on CSM. Once again, test scores and classroom performance began to climb the charts. Excited all over again, I asked myself how many *other* kids in Somerset County's school district might be struggling with toxin-linked learning difficulties of this kind.

All we needed was a bit of simple (and inexpensive) screening, and we'd be able to tell for sure if those nose-diving reading and math scores were due to "teachers who couldn't teach

reading" (a paraphrase of the assessment provided by the Department of Education consultants)—or to the ongoing political
coverup of the learning problems caused by the local *Pfiesteria*
epidemic. How many more Johnny's would be sickened, if the
State of Maryland's public health bureaucrats continued to insist
that "only a few estuaries" had been affected by the toxin-spewing
dinoflagellate, in spite of the fact that hundreds of people along
the watershed were now showing the symptoms of neurotoxin
illness?

After pleading my case vigorously, I scored a quick breakthrough when the superintendent of the Somerset County
Schools—Dr. Michael Thomas—agreed to present my "screening idea" to a closed meeting of the school board. At that point,
the response to my initiative seemed to be very positive.

As you might expect, I had been careful to make my proposal
as straightforward as possible. Why not give every third-grader
in the district my five-minute Contrast Sensitivity test, which is
a highly effective tool for pinpointing the presence of learning
disorders and disabilities? I didn't tell Dr. Thomas that I would
privately make the effort to associate the scores with exposure
to the watershed . . . although I could tell from his probing
questions about *Pfiesteria* that he knew what I planned to do
with the CS data.

Although I kept this strategy to myself, I figured that if a certain subset of the "learning disabled" students displayed other
symptoms of *Pfiesteria*-related illness (along with learning problems), we could at least give parents the option of deciding
whether or not to proceed with CSM treatment.

The "closed session" went well, apparently. Dr. Thomas called
me several weeks later and announced that the board had agreed
to listen to my proposal. Would I agree to make a public presentation before the members on March 16th (1999)? You bet I
would!

A bit of background: Somerset County includes two major
population centers—Princess Anne and Crisfield—and each boasts
its own high school. And because Maryland has been enjoying a

tax surplus in recent years (like many other areas around the country), the governor has been eager to build new schools. As March 16th approached, in fact, a $5 million budget recommendation from the same governor had just finished making its way through the General Assembly. All it needed now was an executive signature. Supposedly, that money would allow the county to build a central high school . . . a move that would reportedly permit large savings on staff costs, while also increasing efficiency and providing more opportunities for county students. This was "better education through building"—a brand-new way of mixing mortar on a mortar board.

How well I remember the muffled phone call from my friend in the Maryland Health Department. It came on March 15 . . . one day before the public presentation.

"Watch out, Ritchie," said the clipped, baritone voice. "They're after you! There will be plenty of state officials at the school board meeting who want you to fail."

Later, I learned that the wires from Annapolis (the state capital) to Princess Anne had been smoking all day long. And the message was everywhere the same: If Ritchie is permitted to proceed with his "screening plan," his findings may very well expose the whitewash of the *Pfiesteria* epidemic now taking place along the Chesapeake watershed. And if *that* happens, you can be sure that your $5 million will go winging out over the Chesapeake, *pronto!*

No, I don't have the "proof" that these threats were made . . . because hearsay isn't admissible in court . . . even if the hearsay comes from independent-minded Eastern Shore folks with a statewide reputation for "telling it like it is." At any rate, you can be sure the board meeting was packed with out-of-towners, marked by their coats and ties, that night in Somerset County.

"Dr. Thomas," I told the gathered assemblage as calmly as possible, "as president of the Somerset County Medical Society, I must tell you that our members are alarmed at the number of children who are being prescribed Ritalin in this county.

"We do not agree with the diagnoses of the new psychology operation down the road, or with the prescriptions written for their youthful patients by the physicians-in-training who are paid 'per patient' by those same psychologists.

"We respectfully request the opportunity to determine the extent of learning disability in this county by testing third-graders with the Contrast Sensitivity test. The test is non-invasive, reliable and portable. It has also been documented to be an effective instrument in detecting particular deficits associated with learning disability.

"If we find that Ritalin truly is being dispensed like candy, we propose that a public educational program be provided to parents regarding the proper use of Ritalin. We will also recruit the experts who will be needed to help parents of affected children make up their minds."

At this point, of course, the Expensive Suits were squirming in their chairs. What would the Board do? The room fell silent, while one particularly irked Member announced that he didn't "like the idea" of "all those statisticians and neurotoxicologists coming in here from the EPA to look at our data." No, he didn't "like those EPA boys at all," because they'd given him a hard time a few years before about "water quality" in some local streams adjacent to work sites in the County.

As soon as this peeved Board Member fell silent, another took his place and quickly asked why there was "any need to question the conclusions of the expert from the State of Maryland?

"If the State says that the learning problems are caused by bad teaching, then let's get busy helping the teachers!"

A moment later I was back on my feet. "Fine, by all means, help the teachers. But why not get a 'second opinion,' at the same time? As you know, many respected educators believe that your standardized school tests simply aren't effective, as indices of learning ability. And what about all those attention-deficit drugs that are now being prescribed around the county? We've got kids taking drugs they don't need, based on the opinions of a group of specialists whose self-interest requires that the children be endlessly 'reevaluated' in their offices at $75 a pop!"

What if the learning problem wasn't due to "teachers who can't teach," but instead to "students who can't learn?" Those same teachers were doing an excellent job 5 years ago. What if the learning disability had been environmentally acquired? Wasn't it time to find out if Johnny's "reading problem" might be connected to the larger public health problem of neurotoxin-illness caused by recent, rapid chemical changes in our environment?

The suits were squirming for real now. Were their hemorrhoids about to burst? But they needn't have fretted; a few minutes later, Dr. Thomas suggested that the Board "table" the proposal for "another time," and the motion carried unanimously.

Near the end of this attempt to really help kids who might be unfairly labeled—for the rest of their school careers—as being learning disabled, I paused to examine the letters of support my proposal had received from parents, teachers and school principals. All seemed to agree that "something is wrong here." Was the "problem" actually the hidden agenda and the "political spin" coming from those Expensive Suits—which even now were exiting the hall and making their way into the drizzly March evening?

Two weeks later, the state awarded the funds for the new high school.

• • •

I went back to work, and within a few days I was treating a 15-year-old girl from Lake County, Florida, whose tragic case provided yet another example of how learning disabilities from environmentally acquired toxins can be corrected, once they've been properly diagnosed.

This bright, personable student had done well academically until the sixth grade, when her learning problems had suddenly taken off. Around the same time, she began to complain of being constantly "tired," while also reporting pain in one joint after the next. The joint-pain moved around a lot, and she also suffered from back aches and headaches. She threw up in the morning some days, and insisted that since she couldn't "pay attention," she shouldn't have to go to school.

As you can imagine, the diagnosis was extremely difficult. Was this child suffering from depression, anemia, endocrine problems, lupus, school phobia, somatization syndrome . . . or some debilitating combination of several of these disorders?

Her parents seemed convinced that agricultural chemicals were to blame. Ag chemicals? What a stretch. Were her folks some kind of eco-wackos? Besides, there was no way to test for toxic effects of chemicals in their child. Next case.

The Professor of Pediatrics whom they consulted had published scholarly papers on the topic, and he was at least willing to entertain the "Ag Chemicals" theory, but only as one line in his six-page annotated report. In the end, however, he concluded that the problem was "pediatric fibromyalgia." Given that the patient's lab tests were all "normal," the Prof's recommendations were reasonably appropriate, as follows:

1) Since the results of the above studies are all normal or negative, we need to do everything we can to reassure the student and her family that this is a benign condition and that permanent disability will not occur;

2) Stress management techniques should be explored;

3) Physical therapy, including active and passive range of motion, exercises, whirlpool and stretching exercises may be helpful;

4) Gradual re-introduction of physical activity is important. Vigorous, jarring or traumatic activity may aggravate her pain but active gentle movement (swimming, walking, bike-riding, dancing) should be pursued.

5) As arthralgias and soft-tissue pains recur, I would suggest the use of NSAID agents like ibuprofen, tolmetin, or naproxen, to help control her symptoms. The "characteristic trigger points" of fibromyalgia and associated musculoskeletal pain

may also be responsive to NSAID treatment, along with stress reduction and physical therapy.

6) The professor didn't add a sixth recommendation, one that would have eliminated the first five, but he should have: Get the child de-toxed from the land now!

The Professor had missed the diagnosis. This patient had told him what was wrong—but he couldn't or wouldn't hear it! She'd described her sensitivity to smells such as cigarettes and paint, and she'd also mentioned her "shakiness" after eating sugary foods. If he had asked, she would have told him about her metallic taste and sensitivity to bright light.

If the Prof had just known to ask the questions that are part of the neurotoxin history, he would have learned about her severe memory deficits with accompanying impairment of "assimilation of new knowledge," especially in situations that demanded attentional ability. Unfortunately, the Professor still writes his misguided opinions for a colloquium of state scientists who make policy in education and health.

A neuro-psychologist eventually identified these deficits, however, (on the initial interview) and documented the girl's math deficits as well. What a shame that the diagnosis took so long —and that it proved to be so expensive. By way of contrast, my bedside screening exam takes less than five minutes and yields excellent results.

The process is quite simple, as well, and patients are merely asked to remember five numbers after an interval of five minutes. I also require them to count backwards, which requires mental manipulation of numbers, and to do some simple math without pencil and paper while I distract them. Example: I'll ask a patient to mentally divide 91 by 7, then record the length of time required to complete that abstract thinking exercise. Next, I'll have the patient perform the same calculation using pencil and paper. The two exercises should take approximately the same amount of time . . . and if they *don't*, the physician should begin testing for the presence of neurotoxins.

In the case of the unfortunate Florida teenager, the results showed that—like most of my *Pfiesteria* patients—she had lost most of her short-term memory capacity. She was slow to absorb new information and needed repeated exposures to test materials (with repeated cues) in order to function at even a "moderately impaired" level. Only when the information was presented to her in a carefully structured manner was she capable of even "average" retrieval abilities.

Faced with these limitations, the local school system had concluded that my patient was afflicted with a learning disability, and had provided her with educational support.

This troubled adolescent was indeed suffering from a toxin-mediated illness that likely had been triggered by the impact of ag chemicals on soil microorganisms.

As later privately commissioned assays would determine, exotic species of toxin-forming bacteria and fungi were flourishing on the land, producing poisons that the child breathed every time she went out to her barn to saddle her show horse.

Indeed, the parallels with the *Pfiesteria* disaster in Maryland were almost eerie. Once again here in Florida, no testing for chemicals had been done by state officials, who were under enormous public pressure and had not approached their task with disciplined thoroughness. In many cases, DEP acknowledged testing was performed with expired reagents . . . even as the levels of detection remained too coarse to detect the minute quantities of offending chemicals known to cause illness.

Incredibly, no microbial testing was done by DEP. In the end, the worried state officials resorted to the Fourth Principle in my "Appearance of Good Science" catalogue, in order to obscure the real cause of this child's environmentally acquired learning disability: They agreed to "study the problem" to death!

By performing the wrong tests at the wrong time on the wrong samples, they also made sure that the burial of truth would take place on reams of white paper printed at taxpayer expense.

• • •

Before concluding this abbreviated chapter on environmentally acquired learning disabilities (a whole series of books on this subject is indicated), I should point out that chronic Lyme disease often creates special emotional barriers to successful school performance. Unfortunately, Lyme children often must endure pronounced mood swings. *Pfiesteria* patients tend to become moody or withdrawn, and those struggling with Lyme toxins do that as well. But they're also subject to bouts of explosive, unpredictable anger, during which they appear to lack cognitive controls.

Whenever I hear reports of children "getting into trouble" from rage reactions or other bizarre, antisocial behaviors, I think first of Lyme disease. If you and your family are struggling with this kind of problem, I suggest you start seeking help by getting a FACT Test for your loved one now.

No, Lyme shouldn't become a "catchall" explanation for all types of sociopathic behavior. But when a stable behavior pattern suddenly shifts into chaotic, raging tantrums, we need to "think Lyme," or some other neuro-toxic cause.

A 20-year-old college student provided a compelling recent example. He and his father had spent many hours on the road, driving to Pocomoke for a Contrast Sensitivity test and a twentieth opinion on his illness. The young man was constantly fatigued, but insisted on working a full shift. He also did his best to ignore the constant muscle pain and headaches that tormented him. He'd tested positive for Lyme . . . but the standard dosages of oral doxycycline hadn't helped.

These symptoms were distressing, of course, but the major reason for this long journey was the father's growing concern about his son's out-of-control anger. The duo had worked well for several summers, but then their relationship had begun to change (as so often happens), when the boy entered late adolescence. Increasingly, little things were triggering his hostility and his penchant for ugly confrontation.

With strong emotion burning in their faces, both men described an incident during the previous year in which a row of plants had been destroyed. When the son realized that his father had not responded to his shouted warnings about a malfunctioning machine (and that the plants would be ruined as a result), he went ballistic. Yet he seemed to have no later recollection of the incident, in which he had attacked his father with his fists.

The same pattern of outbursts continued later that fall, at college. In one episode, the son attacked a varsity football player who "cut into" a cafeteria line. Despite being outweighed by 100 pounds or so, the kid hurled the brawny athlete to the ground and pummeled him. But once again, he could not remember his enraged attack. At this point, the worried father brought the youth to see me.

After testing positive for Contrast Sensitivity, the young man began taking his medication according to the "Herx Preventive Protocol." And he did well. He returned to school, where his grades rose and his bouts of white-hot rage soon disappeared.

In recent years, I've heard many psychiatrists describe similar scenarios with their Lyme patients. Is it finally time to install the CS Test in psychiatric consulting rooms and social workers' offices from coast to coast? And how many of the nearly 2 million men now being held in the nation's jails and prisons are actually the victims of chronically acting toxins from Lyme bacteria?

Pretty disturbing, no? And it's also distressing to hear from chronic Lyme patients—as I often do—that their children now have congenital Lyme. Is there any convincing reason to believe that Lyme toxin can't cross the placenta to affect unborn infants? Increasingly, anecdotal studies suggest that it's beginning to happen.

Over the years, I've prescribed amoxicillin to many young Johnny's who were grappling with respiratory infections . . . only to have Mom call back in two or three days to report that the child "has gotten much worse." In the past, I would always respond by suggesting: "Oh, give it a little more time." But whenever that scenario unfolds now, I find myself wondering: "Is Johnny actually having a mini-Herxheimer reaction?"

Watching kids struggle with learning disabilities is no fun. But these days I take solace in one heartening fact: If a child shows a deficit on my CS Test, I know I can help him or her in the classroom with CSM.

If only our schools would begin to see the light, and start testing these troubled children for Contrast Sensitivity. Such an initiative, thoughtfully carried out, could change the future for an entire generation of young people.

Let's face it: the stakes are simply too high to do otherwise!

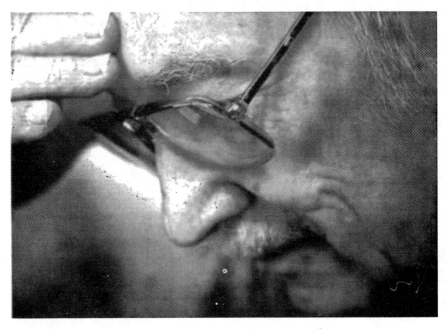

Jack Spurling and the Pfiesteria *salute.*

Even Ph.D.s Die.
Making the Ultimate
Sacrifice for Research.

Snow Hill, MD –December, 1999

*"You must learn to love your fate . . . for it will surely return
to you on some distant day. The sea will cast it up again!"*
—*Friedrich Nietzsche, "The Will to Power"*

His name was George Demas. He was a heroic scientist—a researcher who took the ultimate risk for the sake of knowledge —and he was my friend.

George died after repeatedly contracting *Pfiesteria* as a result of his field studies in Maryland and Delaware, just before Christmas of 1999. He was 40 years old and at the height of his promising career as a soil scientist. Like a figure out of Nietzsche's existentialist philosophy, he chose to continue his research despite the obvious risks involved.

George Demas accepted his fate as a scientist, and his tragic death provides a compelling example of the price that often accompanies new discoveries. Whenever I look back at his odyssey as the first scientist who gave his life during *Pfiesteria* research, I find myself struggling with a host of questions I can't possibly answer.

- Who first determined the safe amount of digitalis leaf to give to a heart patient?

- How does the dedicated zoological researcher find the courage to wake up that dozing grizzly bear for another mid-winter temperature check?
- Who did the original research on shark repellant—and how much did that exercise cost them?

I could spend the next several hours asking questions like those, but I think you see my point . . . which is that all too often, the first one *in* will be the first one *out*—and the man or woman who's the first to try something new might be the first to die.

I know I'll never forget the inscription Dr. Demas wrote to me on a copy of his Ph.D thesis. In a few scrawled words, he thanked me by saying: "When things seemed the darkest, thanks for reaching out a hand and not letting go." Each time I read his words today, I smile again with the knowledge that his work will not be lost.

He understood the dangers that were an inescapable part of his study of the ecology of *Pfiesteria*, since he'd contracted the illness several times during his forays along the threatened estuaries of the Chesapeake Bay watershed. Yet he went right on collecting samples of submerged sediments in clearly identified *Pfiesteria* "attack zones."

"Don't worry about it, man!" he joked to me more than once. "Nobody ever died from *Pfiesteria* toxins, you know?"

Not until Dr. Demas, that is.

George's final act of heroism became a telling symbol of the struggle that had marked his entire life. How well I remember the painful uncertainty that had marked his early career as a scientist. Fresh out of grad school and with a brand-new master's degree under his arm, he'd worked hard during the early 1980s to find the right niche in which to use his new knowledge about soils and ecology.

Like most of us, he'd changed direction a few times . . . before finally signing on as a farm analyst and planner for the U.S. Department of Agriculture's local conservation district in

Maryland. The work had proved satisfying, but George hungered for more. Like every true explorer, he burned to pit himself against the unknown in an authentic struggle to push back the boundaries of knowledge.

Like those ancient, "fated" Greeks who were his ancestors, Demas was driven by a single-minded passion that ruled his life. For him, that passion was "pedology," the science of soils, which are scientifically described as "an organized natural body at the earth's surface." As he went about his studies, George was greatly influenced by several distinguished scientists . . . including Dr. Court Stephenson, a prominent contemporary biologist, and Dr. Marty Rabenhorst, a pedologist who eventually became his doctoral thesis advisor at the University of Maryland.

But the most important single influence on George Demas during these early years was his new bride, Susan. She made him whole in an unspoken way. He explained to me more than once that she had given his life—and his work—a whole new dimension of meaning. Endlessly delighting in her presence, George seemed truly happy as he began his doctoral researches, which centered on a project to map the submerged sediments of the Sinepunxent Bay, a coastal region located near Maryland's Ocean City. George's assignment: correlate soil types and sediment composition in order to define the makeup of "estuarine soil."

As you might expect, Demas took his watershed soils *very* seriously. And if you wanted to rile him up, all you had to do was make the mistake of referring to soil as "dirt!" He began to document first how sub-aqueous soils were the foundation of plant nutrition. Then he focused hard on the complex relationships between submerged aquatic vegetation and sediment. In George's lexicon, "soil" was a dynamic term—and it was an essential part of the complicated biological dynamics that take place endlessly at the interface of water, submerged sediments and functioning roots.

A bold and prescient theorist, George Demas was nonetheless a very practical and down-to-earth scientist. Like Ken Hudnell (See Chapter Five: "Brilliant, Just Brilliant"), Demas was determined to find useful applications for his research, which was based on the "elegance of simplicity."

Example: At one point, George showed me how the oxidation of iron in sediment cores provided clear evidence for his theories of how water and oxygen movement determined the growth of associated vegetation. As I soon realized, his insight had important implications for the relationship between land-runoff and toxic pollution at the water's edge. Indeed, his cores displayed the chemical changes affecting those heavy metals—including copper—that provided the bedrock evidence (oxidation, reduction, and hydration) of the bio-availability of copper in sediment.

I'd never heard of an "N Value" before this discussion with George, and I was all ears as he demonstrated how submerged sediments that held together when you squeezed them (a high N Value) must have once stood high enough above the water line to have been compacted. On the other hand, low N Values were inevitably found among soils that had never been out of the water.

Such distinctions were important, said George, because they provided researchers with a structural indication of the percentage of "fines" (small soil particles) contained in any estuarine sample. This second type of soil possessed no internal structure, he said, and if you squeezed a sample, it would simply liquefy and fall apart. And there was more: if stirred by waves, winds or tides, such unstable soil-configurations would quickly break down into their component particles. Without the fines to fill in the spaces between coarser soil particles, porewater full of activated chemicals would fill the gaps.

It was fascinating to hear George discourse on the wide, wide, wonderful world of estuarine soils. Under his tutelage, I soon learned that soil types were defined by color and presence of aggregates (such as those one might find in a bag of concrete mix), along with the presence of shells, loam, clay and sand. George's work showed that—depending on the dynamics of the local hydrology, or on the soil types of the upland landscapes, as shaped by the topography—soil sediment-types at distances of ten feet or less could differ markedly in the same river.

George was also fond of pointing out that the contents of any particular soil always determined the kinds of vegetation it could support. And that content meant that the soil habitat depended in part on the forces brought to bear on an area by the body of water that adjoined it. The brilliance of George's approach was that it pointed out the weakness of many earlier studies—estuarine soil assays in which samples that had been gathered 500 meters or more apart were not adequately classified, in terms of understanding the impact of physical location on the complex relationships described above.

By sampling these submerged cropland soils more closely (the scientific term is "within a close matrix"), Demas showed that meter-to-meter variations in distance often create dramatic differences in submerged sediment viability. Because of George's work, the entire concept of reduced submerged aquatic vegetation growth had to be revised and became a function of submerged sediments growth-capacity. And the key concept that emerged during this redefinition—for my own research, that is —was his understanding of how soil fertility is always balanced by soil toxicity.

Thank you, George Demas! These days, whenever I hear the "nutrient enrichment mantra" emanating from Maryland's various "public health experts and officials," I also hear the gruff, no-nonsense voice of Dr. D, endlessly repeating: "The reason that SAV [submerged aquatic vegetation] is disappearing isn't nutrient enrichment alone. If these plants could live—which they *can't*, because the sediments are too toxic—they would simply use the nutrients for their own growth.

"The state's explanation is absurd! It's like blaming fertilizers for the failure of plant growth on farmlands that have been used as toxic waste dumps!" As George loved to point out, an accurate understanding of these complex soil dynamics required analysis of many other factors—such as the mobility of soils, the effects of sunlight and animal activity and the depth of water at various locations.

(In essence, the very insightful Dr. Demas was advocating the same approach to estuarine studies that I have employed throughout *Desperation Medicine*: the "Systems Approach!")

George always argued—and quite effectively—that the analysis of any environmental problem involving water must begin with an analysis of sediments. He was convinced that "sediment composition" could tell us the history of what had taken place in the water column over time . . . including the parent type of soil, the deposition of chemicals, the leaching off of those same chemical substances, nutrient enrichment, and the presence of toxic chemicals.

George's approach was invaluable, because it allowed me to understand why attack zones for *Pfiesteria* were always located in areas of palustrine emergent vegetation (areas bordering changing marshlands, that is) where low N Value sediments are changing to higher N Values, and also in deposition sites of loam silts near intruding salt-wedge tongues linked to tidal flow. And indeed, as my own charting of sites of acquisition of human illness soon made evident, a map of these sediments amounted to nothing less than a map of *Pfiesteria* attack zones along the Chesapeake Bay.

Remember, George often worked alongside U.S. District Conservationist Bruce Nichols. And the three of us loved to argue about sediments, soils, ecology and human health. But the key point was something we all could agree on: the fact that submerged sediments enjoy the same diversity as soils *above* water . . . and a change of only a few feet in a river will often be associated with the presence of an entirely different biological habitat, just as in any above-water agricultural operation. George's painstaking and methodical sediment-mapping soon documented the fact that his theory of soil dynamics matched the reality of conditions found in the estuarine environment.

Did the experts in the world of pedology agree with this assessement? Yes, they did—by giving George Demas the coveted Emil Truog National Award, the highest such honor given out by the Soil Science Society of America for producing the best

Ph.D. thesis in his field during 1999. The experts at the U.S. Ag Department could also be heard applauding, as they awarded Demas an $888,000 grant supporting his three-year soil mapping effort along the rivers and inland bays of Delaware and Maryland's Eastern Shore.

Fate! Suddenly, George Demas was both a "brand-new Ph.D." and a "highly regarded, nationally prominent Ph.D." whose scientific future glowed with promise. Because he was so obviously on the "fast track" to the top, Bruce Nichols and I had felt comfortable while teasing him a bit about his presentations at a series of *Pfiesteria* forums in 1998. At that point, George had barely begun to assemble his impressive data for publication, and his nervousness could be seen in the way he introduced each new slide for discussion with the same booming expletive: "*So!*"

"*Hey, George,*" we shouted at him more than once, "*so!*"

He needn't have been so nervous, however, because his work was nothing less than awesome. At that point, no other scientist in the world was engaged in the kind of discovery-making that occupied Dr. D each and every day of the week. And I've always considered myself to be quite fortunate . . . because of the way that George came along at precisely the right time for my own researches on submerged soils and helped open several new windows for me on this key area of *Pfiesteria* research.

Awkward and ungainly at first, Dr. Demas had resembled the Ugly Duckling during his first scientific struggles. But as time passed and he gained increasing confidence in his own acumen, the Duckling became the Swan. How tragic, I told myself later, that *Pfiesteria*-related human illness would eventually prove to be his Swan Song, and would so cruelly subtract him from the ranks of important researchers in the world of estuarine ecology.

George kept sending me articles that helped me develop my theories about copper toxicity and its relationship to surges in the growth of *Pfiesteria's* toxic phase (as an aggressive dinoflagellate) along the Chesapeake watershed. As it turned out, Demas was one of the few academics in the world who had done research on the toxicity of submerged sediments. He knew that toxic upriver chemicals, when deposited in attack zones, could be re-suspended from porewater into a killing zone for algae. He also understood that my ideas about copper and other fungicides made sense—when tested in the crucible of contemporary knowledge about sediments and ecology.

Armed with some of George's insights—and huge amounts of our own research on estuarine sediments—Nichols and I in 1999 had decided to do our best to put a stop to the swirling Maryland controversy over *Pfiesteria* and human illness by performing those experiments that would be required to prove the theory that toxics underlie *Pfiesteria* blooms.

After three years of "AGS" from Maryland State scientists, it was obvious that the State public health officials and the politicians would almost certainly refuse to do the porewater-sampling that was necessary. Nor would they insist on epidemiological surveys aimed at tracking the additional cases involving patients exposed to locations where other *documented* patients had acquired *Pfiesteria*-linked illness. So be it! Undaunted, Nichols and I decided that we'd take on the task on our own time.

Having named our project the "Researcher Study," I asked my longtime Trail Committee friend and fellow-ecologist Jack Spurling to participate. He quickly volunteered: "I'll bring the boat, and [his wife] Marian will make the fried chicken!"

Suddenly, it was like old times again, as I got together with some of the folks who'd created the $300,000 Pocomoke Nature Trail from scratch. And soon we were heading back into battle—this time intent on running experiments in hazardous areas, so that we could expose the truth about toxic levels of copper, fungicides and *Pfiesteria*.

With his "GPS," or "Global Positioning System" at the ready, George could pinpoint our locations down to the very last coordinate. But I didn't have to be told that we had entered *Pfiesteria* attack zones. No, the "peppery" feeling on my arms and the heaviness in my chest and the difficulty I felt in breathing was enough to signal the presence of dangerous toxins at work on my skin and in my lungs. . . .

Our study began on the 19th of July, 1999. All four of us took the CS test, and all of our scores were normal. Then we clambered aboard Jack's boat and started motoring into known attack zones. After anchoring the craft securely, we plunged into the water and began slogging along at knee- and shoulder-depth, as we collected water samples by the hour. Equipped with beer can-sized cylinders, we scooped up dozens of soil and water samples, along with plenty of three-foot-long soil borings, in order to take away many different soil types.

Unfortunately, Spurling did not take cholestyramine properly as a preventive measure, and hadn't consumed a single dose until just before setting out that morning—when he took it with breakfast, which sharply reduced its effectiveness. (He might as well not have taken it, in fact.) I'd taken ample doses in the days before the expedition, but Bruce Nichols was his usual self . . . while declaring that "ticks who bite me fall off dead!" and refusing to ingest any of the toxin-fighting medicine.

To this day, I'm not sure why George said no to CSM that day. Was it because he'd spent so many hours wading through other estuarine zones where toxins were reported to be on the march?

The hand of fate!

All I can tell you is that we had a great time. My notes from that 48-hour expedition are full of references to countless species of water birds and mudflat creatures, along with the soul-deep beauty of the Pocomoke River estuaries and marshes. We watched, cheering, while majestic bald eagles outpaced Jack's boat at full throttle, and diving ospreys arrowed through the summer haze to spear and then carry away their share of perch and bass. . . .

As the hours passed and the sun drifted westwards over the marshland, I noticed that George and Bruce were spending most of their time on the river flats, while taking water samples repeatedly. Along the way, we carefully recorded our exact positions, sediment types, soil types, vegetation, wildlife and the presence or absence of the possibility of blooms at sites where we knew *Pfiesteria* had once lurked. But we also examined many sites where we knew the marauding dinoflagellate had never been present.

Later, we would analyze these "sediment profiles," and Dr. David Oldach would oblige us by running DNA-assays for *Pfiesteria* on them. Dr. Gian Gupta would extract the porewater from the samples, and Dr. Rick Kutz of the Chesapeake Bay EPA Program would arrange to have it analyzed for copper. George pointed out that it would be vitally important to make sure the labs performed the analyses correctly. "We're giving them unknowns, some with a high load added," he said excitedly, "and we have to be damn sure they give us both low and high values correctly [in scientific parlance, that's called 'spiking a sample']."

During our lengthy river sojourn, we went into numerous known attack zones, along with many known "control sites," deposition sides and "dig sides" of the river, in an effort to uncover the sediment characteristics of resident *Pfiesteria*. We'd all been careful to test our Constrast Sensitivity before and after exposure on both days, and everything seemed fine until about 24 hours after we traversed Bulbeggar Creek, located on the Virginia side of the Pocomoke.

Only a few minutes before I read a screaming headline—MASSIVE FISH KILL IN BULBEGGAR CREEK, LOW OXYGEN BLAMED—both Jack and George were on the phone. Both were sick, and it wasn't pretty. (I still have a photo of Jack holding his head with both hands in the "*Pfiesteria* salute"—a mournful image that made the front page of the Salisbury Times.)

Like most of the other *Pfiesteria* patients I've treated over the years, my fellow-researchers had knots in their bellies that loosened only with the onset of each new diarrhea-attack. Racked with pounding headaches, they were also experiencing the new sensitivity to light that marks the typical *Pfiesteria* attack. In addition, both reported that their muscles ached . . . to the point that merely breathing caused them nearly unbearable pain.

Were they suffering from migraine? Had they been attacked by the flu?

Nope. Like so many of my friends and neighbors along the Pocomoke in recent months, these two brave men were battling *Pfiesteria* toxins. Neurotoxins hurt brains; don't forget that important fact!

Bruce and I remained unaffected by any symptoms, however. Our CS scores read "normal" day after day . . . but not George's and not Jack's. (Can you imagine some CDC desk jockey telling me that my treatment was "premature," after *this* experience?)

CSM had literally been called to the rescue! And soon it was helping my two other friends as well. First Jack announced that his headache was lifting (within an hour of his first dose). Then George began a rapid recovery, which he monitored with frequent CS testing.

This medication *worked*; was there any remaining doubt?

Together the four of us had lived through one of those "life on the line" moments that you only see in the movies. And my own self-doubts had also lifted as a result; from this point forward, I would feel completely confident each time I told a patient: "If you get sick, my treatment protocol will work."

Up against the Appearance of Good Science

In the days that followed, the reports from the State of Maryland about "low levels of oxygen" in Bulbeggar Creek causing the fish kills were a laughably obvious misrepresentation of the truth. Health officials scrambled to blame the *Pfiesteria* assault on anything other than the microorganism which had caused it. (Talk about The Appearance of Good Science!)

As usual, the Official State Explanation was a transparent attempt to make the public rest easy about a growing estuarine threat. Question: Why had more than 1 million crazed menhaden swarmed so far upstream that they'd run out of water and oxygen and then perished. (Answer: *In flight from Pfiesteria!*)

Maryland soon announced the unnatural deaths of 500,000 fish . . . but uttered not a peep about *Pfiesteria*. Meanwhile, Virginia officials using the same data, were boldly announcing that the one-celled dinoflagellate had killed 10,000 fish in their state. Did we really need a DNA-assay in order to understand that George and Jack were struggling with *Pfiesteria*—and not a "low-oxygen illness?"

On the 12th of October, George Demas took eight co-workers and USDA officials on a demonstration tour of his proposed work sites in the Inland Bays of Delaware, located in Rehoboth Bay. George worked hard that day, because he knew that his grant was very much on the line. The bosses examined his proposal and liked it—and they agreed to fund the project.

But George paid a price for his victory. Within a matter of 36 hours, he was once again battling the headache, the abdominal pains, the cramps and cough and fatigue that together form the signature of *Pfiesteria*.

Once again, CSM was rushed to the rescue.

George recovered more slowly this time, and one look at him was enough to know that *Pfiesteria* had come to Rehoboth Bay. (These days, of course, human beings provide a far more accurate "marker" for the dinoflagellate than any lab test.)

George got better in about 10 days. And he didn't return to Rehoboth Beach until the Australian Broadcasting Company (ABC) team called on his services in November of 1999. ABC's Geoffrey Burchfield was shooting a documentary on *Pfiesteria* in preparation for an international conference on Harmful Algal Blooms scheduled for Tasmania in February of 2000. Apparently, the Cell From Hell was making a name for itself worldwide!

Burchfield planned to come to the U.S. to interview some of the major *Pfiesteria* players—including Dr. Burkholder, Dr. Glasgow, and several members of the University of Maryland team. While discussing the outbreak with a Baltimore Sun staffer, Burchfield had learned my name. He called me at 3 A.M. (his time) from far-off Sydney.

"They told you no one in Maryland has been sick from *Pfiesteria*? Nonsense! How many patients do you want to interview? Fifty? A hundred? And by the way, the most dramatic *Pfiesteria* story is probably what happened to George Demas."

ABC wound up with some great shots of George taking the CS test. And the soil expert's dramatic description of the symptoms produced by this acute illness have been preserved forever on Australian videotape.

After the filming, George took what can only be described as a "fateful step."

He led the ABC crew back to his work site in Delaware. He splashed back and forth through the affected shallows and attack zones. And all too soon, he had fallen sick again.

Of course, George Demas had beaten this illness twice before, despite cutting his CSM therapy short during the second bout. But now he made a crucial mistake . . . by staying with the cholestyramine therapy for only a few days.

Why worry, however? He felt fine, didn't he? I won't ever forget a moment in December of 1999 when he and Susan drove up beside me in Salisbury. I was returning from a lecture in Washington, and I looked over in their car and saw that he and his wife had just picked out their Christmas tree.

(We must love our Fates. . . .)

Sitting happily behind the wheel, George gave me a huge grin.

"Hey, Ritch, our new house is almost finished. We're building a fireplace in the living room . . . can you give us a rock for it? A brick? We want something meaningful from you, something we can build into that fireplace!"

"George, I'd be happy to oblige. Let me look around and see what I can find."

I was thinking of a piece of petrified wood I'd been given by a college professor, and the words he'd said to me as he presented me with the gift: "Rocks and friendships can last forever."

But then the light changed.

We drove off in different directions and I never saw George Demas again.

He went back to the Rehoboth work site on the 19th of December, and he was soon afflicted all over again with *Pfiesteria*-related human illness syndrome.

Another physician saw him on the 20th, and prescribed antibiotics and bronchodilators for presumed pneumonia. But George didn't take his CSM. He felt a little better on the 21st; he had less cough and no fever. By the 22nd, he was even more improved . . . though still had a dry, non-productive cough.

That night he was snoring so loudly that Susan wound up on the couch in the living room.

The next morning, she found him cold and blue. She dialed 911, but it was too late.

What killed him? It sounded like an upper airway obstruction to me. When the Wicomico County Medical Examiner phoned me, searching for information, I did my best to help: "Sir, I'm convinced this is a *Pfiesteria*-associated death, and it's the first ever. You must have an autopsy performed by the state. This is a Public Health issue."

The next day—Christmas eve—Assistant State Medical Examiner Dr. Joe Pestaner called. He explained that pneumonia had been found in the deceased's lung tissue, although it was patchy and atypical. No bacteria or pathogenic organisms were found. There had been no obvious obstruction of the upper airway. Increasingly concerned, I suggested that the coroner should look more carefully. What about the illness, the snoring? The repeat episodes? There *had* to be a physiologic basis for his airway obstruction—even if the examiners could find no anatomic basis!

Later that day, around 5 P.M., the Maryland State epidemiologist called. He "just wanted to be sure the death was associated with *Pfiesteria* from Delaware and not from Maryland."

That was too much for me. My friend was dead, Susan was devastated, *Pfiesteria* had been unmasked as a killer of human beings . . . and Maryland wanted confirmation that *Delaware* was responsible!

Enraged, I phoned the DNA and bio-toxin laboratories run by Dr. Oldach and Dr. Ramsdell, respectively. Could they perform assays on human tissue, George's tissue, in order to confirm the presence of *Pfiesteria* toxins? Could they assay for *Pfiesteria* DNA or toxin in lung, larynx and bile? Maybe sometime in the future . . . but they also pointed out that all tissues would have to be stored at minus-80 degrees centigrade for an indeterminate period until such assays became available.

Meanwhile, Dr. Pestaner kept looking for answers. In the soft tissue above the larynx, he found an unusual assemblage of white blood cells . . . a medical condition known as "eosinophilia." Listening to his description, I caught my breath; I'd detected the presence of that same abnormal collection of eosinophils in skin biopsies of patients with acute *Pfiesteria* rash! (Biopsies done on chronic *Pfiesteria* rashes didn't show the eosinophilia.) Was this the missing link that might explain the upper airway obstruction? And what about those tissues from bile, brain and lung? Impatient and alarmed, I pushed the medical staff as hard as I could.

A few days later, however, they informed me that the final diagnosis would be "pneumonia and reactive airway disease." But George certainly didn't have reactive airways disease; he wasn't an asthmatic. And yet the autopsy presented no other cause for either the eosinophilia or the upper airway obstruction.

We'll never have a final answer—because George Demas's body was cremated and nothing was saved. When will there be any further investigation into the effects of *Pfiesteria* toxin on human tissues? Without such an enquiry, how can anyone say with certainty that the Cell From Hell killed my friend? At this time, no one can—but I doubt that anyone will be able to convince me otherwise.

No, my hunk of petrified wood won't be going into George's fireplace.

Bruce and his friends built the chimney for Susan, along with a massive stonework hearth for the room George would never see. That room is now full of memories and mementos from George's short life. But the rock I'd wanted to give him now sits on my shelf, a perpetual reminder of the price that some researchers have to pay . . . and of the fact that my own work is far from done.

Footnote: Just the other day, the press reported attacks of *Pfiesteria* at Tuckahoe Creek, near Atlantic City, and the Public Health brass of New Jersey quickly responded with a predictable press release.

"There is no risk to human health!" said the New Jersey official. "We're certain that *Pfiesteria* lives in a non-toxic, harmless state in many watersheds."

What the article in the Asbury Park Press left out, however, was that investigators had *also* found *Pfiesteria* in the same creek the previous September—and that they hadn't even bothered to inform local officials about the possible health risk. Why not? Hey, who needs the bad public relations?

Another key question that never got asked in New Jersey: What chemicals are sprayed daily on the huge farms and blueberry and cranberry fields of this region, and how frequently are they washed into the waters of Tuckahoe . . . to be concentrated in palustrine emergent vegetation sites with a high loam/silt content? How many patients in New Jersey are already suffering from a chronic, neurotoxin-mediated illness that's been blamed on something else?

Final question: how many patients will eventually die with an airway obstruction—blamed on something else—following exposure to the Tuckahoe or other estuaries in which this newly unmasked suspected killer is now multiplying at will?

For my friend George Demas, fate took the form of an illness linked to an obsessive search for scientific truth.

But he died a hero, and we must fight hard to preserve his legacy.

We must make absolutely certain—now and far into the future—that we never stop telling the world about the epidemic of chronic, neurotoxin-linked illness that is now among us . . . and that millions of vulnerable human beings are now at risk for diseases such as *Pfiesteria*, chronic Lyme, chronic fatigue syndrome and Sick Building Syndrome.

If we are to properly honor and embrace George Demas' mysterious fate, we must start by telling the world honestly and openly about the new family of fast-spreading diseases that killed him on December 23, 1999.

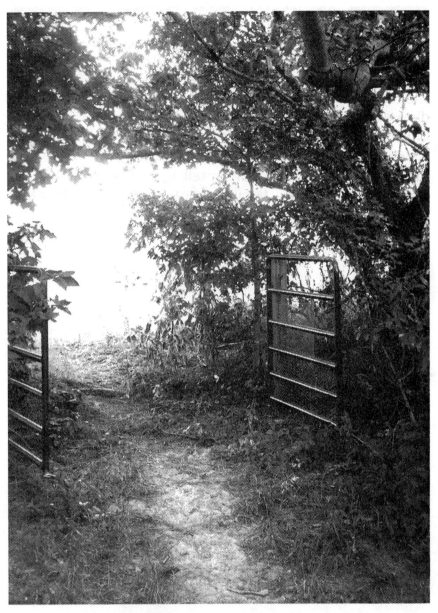

"Welcome to Wonderland,"
Sally Shoemaker, September 1999
Opening a window onto a new world of medicine.

chapter 29

Reflection

Struggling Towards the Light

Pocomoke, MD –September, 2000

Remember when the focus of medical care was on the patient alone?

In those earlier, halcyon days of treatment—long before the 1926 "Flexner Report" called for shifting medical school education from the patient's bedside to the university lecture hall and laboratory—good medical practice placed a high value on encouraging patients to describe their problems to the doctor. Before all else, in that now vanished world of the early Twentieth Century, an effective doctor was a "good listener" . . . a humane and open-minded observer who earned his professionalism by letting the patient talk. Before anesthesia, antibiotics and safe intravenous fluids (including blood), the term "listening" would have served nicely to describe the goal of the Hippocratic oath—a vow which first and foremost embodied the maxim: "Do no harm."

The physician of that earlier epoch learned his medicine from his patients and he communicated his knowledge in thick books and sparse journals that enjoyed little distribution. Back then, proprietary medicine was patient-oriented and featured an "observational" approach to research and teaching.

Bedside physicians in those simpler times understood that the key to successful treatment is taking a full history, and that careful interviewing of patients actually comprises more than 80 percent of the diagnostic process. But then, gradually at first, everything began to change. After the Flexner Report—as the inconsistencies, inaccuracies and lack of rigorous scientific research of bedside medicine gave way to medical centers, research labs and high-tech medical machinery—communication on the topic of medical and scientific progress began to be dominated by practitioners who saw relatively few patients.

In short, the teaching pendulum swung away from the bedside toward the conference room . . . and away from primary care offices toward tertiary care clinics.

Is there any remaining doubt that the outdated "patient-centered" approach to illness has been replaced today by our growing emphasis on "high-tech" diagnostic tools and treatment protocols—along with the "publish or perish syndrome" in which medical educators spend most of their time working on minutiae-filled journal articles?

These days, the neurosurgeon and the orthopedist are usually far more intent on examining the results from the MRI or the lab test than on looking for subtle clues that might emerge from a thorough physical exam. And the result? All too often, the medical receptionist winds up telling the physician: "The hand injury is in Trauma Room 4," instead of "The patient with the injured hand is waiting for you in Room 4."

Although most public relations-minded clinicians will insist that medical care today is "better than ever before," the blunt fact remains that in most doctors' offices the emphasis has shifted from the living, breathing patient to the high-tech gadgetry and the powerful new pharmaceuticals that increasingly dominate the world of medicine.

And what about the ever increasing pressure from managed care, which all too often dictates that physicians spend as little time with patients as possible—before "getting them out the door" and moving on to the next "HMO enrollee" for that next 9-minute "consultation?" (The HMO *patients*, meanwhile, will be pressuring the doctor as hard as they can to extend that 9 minutes . . . in the hope of getting some extra value out of the thousands of dollars they've paid in insurance premiums!)

As many commentators have noted in recent years, this loss of the "personal touch" now forms one of the most alarming and disheartening trends in all of medicine. But one area of medical practice has remained relatively invulnerable to the dehumanizing effects of the "new medicine."

Talk to the older "rural docs" who operate family practices in America's small towns, and you'll discover that many of them have been able to keep Sir William Osler's philosophy of treatment ("Listen to the patient!") alive in their more down-to-earth country practices.

For many of these older practitioners, living and moving among their patients daily has provided an effective defense against the temptation to start seeing human beings as numbers. That continuing interaction with patients has also allowed the older practitioners to cling tenaciously to their identity as physicians—and not as mere "health care providers." More so than their counterparts in the big group practices and the university med schools, the "country docs" have been required to maintain a close, intimate connection with most of their patients.

According to many of these smalltown physicians, there are no sweeter words than those of the patient who tells family and friends: "I always feel better, just by going to see him!" Family practitioners beam with pleasure when they hear this kind of compliment, because it tells them that the patient sees the "doc" as a caring, trusted professional who's authentically interested in helping patients achieve good health.

During more than two decades of caring for patients in my little corner of Maryland, I've been saddened—and frequently angered—by the increasing dehumanization of medical practice.

I've also seen how our growing failure to listen to our patients often prevents us from making an accurate diagnosis . . . or recognizing the presence of new kinds of disorders and diseases in our increasingly pollution-stressed human habitat.

Make no mistake: many of these chronic, neurotoxin-mediated ailments (such as Lyme and ciguatera) aren't really the "emerging diseases" we hear so much about. As a matter of fact, they only *seem* to be emerging illnesses because we physicians have barely begun to recognize and understand how widespread they really are. Fortunately, however, one of the great blessings of the Information Age is that e-mail and fax and most other modern communications tools move with lightning speed.

Today they're rapidly replacing meetings and correspondence —which means that it shouldn't take long for the scientific validity of the principles and concepts presented here to be rigorously evaluated.

It's now time to swing the pendulum back to primary care— while arming the bedside physicians with access to better communication and high-tech tests such as FACT. Such a shift will restore some balance to the treatment approaches now being applied to the newly recognized chronic, neurotoxin-mediated illnesses. And here's the good news: as information-control becomes more and more primary care-oriented, the power of the previous controlling elements of communication of medical information will be lessened dramatically.

But you can be sure that better communication about chronic, neurotoxin-mediated illnesses will pose a major threat to the established, hierarchical system of medical decision-making!

No matter how solid the evidence for this new family of diseases, you can expect a great deal of determined resistance to the discovery from state scientists whose opinions are usually controlled by the politicians—and by corporate interests which might face liability for habitat alteration that contributes to the spread of illness, as news about neurotoxin-linked illnesses increasingly makes the front page.

Another source of resistance, of course, will be the well entrenched medical bureaucracy—which continues to insist that such widespread diseases as chronic Lyme do not exist. How will these powerful entities and agencies react to the challenge to their grip on the communication of medical information?

As I pointed out in the earlier Reflection, "The Appearance of Good Science" (See Chapter 10), one of the most effective techniques employed by those in power is to simply ignore new evidence (no matter how compelling) for theories that lie outside the current "scientific paradigm." Whenever new ideas threaten the status quo, send in the AGS Team to bury them!

One of the major problems with the AGS approach to public health issues, however, is the way it increasingly distorts our national priorities—an outcome that takes a toll on all of us. For that reason, we really can't afford to ignore the ways in which political influence today dictates the "national research agenda," while also controlling most of the government dollars that are spent on investigating health issues. We certainly can't afford to let research dollars and public health policies be influenced by private entities.

Whenever public health becomes "politicized," you will hear such familiar refrains as "The river is safe!" or maybe, "Nothing in the building can cause harm, since all of our tests were negative!"

Remember the endless stonewalling that took place in Florida, after toxic chemicals and blue-green algae combined to wipe out hundreds of alligators and birds? Well, things haven't changed much in the Sunshine State, and the current news media-refrain from "concerned public health officials" sounds hauntingly familiar: "Look, those 400 pelicans were killed by Newcastle Disease. We now know it wasn't toxaphene, after all. And don't worry: we've set up watch lines to scare away any pelicans from the disease area." The idea that organic toxins might have been involved—that simply isn't on the list of probable causes!

Florida: Anatomy of a Coverup

After many years of watching public health issues unfold, I've learned how to recognize the exact moment when the key AGS Consensus Statement gets flushed from Whitewash Lagoon and sent streaming out into the news media for dissemination to a seemingly gullible public. (The key statement, of course, is the one that firmly establishes the government/corporate coverup of the issue as the "conventional wisdom" on that particular topic!)

Like those mighty thunderstorms that boom along Florida's Gulf coast each afternoon, the Arrival of the Consensus Statement is utterly predictable. But so is the behavior of the scientific panel that rubber-stamps the Consensus, whenever the actual facts about a public health issue do manage to emerge. (Veteran journalists refer to this situation—a moment of real news coverage that actually reveals something new and important about an issue—as "an unfortunate slip of the truth.")

It's always the same story: When the truth slips out, even for a few moments, the esteemed members of the blue-ribbon scientific panel will turn tail and run for the cover of damage control. And that's precisely what happened during the massive bird-kills at Lake Apopka, located only a stone's throw from the wonders of Disneyworld in central Florida, near Orlando.

If you remember, the public health officials at Apopka first blamed the pelican deaths on outdated pesticides, including toxaphene. But the data "supporting" that conclusion finally were proven to be flawed, and eventually gave the lie to the prior formal explanation . . . a transparent assessment that anyone could have identified as contrived, absurd and outrageous.

Although the State of Florida's explanation for the pelican catastrophe defied logic and good sense, such apparently well-intentioned groups as the Florida Audubon Society participated willingly in the obfuscation. (Is that why my calls to officials at the Society were never returned?) Still, a number of other environmental groups with political clout did manage to keep the pressure on State officials to continue searching for the causes behind the slaughter of the birds.

In a startling report issued July 27, 2000, the Florida officials acknowledged that their consultant had concluded that the toxaphene data were worthless—but that the afflicted birds probably died from Newcastle Disease. Buried deep in that report was the truth: "The etiological and pathological evidence of the mortality event are not sufficient to identify the specific cause of death of the birds."

(In the absence of proof, of course, the *name* of the disease hardly mattered; why not blame the disaster on avian cholera, a hailstorm, or maybe even the ozone hole?)

Like most scientific researchers, I spend a lot of time making theoretical models. Many are shown to be flawed in one way or another, as testing of the model proceeds. Nonetheless, I do hope they emerge from logical, down to earth efforts at finding reasonable answers to reasonable questions. But that's not what happened in Florida—where the public health bureaucracy embarrassed itself again with its disingenuous attempt to blame the pelican deaths on a wild-blue-yonder virus, based on several low-level antibody tests in a few birds.

Like blaming "pesticides," the Florida attempt to pin the disaster at Lake Apopka on a virus was a smokescreen . . . a strategy designed to make sure that no State agency (and no private corporation) would be held responsible for causing the environmental havoc that triggered the pelican deaths. Meanwhile, the test for blue-green algae toxins remained in a box, unused. Once again, AGS was in firm command: *When you find yourself caught in the environmental spotlight, test for everything except the likely cause!*

Appalling as it now seems in retrospect, the public health foot-dragging at Lake Apopka was soon matched by recent events in the nearby Lake Griffin region . . . where the Florida Fish and Game Commission recently acknowledged that the levels of blue-green algae toxins found in many lakes and rivers used as sources of drinking water are lethal for mice. Alarming? You bet. And the *next* question for the experts at Lake Griffin ought to be obvious: are those same levels also lethal for alligators?

How about other aquatic species, including invertebrates and competing species of algae? How about children mixing their summer cooling drinks with water, fresh from the tap, coming from unknown reservoirs?

The time to stop the scientific stonewalling over these issues is now.

Remember: when it comes to evaluating and then making decisions about public health threats from emerging illnesses, silence kills.

As the Chemical Age advances and the impact of toxic substances on our environment increases daily, conscientious physicians must do their best to understand how that same impact is affecting their patients' health from one moment to the next.

Don't let the public health bureaucrats and the politicians get away with covering up the facts!

Maybe there's another way? In addition to demanding "full disclosure," patients can insist on a FACT exam in situations where they suspect a chronic illness linked to neurotoxins. And if their doctor doesn't know about Contrast Sensitivity—or if he says the test isn't reliable, based on a snap judgment and no knowledge about the procedure—then a patient can always obtain another opinion.

For millions of suffering people today, the good news is that the groundswell of patients asking for an objective new approach to the diagnosis and treatment of chronic disease has really begun to take off. And you can be sure that these tens of thousands of patients who increasingly describe illness symptoms linked to environmentally acquired toxins are going to be *heard*. At the same time, even the specialists from the CDC are starting to pay attention, as are public health officials in such states as Florida, North Carolina, Delaware and New Jersey.

The bottom line is quite simple here, and the bottom line is that our environment *can* poison us. (Nor will an illness go away merely because an authority figure says, "The water is safe.")

But how will the public learn about the very real risks involved, if the sources of news about public health are contaminated by increasing concentration of ownership? Obviously, the recent mergers of giant-sized communications companies and equally large pharmaceutical companies raises the sinister specter of "information control."

Ask yourself: If a pesticide manufacturer has access to the results of a state investigation into harmful effects related to the use of that pesticide before the affected farmer does, can we really expect a "fair, even-handed probe" into the harmful effects?

That's one example of how political favoritism can degrade public health policy and public health regulations.

And what about the highly dubious situation—all too common, these days—in which a major university's academic health center winds up being controlled by regents who also happen to control the most powerful newspaper in the state?

Can we really hope that the shortcomings of the university will be reported under such circumstances? And will the typical newspaper be willing to take a stance that conflicts with the large regional university's position?

To make matters even worse, what happens if the reigning political opinion in the state gains the full support of those same regents . . . so that the latter can cozy up to the elected officials in their relentless quest for more public money for their own academic fiefdoms? (And does anyone out there really believe that such public funds *won't* ultimately be used to expand private operations?)

The uneasy relationship between public health and our politicians seemed all too evident last April 8 (2000), when Senator Rick Santorum (R-Pa.) addressed a noisy rally of Lyme activists that had been billed as "The Second Battle of Gettysburg."

The activists had gotten the senator's attention with their urgent demands that the federal government do more to help the few "Lyme-Literate Physicians" (LLMDs) working in the mid-Atlantic region. They also wanted to see much more research on (and research funding for) chronic Lyme disease. Before the rally, Santorum had been fully informed about the attacks on the licenses of the LLMDs by health bureaucrats in Connecticut and New York. Those attacks had been aided and abetted, some observers felt sure, by researchers with a vested interest in maintaining the status quo in Lyme.

By April of 2000, the non-stop attacks had already claimed a few practitioner-licenses in the region, and had persuaded many other docs to stop treating the disease entirely. (The CSM/ pioglitazone protocols should put an end to such needless persecution of treating physicians.) Rather than focusing on the plight of the victimized doctors, however, Santorum drew his loudest cheers of the evening by pointing out that "more than $40 million will be added to [federal programs] to fund additional Lyme research!" (Got a problem? Throw money at it!)

And where would all those greenbacks eventually wind up?

According to the senator, $5 million was earmarked for the CDC. Another $5 million would be headed directly toward the NIH . . . where it would undoubtedly end up funding more studies that could lead to more researchers forming private corporations—after appropriating key aspects of the studies and then taking such dubious steps as selling "Lyme Test Cards" on the open market!

But what about the remaining $30 million? As usual, the Pentagon heavies would end up with the largest slice of the Lyme pie. That outcome was easy to understand, however, since the DOD had known since 1990 that Lyme was a "major threat" to its own personnel. In earlier tests, the U.S. Army had collected samples from 100 deer near Ft. Meade, Md., and had found that essentially all of the animals were carrying Lyme antibodies. (So do horses in New Jersey and dogs in Long Island, by the way.)

In addition, 85 percent of the deer in Maryland had nymph or larval stages of ticks feeding on them . . . while 14 percent of the bugs were carrying the actual Lyme spirochete, *Borrelia burgdorferi*. But who knew about this U.S. Army report, which had to be pried out of the government's hands by using the Freedom of Information Act?

Although the American military hasn't necessarily been eager to share its findings with the public health sector, the fact remains that the Department of Defense may be the most progressive and open-minded government agency to have studied the growing epidemic of Lyme disease.

Example: in recent years, the U.S. Army has conducted numerous field tests aimed at determining whether or not deer and deer ticks on their far-flung bases are carriers of the Lyme bacteria. Their conclusions, contained in a recently obtained Pentagon document—"Addendum, Lyme Disease and Risk Assessment"—left no doubt that Lyme disease is thriving on military installations all across the country:

- "At Ft. Stewart, Ga., the U.S. Army has conducted at least 4 Lyme Disease Risk Assessments—1991, 1992, 1993, and 1994. These assessments found the Lyme disease tick, Lyme disease bacteria in the ticks, and the Lyme disease bacteria in mammals at the facility."
- "At Ft. Benning, Ga., the U.S. Army has conducted at least 3 Lyme Disease Risk Assessments—1991, 1992, 1993. These assessments found the Lyme disease tick, the Lyme disease bacteria in the ticks, and the 1991 study found the Lyme disease bacteria in mammals at the facility."
- "At the Marine Corps Logistics Base in Daugherty County, Ga., the U.S. Army has conducted at least one Lyme Disease Risk Assessment and found the Lyme disease tick and the Lyme disease bacteria in the ticks at the facility in 1994."

Responding to these three studies, a thoughtful scientist who remembers the CDC's position on this issue during the past ten years can only ask:

- No Southern Lyme?
- No Southern Lyme?
- No Southern Lyme?

The CDC says there *is* no Lyme in the south! What happened to "communication?" The military already knew what the CDC acknowledged only after ten years of acrimony! Couldn't the military have informed the CDC about its positive tests for

Lyme, and thus have saved the taxpayers a huge expense . . . while also eliminating paralyzing uncertainty about the spread of this obvious epidemic? Wouldn't this Lyme data from the Pentagon have brought the ongoing argument over the "reality" of fast-spreading Lyme disease to a crashing halt?

Why didn't the CDC experts ask the military what it knew about Lyme disease?

If the military demands command control, the CDC seems to demand communication control.

Communication costs money, of course, and it's true that federal dollars for health research have been extremely difficult to come by in recent years . . . which makes the recent decision by Congress to hand the Center for Discussion Crushing $100 million for better public relations rather difficult to understand! More funding for the "CDC spin" on communication about health issues?

Yes, you read that last paragraph correctly. While federal funding for research on such chronic and misery-inducing diseases as asthma, diabetes and Alzheimer's is hard to obtain from year to year, the folks on Capitol Hill recently authorized the release of 100 million Big Ones for *"improved communications!"*

Hard to believe, you say? But it's all true . . . and it was all reported in September of 2000 by an international, Internet-based news service (FedBuzz.com) that presented the facts in shocking black and white:

CDC's New Communication Plan
A $100 Million Voice Change:

Hoping to help consumers buffeted with tidal waves of confusing and sometimes conflicting health information, the federal government plans to spend up to $100 million to strengthen the voice of its health promotion agency—the Centers for Disease Control and Prevention (CDC).

The two-pronged effort allocates up to $50 million for health communications market research and evaluation plus another $50 million for actual production of various health information programs. Seven private contractors have been chosen to do the work. (See list page 446.)

The long list of new communications projects includes:

- Revamping of the entire CDC web site and development of a web page for children.

- A program encouraging the writers of tv soap operas and prime time shows and Hollywood screen writers to embed positive health behaviors in their creations.

- A national effort to bring safer needle devices into the nation's hospitals and reduce health worker exposure to blood-borne pathogens.

- A video/workbook program to help men decide whether they should undergo the PSA blood test for prostate cancer, a test whose effectiveness is under considerable debate.

In recent weeks, some 23 separate projects have been readied for award through the task order process, a rush of communications for Christine Prue, Ph.D., coordinator for creative services at CDC's Office of Communications.

"If there is a sound bite, it is this—strategic communications —there is a strategy behind the words and ideas we present," said Prue. "There are a lot of people in the marketplace trying to influence people about health, either for the good or bad, and it's getting more confusing. We want to be an objective but also an effective voice with all those other voices out there."

Prue and other CDC officials said the agency's new focus exploits its traditional science and research strengths, which are highly-regarded among physicians and health professionals, by applying strong research to the emerging science of health communications.

Galen Cole, CDC coordinator of communications research and evaluation, said the agency aims to not waste its health messages. "We're not cluttering the airwaves with things we don't know work," he said. "When you just shoot a message out there without having tested your various audiences, you don't know what harm you might be doing."

He said the CDC is better suited to research its messages than private organizations with less of a science base. "We do a better job and there is a lot more riding on our research," he said.

"For example. We have low immunization rates in a couple of cities. We want to find out why parents are not getting children immunized. We'll do research, maybe focus groups, talk to providers to find out what is unique about the population. We might design a computer-assisted interview, then design a program to get the message out. We need to combat misinformation about immunization—that shots don't work, for instance—and make sure we develop a clear message."

Cole said the contracts for evaluation were developed so the same contractors that produced health communications materials did not evaluate them. "That's where we probably have an added advantage over the private sector," he said. "We don't have the fox guarding the henhouse."

One of the companies doing the research and evaluation, Macro International, has done previous CDC work, including research on a program to help parents avoid water-born parasitic diseases that could strike children at water parks.

"The whole area of health communications is a burgeoning area," said Doryn-Davis Chervin, director of health communication evaluation services for Macro. "The CDC is really looking at how you communicate to an audience, how you communicate scientific information. How do you understand what people need?"

Her company is involved in researching a program to promote safer needle-handling in hospitals, she said. "We're trying to understand the decision making process, so we'll probably do a web-based survey of hospital infection control managers."

She said other CDC programs include such things as a project dealing with the use of fluoride in children, another to reduce the burden of arthritis, research into the school food safety program and a communication program involving the condition of excessive iron in the blood.

"At the same time work goes out for evaluation, there is also a contract going out for the creative contract which involves implementation of the campaign," she said.

"Health communications really is changing," said Chervin. "In the past, the decisions might have been, well, let's send out a brochure. Now we ask who needs it and why, what is the approach? How do we evaluate it?"

Echoing the thoughts of many at the federal agency based in Atlanta, Chervin noted that the CDC has tremendous credibility. "The task now is to present health information to a lay audience," she said. "There are many very complex health issues and they are being very thoughtful about it."

One major communications channel for the CDC is its web site, which "is actually one of the best kept secrets of all health sites," said Susan Robinson, who focuses on multimedia development for the site. "We get a tremendous amount of traffic." (The agency said it got 1.7 million unique visits in the month of July.)

Robinson said a contract was soon to be awarded to one of the designated contractors for evaluation and revamping of the site.

"We're a first-generation site that has grown quickly over the last few years," she said. "Now we'll revamp the site to be more nimble in a very busy marketplace. We have a huge advantage because credibility has surfaced as a major issue in health communication and the CDC name is very credible because of all the good work we do."

Introducing ... The CDC
Health Communications Players

The CDC health communication initiative is a five-year plan, with separate tracks for evaluation and production. Each track will spend up to $50 million over the five years.

Three companies have received contracts to evaluate health communications in the first year. Because each of them will be invited to bid on all task orders, each has been give a one year contract (with options for future years) for a maximum of $10 million.

The three are Macro International, Atlanta GA; Affect Inc., Lake Forrest IL; and Westat, Rockville MD.

Four companies have received contracts for health communications creative productions, with similar $10 million contracts each for the first year. The CDC said it expects to spend up to $50 million over five years on this creative side.

The contractors are: Ogilvy Public Relations, Washington DC; Porter Novelli, Washington DC; Prospect Associates, Silver Spring MD; and AED, Washington DC.

•   •   •

Question: Why are we spending $100 million to help the CDC communicate Consensus Statements better to the public . . . when it's quite obvious that the Atlanta health experts are unable to communicate with other agencies inside their own *government?* Let's face it: what's needed here is for the primary researchers—real doctors who see real patients—to step in and help Washington's Beltway-based think tanks to understand real medicine and real health care issues. And spending millions on revamped PR operations won't help that process in the least!

As a reminder for the CDC type information control, look how the U.S. military long ago concluded that Lyme disease now represents a significant health threat in most areas of the country. They didn't need $100 million to cut right to the truth.

Even better, the military will talk to the private sector even if other government agencies don't ask the right questions.

For example, after visiting the U.S. Army Centers for Health Promotion and Prevention (USACHPPM) and conferring with key military leaders about the problem, one of America's top Lyme disease activists—Pat Smith, executive director of the Lyme Disease Association—issued a startling report noting that the generals and the colonels were, indeed, gravely concerned about the illness and saw it as a major threat to the health and safety of their troops. As Smith noted in a voluminously detailed summary compiled soon after the meeting with the Army command:

"Why are Lyme and other tick-borne diseases (TBDs) seriously considered threats to the troops who defend our country, yet not considered threats to the civilian population? Why are military installations mapped and rated for tick densities and rates of infection, while public parks are not even posted with warning signs?

"Why would PCRs be reliable 'in the field' and not at commercial labs? Why is the government impregnating uniforms with permethrin, when we all know that the civilian population is creating a climate of 'Lyme hysteria' and that Lyme is 'over-diagnosed and over-treated?'

"To quote the report: 'In addition to directly transmitting disease, the adverse impact of psychological factors associated with tick attack, including fear, discomfort and distraction, as well as indirect medical complications such as secondary infections, dermatitis or allergic reactions, should not be overlooked.'

"The Army has not labeled this 'hysteria' but normal 'complications' of tick attacks.

"Why is the vaccine promoted to the civilian population, yet the report states: 'Questions and concerns linger regarding the new vaccine's safety . . . effectiveness . . . age restrictions . . . frequency of boosters . . . and the known limitation that it is ineffective against European strains of the Lyme disease agent.

"'Confident decisions as to its value and use within the military cannot yet be made.'

"Why does this double standard exist? I do not have all the answers, but I think we need to work more closely with government and the military to get all the answers so that we can solve this enigma that has been called Lyme disease."

Amazing, isn't it? The CDC didn't ask, the military didn't tell, and now we're going to pay $100 million for more control of information going into every school, TV show, movie and newspaper . . . all of which will bear that increasingly familiar label: "According to the CDC!"

• • •

Diagnosing Lyme: How Much Should It Cost?

The Pentagon study quoted above demonstrates beyond a reasonable doubt that Lyme disease is widespread throughout major regions of the United States, and that the public health establishment will soon be required to face up to that fact.

But what's the best—and most economical—form of treatment for those unfortunate enough to be bitten by a Lyme-carrying tick?

In a study reported in the New England Journal of Medicine less than ten years ago, an investigator was able to show that if the incidence of spirochetes in ticks was more than one percent, it becomes cost-effective to treat everyone who experienced a tick bite with doxycycline for three weeks—and thus avoid the need for serologic (blood) testing on anyone.

Even a brief look at the economics involved in treating chronic Lyme is enough to show the wisdom of the NEJM investigators on this topic. For starters, the standard ELISA test for Lyme costs $60 and has a 60-percent "false negative" rate. (Of course, it also has a 60-percent "false *positive*" rate.) Meanwhile, the more complicated "Western Blot" test currently retails for $120 . . . since the CDC now insists that a high number of "bands" (positive antibody tests) appear in the results, in order to make sure the "false positive rate" isn't too high.

(Or is the *real* reason—as suggested by one Lyme activist I recently interviewed—to make sure that the *true* positive rate doesn't climb too high?)

What is the health dollar cost and human cost of a case of untreated Lyme? Whose dollar are physicians spending? Theirs? When it comes to sick children, parents will demand treatment and forget the cost. It's helpful to remember that our "Lyme I" study demonstrated how the FACT assay for Lyme is far superior to any blood test for diagnosing the effect of both the Lyme toxin and the chronic illness.

Our research proves there's a better way! Spend five minutes taking a FACT at your doctor's office (or maybe at our website: *chronicneurotoxins.com*) and get a head start on a Lyme diagnosis that leads to *effective* treatment.

A Helping Hand from FDEP

Although *Desperation Medicine* has often been critical of state public health departments and the bureaucrats who run them, the State of Florida deserves credit for bucking the trend and actually taking steps to investigate reports of chronic, neuro-toxin-mediated illness possibly caused by mutation-inducing toxic chemicals.

Florida's Department of Environmental Protection consists of several different pollution-fighting units—one of which is charged with cleaning up hazardous waste sites and investigating toxic leaks on land.

Despite some early hesitations and mis-steps, the FDEP acquitted itself honorably in the investigation over alleged toxic pesticide residues at Frank Fuzzell's nursery near Orlando. What happened in Florida, thankfully, was that several state officials who had tuned into my conference call with the CDC in February of 2000 were struck by my final remark: "This problem exists all over the State of Florida!"

Because they felt my statement was accurate, the Sunshine State officials immediately went to work on the problem. Led by Bill Martin, a team of FDEP investigators began assembling a plan that would create the chemical and microbial investigation I had called for.

I had my doubts about the FDEP initiative, but I got a very pleasant surprise when the Martin team actually delivered a work plan containing more than 300 pages of documents. The project included plant disease experts, detection specialists and microbiology labs. And most surprising of all . . . I was named to review the human health data that would be generated by the investigation.

At first, the whole thing seemed too good to be true. Hadn't the Florida Department of Health gone out of its way again and again to slam my credibility throughout the state? Yet the FDEP kept insisting that any health investigation would have to start with the Fuzzell site . . . and with the lengthy epidemiological research I'd already conducted in the region, as I went about the task of recording the cases of patients who were clearly suffering from chronic, neurotoxin-mediated illness.

Against all odds, the work plan was eventually approved. Let freedom ring! Here was a chance to get out there and *document* the human health effects from what appeared to have been an agricultural disaster. I was thrilled with the news, because I knew our findings in Florida would eventually be applicable to other human populations suffering from neurotoxin-linked diseases around the world.

As the team began to prepare for the upcoming investigation, I asked myself a couple of key questions. First, was there a link between the land and the *cylindrospermopsis* blooms in the nearby lakes? And second, why were so many people blaming the chemical company that had supplied the allegedly habitat-altering pesticide, when the investigation hadn't even begun?

I wasn't interested in the blame game, because I had long ago observed that as soon as a corporate entity is accused of causing health problems, angry lawsuits spring up like Theban soldiers from buried dragon's teeth—and then the entire debate becomes a squabble over "compensation" and "punitive damages."

Instead of quibbling with lawyers, I wanted to attack the public health issues that now loomed over the Florida landscape. And that's why being named to the FEDP investigative team (and then permitted to study the impact of chemicals on chronic, neurotoxin-mediated illness) was for me a dream come true.

Clean up the neurotoxins, I told myself, *and the questions about where they came from will be answered later!*

The good news, of course, is that such questions are now beginning to be asked in several areas of the country where neurotoxin-linked illness has been identified. In Florida, for example, 40,000 people recently signed a petition insisting that state public health authorities address the dinoflagellate problem and the lesioned-fish problem in the St. Lucie River (near Stuart on the East Coast). Their message was clear—"Stop stalling!"—and the politicians were listening. Money was appropriated for river cleanup, and a supplemental one-percent county sales tax was imposed for three years to raise funds for purchase of farmland that would soon be returned to its prior state as protected wetlands.

In Maryland, unhappily, the official response to habitat contamination and resulting illness was far different. There the governor supposedly "saved the Bay" by restricting nutrient-usage among farmers. In contrast, the Chesapeake Bay EPA Program published a "Toxics Inventory" for the Bay in 1998. That document showed that the EPA investigators had found a huge amount of copper in the Bay . . . but their official report noted the presence of only *nine pounds* of DTC fungicides.

Nine pounds! What about the 6,000 acres of tobacco lands that had been treated that year with ten pounds of DTC for each acre . . . *during each week of the growing season?*

The good news for the State of Maryland is that the CDC has finally begun hearing the very loud voice of our data on the *Pfiesteria* health issue.

Indeed, by June of 2000 word was beginning to filter down that the Centers for Discussion Crushing might be ready to flip-flop on this issue. Then Bob Venezia called: could he visit my office along with several colleagues from the North Carolina *Pfiesteria* team? Incredibly, they now wanted to learn what I was doing, and they wanted to "work cooperatively" with me. And because they were closely linked to the CDC, I knew that I'd probably be able to get my cases onto some executive desks in Atlanta, where they would matter most.

"Sure," I told Dr. Venezia, "come one down as soon as you can. But you're going to have to go with me into the attack zones and do some sediment-testing. Get your toes into that river bottom, and find out what the locals know—the truth about *Pfiesteria* habitats. Compare for yourselves the difference between silty loam sediments adjacent to palustrine emergent vegetation and sandy silts in the same areas.

"Discover why deposition sites of heavy metals provide nothing less than a map of *Pfiesteria* attack zones in all the rivers of the lower Chesapeake Bay!"

Dr. Venezia instantly agreed. But what he hadn't counted on, perhaps, was that his arrival on June 22 of 2000 would be preceded by several fish kills in the Pocomoke. (The state public health officials remained silent about the kills, of course, although they would later release evidence of *Pfiesteria* isolates in the river during that same period.)

Accompanied by Amy Chapin of Maryland and Paul Webb and Kathleen Buckheit of North Carolina, Bob Venezia appeared in my office right on schedule. But he looked a bit pale, as I described fish lesions and showed him pictures of rashes on patients from Florida to Delaware. The photos must have been powerfully effective, because he soon began to perspire and then even to retch violently. As a matter of fact, he became so ill that he couldn't accompany us into harm's way on that particular day. Was it something he had eaten the night before? Or was it simply fear? (He needn't have fretted, however; CSM works wonderfully as a medication for clearing organic toxins from the human body!)

Although we missed Dr. Venezia, it turned out to be quite a day. Jack Spurling ferried us to Fair Island, then to Pitt's and Bulbeggar Creeks. The weather seemed ideal, and we all learned a great deal about each other. Paul and Kathleen promised complete cooperation, as did Amy.

Soon after the excursion, Gary Mayo called me from Rose Bay, N.C. He was a well-known *Pfiesteria* victim, having been exposed in 1996. Gary had consulted all of the North Carolina experts, but he was still markedly affected and displayed all of the symptoms of the illness. Paul had spoken to Gary, and while being careful to observe conflict-of-interest strictures, had let him know that I was treating *Pfiesteria* patients.

Unable to drive long distances, himself (he feared getting lost), Gary managed to find a friend to chauffeur him the 250 miles to Pocomoke for diagnosis and CSM treatment. Three weeks later he drove himself to my office. His symptoms had abated, and he was toxin-free. His 18 different PEAS symptoms had vanished, and he was about to enter the record books as the first official PEAS case from the Tar Heel State. But the experience had taken a psychological toll: now Gary was planning to sell his businesses and move far away from his boyhood home. "I don't want this to happen to me again," he explained sadly, "or anyone else in my family."

Another key *Pfiesteria* patient during this early period was Norman Tarr, who became ill after cast-netting among fish later found to be lesioned at Ayers Creek, located on the ocean side of Maryland's Worcester County. After the toxic dinoflagellate was discovered at his fishing site, Norman drove over to Pocomoke to consult with me. He took the Contrast Sensitivity test, and it confirmed what we suspected: he was struggling with the symptoms of *Pfiesteria*-related human illness syndrome.

Norman had already contracted the disease once before, in 1997, but after being exposed at a different location—again on the ocean side of the Eastern Shore, right next door to the populous summer resort, Ocean City.

As promised, I quickly telephoned Venezia and Chapin in order to report Norman's situation. I also noted that this case was right then receiving TV and newspaper coverage as part of the *Pfiesteria* story, statewide. The Maryland Health Department had been told about Tarr's illness, but the response so far had amounted to nothing more than: "We're aware of Dr. Shoemaker's work, but this client's [sic] illness hasn't been confirmed."

Ken Hudnell was outraged by the foot-dragging and denial in Maryland. "They don't have a *positive?*" asked the EPA expert. "Yes, they do. You reported it, exactly as they asked. This case meets every PEAS criterion! In effect, they're overturning the surveillance process . . . and they need to retract their statement on this. We should notify the CDC and every state that could be affected, and we should point out exactly how the surveillance process is supposed to work—and how it has been subverted by the State of Maryland."

Fortunately for the affected public, however, the Delaware approach to the problem differed radically from Maryland's bury-your-head-in-the-sand strategy. There the key officials involved in monitoring *Pfiesteria*—Dr. Sergio Huerta and Dr. Bruce Richards of the Center for the Inland Bays environmental group—were intent on tracing possible links between recurrent, massive fish kills in the Indian River and Rehoboth Bay and increasing reports of human health-effects in the region.

(It should also be noted for the record that the kills and the *Pfiesteria* isolation took place in areas where Dr. George Demas had been working just prior to his death in December of 1999.)

In short, these Delaware officials were determined to confront the problem head-on, and they soon invited me to attend a board meeting of the Center for the Coastal Bays. Also attending were the Secretaries of the Delaware Departments of Agriculture and Natural Resources . . . both of whom were intent on learning more about neurotoxin-triggered illness, diagnosis and treatment.

Because they were doing their best to come to grips with the *Pfiesteria* threat in their own state, the Delaware officials were curious about Maryland's refusal to do the same. No sooner had I finished my talk than one of them asked, "How is Maryland working with you on some of these issues you brought up today? Are your state officials cooperating to solve the public health problem?"

"Well," I said, "let me give you an example." As it turned out, a threatening bloom of *microcystis*—a toxin-forming blue-green algae—had recently begun to choke several rivers emptying into the northern reaches of the Chesapeake (See Chapter 11, "The Monster In the Lake"). The incursion was so serious, I told the Delaware officials, that I'd already received several calls from alarmed officials at the Maryland Department of Natural Resources about these potentially toxic algae.

Meanwhile, the Maryland Department of Health continued to croon its familiar old refrain: "The river is safe. There is no cause for alarm!"

Déjà vu all over again!

After I gave the Delaware officials the information I'd collected about a 17-month-old patient and three dead dogs that had reportedly been exposed to *microcystis* along the Elk River, I told them (hearsay, of course) how a top Maryland DNR administrator had attempted to "solve" the problem by reportedly announcing: "It's nearly winter, and it's getting cold . . . the situation will take care of itself before we can act, anyway!"

Looking back later on the lecture I gave at the Center for the Inland Bays, I was struck by the aggressive determination to face up to the epidemic that I found in Delaware's public officials. Why did they feel such strong motivation to confront this issue? When I asked that question, one of the Center trustees pointed out that "my own nephew has been sick for several months—he goes fishing on the Elk River nearly every day!"

According to the trustee, the nephew had complained frequently about "the green pond scum all over the water," only a few days before becoming ill. "He has headaches, muscle aches and undiagnosed liver abnormality," said the trustee.

I responded by telling him: "Make sure the doctors test the boy for *microcystis* toxin . . . and break out the cholestyramine!"

But this was hardly the first "public health horror story" to unfold in Maryland during recent years. Ironically enough, 51 weeks after the Copper-*Pfiesteria* Conference, the health officials in the Old Line State issued a report (but "not for publication") on the invasion of local estuarine waters by the Cell From Hell. Their bottom-line conclusion: *Copper appears to be a potential factor in the blooming of toxic Pfiesteria, and its role should be investigated!*

In other words: despite all the manipulation of data by some Maryland state scientists, the investigators had finally come to the right conclusion.

And indeed, the very same conclusion would soon be reached by Virginia Tech researcher Dr. Andrea Dietrich. In June 2000, she and her co-workers presented data to the American Chemical Society meetings (at Washington, D.C.) confirming the enormous impact of bio-available copper contained in watershed run-off. In spite of the increasing use of sedimentation ponds and other improved agricultural techniques in our region, copper from tomato crops continued to act as a major poison for some invertebrate creatures inhabiting estuaries.

Although Dr. Dietrich's work carries major scientific clout, it seems likely that the State of Maryland won't do much about toxic chemicals, except to study them in some under-funded manner (AGS—by means of "burial!"). Wouldn't these *Pfiesteria* nay-sayers be better off if they admitted their various mistakes, deletions and distortions and got on with the business of trying to clean up the Chesapeake Bay?

Let's face it: Even the Inquisition was finally forced to admit that poor Galileo had gotten it right! The Earth really does revolve around the sun, folks. But I don't expect to hear the public health Inquisitors of the Old Line State recanting anytime in the near future . . . even if some of them have taken to admitting publicly of late: "We have been testing the wrong chemicals in the wrong places at the wrong time."

Remember: Nutrients aren't the only issue!

How FACT Can Help

I learned a long time ago that the courtroom is hardly a place in which to expect the truth. All too often, it's actually a place where the "spin" of a hidden agenda gets placed on words and deeds by skilled public speakers. And I also learned a long time ago that the skilled public speakers we elect to office will pursue *their* hidden agendas tenaciously—with the spoken word usually a victim of political expediency.

For a refreshing change of pace, why not attempt a bit of truth here? We've entered a new era of "chronic illnesses" in America. These maladies cause similar, persistent symptoms. But with a simple, inexpensive test like the FACT, your doctor can make an accurate diagnosis in five minutes. If you have neurotoxic symptoms, *demand* a FACT! (And don't fret: we can arrange the test for you, if it turns out that your own physician doesn't have the $500 diagnostic tool necessary to perform this basic procedure. Just click on our website (chronicneurotoxins.com).

The most encouraging aspect of the FACT is that it will serve as a highly reliable compass to help guide you and your physician through the rough spots and potholes that are part of CSM treatment. For this guidance we thank the EPA's Dr. Ken Hudnell, Ph.D., who first conceived of using FACT in *Pfiesteria* patients. For millions of long-suffering chronic patients around the country, Dr. Hudnell has turned on the light at the end of the tunnel.

But it's also important to remember that a CSM regimen can cause serious "intensification reactions" for patients with chronic Lyme disease. Because these reactions occur so frequently, I strongly recommend against "taking CSM just to see if it will help." Instead, obtain professional advice from a clinician experienced in CSM use in advance, so that you'll be able to understand and prepare for such reactions. Then, once you've obtained a diagnosis and have begun to feel better, stay abreast of new developments in this fast-changing field. (We're working steadily on improved versions of CSM, for example.)

You should also remember that endogenous neurotoxins will make you sick again, as soon as you stop taking this medication. Although science doesn't fully understand the structure of those toxins yet, we *do* know how to help patients cope with them. And no, it is not "premature" to begin feeling better—even if we don't yet know every detail regarding the morphology and functioning of the toxin.

The point is that the "mechanism of action" makes sense, and the hypothesis has been carefully thought out.

Just a Model

Whenever I speak about these matters with such renowned research scientists as Dr. Hudnell, Dr. John Ramsdell and Dr. Thomas Tosteson, it seems quite clear that the final answers to most of my questions—and especially those involving the mechanism of toxin effects, the interaction of toxins, the relationship between receptors and cell function and the actual mechanism through which CSM provides its toxin-clearing benefit—will have to come from their laboratories and not mine. (As a matter of fact, I don't even *have* a fully outfitted laboratory!)

Once the scientific "testing" has been completed and the model has been reshaped, the evidence will tell us if my approach to treating these illnesses really works.

But I can't afford to wait for the pure science to be finished —not when patients such as Frank Fuzzell and Rhonna Smith and hundreds like them are desperate for relief.

Unfortunately, the Saga of the Invading Chronic Illnesses has only just begun. As we continue to alter our environment with habitat and lifestyle changes in the years immediately up ahead, you can expect more microscopic monsters to come crawling up out of the mud. They'll live among us quite contentedly . . . even if the alligators and the brine shrimp in our ecologically threatened wetlands have all expired.

The older medical model of infectious diseases must be expanded in order to include toxin-mediated illnesses in which antibiotics, antibodies and the immune system do not play a major role in the body's defense.

One major difference between toxins and infections, of course, is that re-exposure to a toxin will likely make you sick again (if you've already taken a course of CSM), or it will make you sicker, molecule by molecule (if you haven't been treated). The painful fact is that if you live, play or work in a toxin-infested environment you have two basic options: getting treatment, or leaving.

Remember, also, that if you do live or play in an infested environment, you have the right to demand cleanup. And if you work in a contaminated zone—a sick building, for example—you should remember that you have legal recourse, if your employer starts playing games with truth.

I've outlined the key ingredients of the Appearance of Good Science in Chapter 10—so don't let anyone deprive you of a safe workplace by using the AGS!

As we continue to trigger changes in our environment, the new creatures who come along will usually be thought of as "bad for us." But if we take a broader view of these changing ecological patterns, we soon realize that our environment can't really be described as "poisoned"—not if some of these new life forms are quite happy to ingest environmental poisons as their food (in the way that some scary new bacteria actually eat cyanide as fertilizer).

In biology, remember, one creature's carbon sources are another's toxins—so that determining the ultimate purpose and value of any life form becomes quite difficult and depends almost entirely on your point of view.

Consider the curious fate of the gypsy moth plague which infested Maryland's Eastern Shore a few seasons ago. After raging unchecked for a while, the plague was stopped cold in the Pocomoke River Forest, when a slow-growing fungus, entomophaga, obtained a selective advantage . . . possibly from the *Bacillus thurigensis* that the state was spraying to kill caterpillars.

The fungus thrived on gypsy moth caterpillars, and it wasn't long before many of the human residents were exulting: "Goodbye, gypsy moths, here's hope for the oak trees."

But when the caterpillars died and the spraying stopped, the entomophaga fungus population returned to normal. Like the bacterial infections that wiped out the invaders from Mars in the H.G. Wells classic, "War of the Worlds," our normal and unchanged populations of life forms can often be quite helpful in restoring the balance among living creatures. And they will undoubtedly help us to contend with the mutant life forms that are created by our relentless pollution of the environment.

Still, there's a finite limit on our altering of the habitat, and if we cross the "point of no return," we will do so at considerable peril to our species. I fear that the many ornamental nurseries which recently experienced crop damage in Florida did go beyond that point of no return, in fact. At the Casteen Roads site, for example, no chemicals of any sort have been applied since 1995, yet the local soils still make neighbors and state inspectors quite ill at times with the same group of neurotoxic symptoms. The same fear holds true for the cylindrospermopsis infested lakes of Central Florida.

Such problems are enormously compounded by the fact that the American medical community has historically refused to take a leadership role in environmental activism. In the past, no doubt, there were many good reasons why practicing doctors felt they should stick to medicine, and leave advocacy to others.

But we have now entered a new era of illness, in which our traditional role as public health advocates has virtually evaporated . . . in large part due to pressures from managed care, which loudly insists: "You, Mr. Doctor, are no different from any other public utility; take it or leave it!"

These days, the busy physician (and especially the managed care physician) needs to take the lead in diagnosis of environmentally acquired illnesses. And the task will not be that difficult. Getting it right under these new medical conditions usually requires little more than the willingness to ask a few additional questions.

The next time you see your physician, ask him or her about the possibility of doing a "neurotoxic history." If the practitioner doesn't know what you're talking about, or says there's "no time for that kind of complicated interview," go ahead and gently push him, as follows:

Doctor, how long does it take to ask me about chest pain? Ten questions, perhaps? We all agree that a good history is important. If you were treating a heart patient, I think we'd all agree in a court of law that you'd be negligent if you didn't ask the standard "chest pain list" of questions . . . even if that meant asking *twenty* questions.

Doctor, I know you try to define my illness carefully, before you send me for an EKG or a lung scan or a $2,000 Persantine-Thallium Stress Test. So, doctor, what makes it so hard to ask me about a problem that's almost as common, lasts forever, and saps the vitality of my life, even if it doesn't kill me? So let's attempt a new kind of drill, shall we? *I'll* be the patient, and you be the doctor.

I will tell you that I've been tired for eight months, and you are the third doctor I've seen in the last six weeks. I rarely got really sound sleep. Here are copies of the CBC, sed rate, metabolic profile, thyroid test and Lyme ELISA. And they all are normal. I can also tell you that if you start asking the right questions—unlike those last two doctors —you will quickly begin to see that my symptoms point towards a chronic, neurotoxin-based illness.

And finally, let me emphasize one last point: My problem is *not* depression. All set, then? Great. Here we go!

1. DOCTOR: Are your eyes sensitive to bright light?

PATIENT: Yes. Excellent start. Especially at night, doctor. Headlights really get me!

2. DOCTOR: Do your muscles ache?

PATIENT: Oh, yes, and especially the day after I do normal physical activity-things. Good question! The other doctors all said I had fibromyalgia. (But fibromyalgia is usually just a symptom of a much larger neurotoxin-mediated problem—it isn't a final diagnosis!)

3. DOCTOR: Do you have irritable bowel disease, or abdominal pain?

   PATIENT: Oh, yes. One other doctor wanted a barium enema . . . and another asked for a gall bladder sonogram—even though my gall bladder had already been removed.

4. DOCTOR: How about diarrhea that wakes you up at night?

   PATIENT: No . . . but what a great question! It shows that you're looking for *Pfiesteria*, ciguatera and *cylindrospermopsis*. The symptoms for those conditions often include secretory diarrhea.

5. DOCTOR: Do you cough?

   PATIENT: Oh, yes. But I don't smoke, and nobody in my family has asthma. I feel short of breath a lot, but my pulmonary functions are normal.

6. DOCTOR: How about your memory?

   PATIENT: A perfect time to ask, Doc. Don't hit me with that one right off the bat. (I'm kind of defensive about that one!) But you bet. More and more, lately, I find that I have to write down a list of what I'm going to do. I know I'm losing it, but I just don't want to admit it. My friends and loved ones will tell you quicker than I will that my memory is going bad!

7. DOCTOR: Okay, I think I see how easy this is. Tell me about your headache.

   PATIENT: How did you know I had one? Very good, doctor. It's a pounding headache most days. But I get one almost every day, at around ten o'clock in the morning. And by the way, Doc—that's the first clue that I have sick building syndrome and not Lyme disease.

   As you know, the ELISA is worthless.

8. DOCTOR: Do you have stiffness in your hands in the morning?

PATIENT: No, but that's a good Lyme question.

9. DOCTOR: Are you real dizzy if you stand up quickly?

PATIENT: No, I don't have chronic fatigue syndrome.

10. DOCTOR: Did you have a high-velocity auto accident before you got sick?

PATIENT: No, but I think you've got it now. Let's go do a FACT, then focus in on possible sources of water intrusion in my office at the bank—the building with the leaking roof. Then we'll do some pulmonary function tests. I'll be better after two weeks of CSM, but I'll relapse quickly when I go back into the building without CSM to save me from the mycotoxins. Remember that we can use the HRF data at every step of the way to remove the artificial objections to Contrast Sensitivity.

There are 14 of us in the building who stay sick, although four others remain unaffected. And a lot of the people who come in every day with deposits or checks are sick too, doc. Thanks to you, a whole lot of people aren't going to feel miserable all the time! That building is going to be fixed, and none of us will develop multiple chemical sensitivity syndrome. (But I'll show you how to fix *that* some other day.)

DOCTOR: Ten questions in less than three mintues! And four minutes remain for the FACT, along with an additional two minutes for prescriptions. The HMO won't kick about that!

PATIENT: Well, just think about it. There are at least 5 million people out there with sick building syndrome and 2 million with chronic fatigue. We've also got at least 1 million with chronic neurotoxic Lyme disease and 2 million with chronic soft tissue injury. As for the remaining victims, their numbers may still be small, but they're growing fast. Let's face it: Hawaii, Australia and Japan are hot spots for ciguatera. And what about our old pal, *cylindrospermopsis*? It's chewing a path right through central Florida, as we speak.

Just wait until the Manatee kills get started. Those Florida politicians might be able to cover up the slaughter of migratory birds and alligators—but everybody loves the Manatees. Just watch the politicians scramble and the concerned citizens scream, when the last sea cow dies a neurotoxic death!

DOCTOR: You do know a lot about all this neurotoxin stuff. But aren't you being a little shrill here, talking about the "last sea cow?"

PATIENT: Sorry, but "shrillness" was what it took to get people's attention, back when DDT was close to killing the last bald eagle and the last osprey.

DOCTOR: I want to help.

PATIENT: Great. Learn that chronicneurotoxins.com is your ally. Use it often. Speak to your physician colleagues. I'll be glad to serve as a "teaching case" for you.

DOCTOR: You know, when you started talking about being tired, I was getting ready to write a prescription for the new SSRI antidepressant. But your symptoms, when put together as a distinct syndrome, have nothing to do with depression. Each symptom taken individually is not diagnostic of the illness. But the group of symptoms, when taken together, is incredibly powerful. They are part of a new syndrome that's easily recognized.

It's remarkable, but I now realize that I would have spent more time doing a "depression history" than it took to complete your neurotoxin history . . . and I would have given you an incorrect diagnosis in the bargain!

PATIENT: Now hold on. You must remember that neurotoxins cause cognitive problems more unusual, more severe and more diverse than any described in the DSM IV R Handbook. Sure, you'll find classic symptoms of depression in some neurotoxic patients—but don't be misled if they feel guilty that they can't function as well as they did before becoming ill.

"Oh, it's my own fault," is the kind of thing they'll often say. "I'm tired, fatigued. Who has energy for intimacy, or the extra driving required to get to the ballgame?" Family disruption is common and suicide ideation is routine. You will see patients with road rage and panic reactions that go away when their Lyme is treated. You will see fibromyalgia, anxiety, mania and frank psychosis in *Pfiesteria* and sick building patients, but even more often in Lyme.

When you're ready to write a Ritalin prescription for a child or an adult with ADHD, think again. The FACT takes so little time. Of course, you'll also find some patients with neurotoxic illnesses and a normal FACT, even if that group comprises only a small percentage of the total neurotoxic population.

At this point, there's simply no doubt that FACT is light years better than any other diagnostic test. Use it as an important part of your diagnosis—but not as your only diagnostic test. Remember that you must have symptoms and exposure that make sense, in order for the FACT Test to make sense! After all, the neurotoxic history is simply an embodiment of the "systems approach" to medicine—an approach based on the idea of "getting the big picture."

DOCTOR: You know that I'm skeptical. It's hard to believe this simple tool can help as much as you say it will.

PATIENT: Is the reflex hammer a fancy bedside machine? How about a pin for detection of pain, or a feather for detection of light touch? Using FACT will soon become a reflex for you, as subtle as the wisp of a feather and as sharp as the tip of a pin.

• • •

There's no denying that FACT and CSM are new tools in medicine. But penicillin was once new, as well. What's needed now is "continuing education" on the use of these disease weapons, and the way to get started is by disseminating the opinions of enlightened experts on ophthalmology, toxicology, rheumatology and neurology to their colleagues. Once a few specialists recognize the value of FACT in diagnosing these illnesses, then the primary care movement can begin to respond to patients' demands for help.

The medical profession may move slowly—but once the movement starts, the dam will burst. It's time to acknowledge the reality: FACT is here to stay (along with CSM and the Shoemaker treatment protocol) for as long as toxin-formers make us sick.

Physicians are more likely to accept a new idea if it proves useful in the effort to improve the quality of patient-care, or if it helps increase revenues. FACT-testing accomplishes both of those goals—but you, the patient, will have to become an advocate for your doctor, at first.

In many ways, physicians in Maryland have been more proactive than those in Florida. Of course, the vicious political infighting of the *Pfiesteria* epidemic kept some physicians from speaking out at first, but now many doctors in the Old Line State are referring cases to the *Pfiesteria* Illness Center here in Pocomoke, while also treating some on their own.

A Helping Hand from Glaxo?

Another potential source of hope in the battle against the new microbial invaders is the pharmaceutical industry. If America's doctors are going to change their practice patterns, the drug manufacturers are strategically positioned to serve as the "switching stations" where new diagnostic and treatment strategies can be assembled. Ask yourself: to whom do working physicians listen most? Answer: the drug detail reps, of course. (Of course, most of the docs *also* pay careful attention to the latest information provided during company-sponsored dinners, all-expenses paid "thought-leader seminars," and free-of-charge "information updates" in the "spirit of continuing education!" The giant drug companies don't blink at spending $100 million for "information and communication control." As far as they're concerned, that's just a standard marketing expense.)

That fact took on compelling clarity for me in April of 2000, when a rep from GlaxoWellcome visited my office in Pocomoke.

I half-listened to the latest news from the pharmaceutical world, then offered a few insights of my own. "You know, your company is missing the boat on Lyme disease," I told my visitor.

"You've got this great drug—Mepron—that works well against Babesia. We use it all the time with our Lyme patients, even though it isn't FDA-labeled to treat Lyme-sufferers who also are infected with Babesia.

"I think it would be quite easy to recruit 50 or 60 known Lyme-Babesia co-infected patients, then run tests that would demonstrate the role of Mepron when the combination of Lyme antibiotics and CSM doesn't work. The study would record symptoms and CS scores, along with HRF laser Doppler recordings of blood flow rates in the capillaries of the optic nerve head. Next step: prescribe Mepron with CSM and watch the symptoms clear up. The next study would bring in the laser Doppler and CS to diagnose those Lyme patients whose blood tests don't show the Babesia antibody (and most won't), but who don't get better when Lyme, alone, is treated.

"I'm certain the FDA would approve of a properly designed study. This would be huge market for you.

"Even better, we could then go into known endemic areas of Lyme and Babesia and examine children with learning disability. I'm sure we'd find a significant number of kids who are taking Ritalin daily—when they're actually struggling with a sub-clinical chronic Lyme and Babesia co-infection. If you think about, their situation parallels that of the *Pfiesteria* kids and the Sick Building kids and the toxic-fungus kids who live along Casteen Road. Just look at all the good your company could do. . . ."

The Glaxo rep took it all down, and within a month the pharmaceutical giant had sent me to Boston to meet with some of the top Babesia experts in the world. Eight weeks later, the company funded a study to test my CSM hypothesis and its vital links to Mepron, vision-testing and Babesia.

The Babesia conference (June, 2000) turned out to be a key step on the road to helping patients co-infected with Lyme and

Babesia. As a newcomer to this group, I found myself reflecting on my promise to Marie Moore—made a year before—that I would not rest until I'd untangled the bio-chemistry underlying the Babesia co-infection problem. Marie's condition had improved dramatically, you may recall, but her illness had not left her completely . . . and I knew I would never be satisfied until it did.

Among the distinguished scientists on hand were Dr. Andy Spielman (See Chapter 18: "Escape From Naushon Island"), a Harvard professor who had authored ten of the papers in my stack of Lyme references. Like the DA on "Law And Order," the pleasant and low-key Dr. Spielman seemed to know everything. When I bombarded him with questions about TNF, malaria, hemazoin, schizonts, merozoites, chronic Babesia and immune interactions in co-infections, he never missed a beat—and answered every question in the same understated, easygoing manner.

The panel also included Dr. Peter Krause, a pediatrician at Connecticut General and also an expert on Babesia. Dr. Krause had been publishing high-quality research on the topic for years. He was eager to learn more about Contrast Sensitivity and chronic, neurotoxin-mediated illnesses. He also pointed out—correctly —that my disease theory was too new for public dissemination. After listening to my presentation and examining my data, he agreed to help on the research project along with Dr. Spielman.

Dr. V.K. Sikand was also in attendance. Although many regarded him as "Mr. Lyme Vaccine," he was quick to give the credit for his breakthrough discoveries to others. I'd attended several of his lectures in the past, and remembered spending a memorable hour discussing toxins with him in a Philadelphia airport. I'd later sent him a rough copy of my Lyme paper for review, and he'd reported finding my approach novel and interesting. Still, he said he needed to know more about CS and CSM. Because he was busy working on his pediatric Lyme vaccine project, I did not to ask him to be a collaborator.

The roster of luminaries on the panel also included veteran Babesia-treating physicians such as Joe Gadbaw, an infectious disease specialist from New London, Conn., and Peter Brassard, a Family Practice doctor from Block Island, R.I. They asked some tough questions . . . but I could also see that they were seriously considering the points I had to offer.

Tim Lepore, a general surgeon from Nantucket Island, came in a little late. He is a striking figure with his shaved head and his boxer's physique. He listened quietly as I talked about learning disability caused by environmental toxins. Then he said: "You know, on Nantucket, many of the children are on Ritalin—and many who *aren't* suffer from learning disability."

I took a long look at him. Then: "Is there any reason why we should not be blaming Lyme and Babesia for the difficulties faced by the children of Nantucket Island?"

He had no answer for that question.

The panel discussion went well. If these treating physicians —along with the secondary and tertiary care specialists on hand —were willing to work with an outsider like me, I felt sure the Babesia puzzle (like the Lyme puzzle before it) would be easily solved. *This one is for you, Marie Moore!*

I was particularly struck by some of these case histories. Many of the patients discussed at the conference seemed to have been struggling with a more severe infection. Or was it actually a recurrent infection of the type I'd seen in Lyme . . . except that it "stair-stepped" to catastrophe after the patient experienced yet another tick bite? Babesia was "just beginning to spread beyond a few island relics," according to Dr. Spielman.

Yet the areas where they'd reportedly been infected didn't seem to match the infection-zones of Babesia that the Harvard expert had charted. What if the patient's information proved to be incorrect . . . wouldn't that mean that over-treatment had taken place?

Or more specifically, what if Babesia were moving faster than we thought—and Dr. Spielman hadn't been sent enough clinical material to show the speed of the advancing epidemic? What if the "Babesia spread" had begun to accelerate? Will it soon be coming to a town near you in Maryland, Pennsylvania or Texas?

If so, we need to be *ready*.

After a couple of hours, the discussion with the panel began to sound some familiar themes. For starters, these experts were still grappling with the problem of what to name the offending ixodes tick. Should it be *Ixodes dammini* or *Ixodes scapularis*? (Rumor had it that the choice carried political ramifications . . . as in, should it be *Pfiesteria major* or *Pfiesteria minor!*) Resigned to the inevitable, I waited patiently for the "MRO" (morphologically related organism) or TCO (toxin-complex organism) tag to be applied to *Borrelia*-carrying ticks in the same way that it had been applied to *Pfiesteria*.

My train of thought was disrupted. Seemingly unrelated thoughts crowded into my view like slides clicking onto new subjects.

Remember that the deforestation of the east in the late 1880s upset the normal food-chain relationships . . . an event that virtually wiped out the white-tailed deer population, in the same way that chemical alteration of Lake Griffin destroyed the bass population and tropical pollutants changed the world of reef organisms forever.

Click.

Of course, it seems quite likely at this point that the CDC will argue about the "case definition" of co-infected Lyme-Babesia patients . . . just as the agency dragged its heavy feet on Southern Lyme, the Florida nursery workers' illness and Sick Building Syndrome. What, finally, *is* Lyme disease? And what should we call "ciguatera"—when we know quite well that multiple toxins and multiple organisms are involved?

Click.

It's interesting to think for a moment about the purely fortuitous discovery of the CS deficit that occurs in chronic Lyme and also in *Pfiesteria*. Was that sequence of events any different, really, than those which unfolded when the *Borrelia* spirochete was discovered by Dr. Willy Burgdorfer, a bacteria expert who had actually been searching for *Rickettsiae?* Dr. Burgdorfer just happened to have been a bacterial researcher who always used a dark field condenser on his microscope. His almost random discovery raises a provocative question: How many other investigators had looked right at the Lyme spirochete—but *never saw it because they weren't using special equipment?*

Click

It's going to be very exciting to watch what happens next. As soon as the pharmaceutical industry understands that 20 million patients can benefit from their medication, a dramatic change will overtake American medicine. Stand by for the era of *Desperation Medicine,* in which physicians will be talking about chronic, neurotoxin-mediated illnesses day in and day out.

Click.

Will they remember where they "heard it first?" Maybe. Recognition is fine and validation is even better.

Best of all, however, is caring for patients!

Click.

•   •   •

One highlight of my earlier efforts had been the Lyme II Study, during which I'd worked with physicians in 25 states in the U.S., as well as practitioners in Canada, Belgium, France, Switzerland and Italy. And the results of that broad-based inquiry had been thoroughly encouraging: they showed that I'd been able to block the "Intensification Reaction" (See Chapter 15: "Solving The Herx") and watch patients improve clinically in fully 90 percent of chronic Lyme patients. These were the "most difficult of the most difficult" Lyme sufferers, and I was thrilled to see that most of their lives had significantly improved as the result of symptom reduction and enhanced quality of life.

Still, a disturbing 10 percent of these patients had failed to improve, and many of the others had not been able to recover 100 percent of their good health. The culprit? According to several authoritative studies, at least 10 percent of Lyme patients are co-infected with Babesia. A careful look at many of these challenging cases soon revealed that the patients involved were refractory to both antibiotics *and* CSM therapy. What to do?

While I struggled with that question, the endlessly energetic Tom Judy made a very important phone call to Heidelberg Engineering on my behalf. An outstanding high-technology optical firm, HE makes state-of-the-art computerized laser Dopplers that image the red blood cells flowing through tiny capillaries in the optic nerve head. This incredible tool generates a series of graphs that show how quickly blood travels through the areas of nerve tissue most vitally affected by hypoperfusion.

Why not try it on some of my refractory Babesia patients?

Most of them quickly agreed to take the test on a "what have I got to lose?" basis. You can imagine the surprise I felt when each registered a neurotoxin deficit, and when I understood exactly what that meant. The laser Doppler results showed beyond my doubt that these patients had to be carrying a Babesia neurotoxin —yet there were no papers on Babesia-manufactured toxins in the world literature.

Fascinating! After studying some related literature, I knew that a similar intracellular parasite—the *Plasmodium* of malaria —produced several chemicals that activated TNF. Did Babesia also produce a TNF-provoking substance, and was that ability the key weapon in its toxin arsenal?

If so, treatment of these patients with a specialized parasite-killer (atovaquone) and CSM would surely resolve the TNF-associated hypoperfusion, while also returning both Contrast Sensitivity scores and symptoms to the "normal" range. And it didn't take me long to understand why: obviously, the Babesia hadn't been killed the first time around and residual toxin was still being manufactured.

In order to confirm that thesis, I proposed to take known Lyme patients with Babesia co-infection and enter them into a double-blinded, placebo-controlled crossover clinical trial. I knew that if I could show a deficit in optic nerve blood flow from Babesia similar to the Lyme deficit, I'd be able to treat patients carrying both bacteria and toxins. And if I could just accomplish that—binding and eliminating the neurotoxins—then I knew the FDA would have to consider my data and possibly provide the manufacturer of atoquovone (Glaxo) with an "IND" (Indication For Treatment).

"Struggling Towards the Light": The Concept

After enjoying more than 20 years as a fulltime family physician here in smalltown Maryland, I'm convinced more than ever of the crucial role that will have to be played by America's "family docs" in confronting the rapidly accelerating epidemic of chronic, neurotoxin-mediated illness.

I'm pleased to report that the Maryland Academy of Family Physicians has recognized the central role of the family practitioner as both a patient advocate and a community leader by recently naming me the MAFP "Family Physician of the Year, 2000"— despite my growing reputation as an outspoken critic of Maryland's public health policies in regard to *Pfiesteria*.

As our environment continues to change (and we mustn't forget that "deteriorate" isn't an "evolutionarily correct" verb!), the profound "cascade effects" of simple alterations on food webs and habitat will continue to have unexpected results.

I wrote *Desperation Medicine* in order to warn people everywhere about the rapidly growing threat from toxin-based disease mutations—while also holding out the promise of new treatment strategies that will lift the burden of suffering from millions. But I also wanted the book to serve as a "call to arms" . . . a clear and compelling summons to the terrific struggle that lies ahead, if America is to confront the public health menace that now looms directly before us.

•   •   •

Diagnosis and Treatment: Some Perspectives

The medical and scientific disputes generated by the debate over *Pfiesteria* were long and exhausting. But they were also key steps on the road to the discovery of "chronic neurotoxin-mediated illness," which now seems certain to become a major area of American medicine in the years immediately up ahead.

Interestingly enough, *Pfiesteria* taught us both the chemistry of toxin-linked human illness and the political/social dynamics by which large public health bureaucracies (in concert with the information controlled media, some corporations and some politicians) increasingly distort health issues and deceive the public about their underlying causes. Perhaps the most important thing we've learned from *Pfiesteria* is that in order to turn back the threat of toxin-based diseases in the years ahead, we're going to have to battle the "health bureaucracy" just as hard as we struggle against the organic invaders who bring us diseases such as chronic Lyme and chronic sick building syndrome.

Make no mistake: the path that lies ahead will be steep and arduous. And the battle to regain control of our own public health bureaucracy will require painful sacrifices at times. What happened in Florida in the late 1990s will serve as a useful model for medical professionals—who must find the courage to lead a reform of public health policy, while also demanding new political responses to new epidemics such as chronic neurotoxin-mediated illness.

In many ways, the story of the discovery of this new family of modern illnesses can be found in the dramatic stories of three women—Marie Moore, Diane Stephenson, Rhonna Smith (See Chapter 13: "Healing Chronic Lyme Disease")—whose struggles over many years provided much of the inspiration for *Desperation Medicine*.

These unique and courageous women stand out in their individuality. In many ways, however, their medical histories parallel the histories of hundreds of other neurotoxin patients with whom I've worked over the years.

Yes, the human illness symptoms differ somewhat, as we move from dinoflagellate toxins to the disabling poisons generated by rapidly evolving species of fungi. But the dynamics of these pathologies remain fundamentally the same. And whenever I listen to the so-called "experts" describe their insights about the diseases (such as fibromyalgia) that actually belong to the neurotoxin family, I feel like I want to jump out of my chair and interrupt the proceedings! Yet the party line continues. If you are a researcher and want academic grants, don't rock the boat.

For many years now, under-reporting of Lyme, *Pfiesteria* and similar diseases has been a common phenomenon in American medicine. In the end, far too many patients with chronic symptoms wind up pleading for treatment from physicians who have simply decided: "You aren't a case!"

The recording of symptoms presents other problems, as well. Most physicians will readily admit that taking a good history is the key to making an effective clinical diagnosis. Yet far too many researchers routinely delegate this vitally important task to a research assistant who merely reads a list of symptoms from a four-page checklist.

Sorry, but that's the wrong way to take a history. Record symptoms properly and completely, and the symptoms of chronic Lyme, ciguatera, Sick Building Syndrome and related illnesses will overlap as if on tracing paper. Failure to record symptoms properly also leads to a tracing paper conclusion "nothing is wrong." Example: One of my *Pfiesteria* patients from South Carolina presented with a chronic cough following his toxic exposure. The public health official who first examined him read from a typical checklist and asked: "Immediately after or during your exposure, did you have a cough?"

Answer: no, the cough appeared two days later.

Conclusion: no instantaneous cough, and no, not a PEAS case in the eyes of the State. The patient, however, knew better, took CSM, and *was* better in 2 weeks.

Looking back on that inadequate and desultory question, I considered the possibility of adding a fifth parameter to the Appearance of Good Science. This category would be named after that famously notorious legal question: "When did you stop beating your wife?"

It's a fact: the one thing that all of these exogenous neurotoxin illnesses *do* have in common is patients who get sick after being exposed at a worksite or residence or recreational area. But physicians now have a good working model of how to help them. When these sufferers don't get better (they don't fit the "model!"), however, there's a strong tendency to blame *them* for the intractability of the illness. Are they suffering from *Pfiesteria Hysteria*? Are they kookaburras (Lyme patients?) The list goes on.

But instead of "calling names" in this situation, we should be constructing a new model!

The most telling single example of what can go wrong when under-educated physicians confront chronic disease symptoms occurs during cases involving learning disability among children. (I've named that scenario the "Somerset County Schools Model!") In this situation, toxin-exposed children struggle along in schools whose administrators have done nothing proactive to defend against environmental hazards that can trigger learning disorders.

Do the children in the Nantucket public schools have a problem? Is that problem correctable? How about those attendees of the Hill School in Austin, Tex., many of whom wound up as victims of the noxious *Stachybotrys* fungal toxin? If we really want to understand how toxins can impede learning, let's journey to Mayaguez, Puerto Rico, and try to find out why kids who eat fish at risk for ciguatera don't seem to learn as well as those whose diet contains no such fish.

Correlation and Confirmation

Here's my suggestion: let's provide a Contrast Sensitivity exam for every child in this country who's currently being given drugs to control behavior. How long would it really take the nation's school districts to test those students who show up at the nurse's station at lunchtime each day for their "mood meds?"

Based on what I've witnessed in three years of research, the patients we've already identified as suffering from toxin-mediated illnesses are just the tip of a public health iceberg. It's a fact: the base of the problem is much wider than I imagined back in 1997, when I started the research that led to this book. And my study of the *Pfiesteria* epidemic is just one example of that reality.

It's time for all of us in the medical community to go on "red alert" for this insidious new family of diseases. It's also time to begin asking healthy-seeming patients with low CS scores some telling (and clearly stated) questions. At present these symptoms are cloaked by the darkness of silence. Well, bring on the spotlight! These offending toxins might be "cloaked" from our immune systems—but that's no reason why the illnesses they cause should remain hidden.

American medicine, stand by. Prepare for a sudden cure (with improvement beginning literally overnight) for all sorts of chronic, nagging conditions . . . such as age-related muscle aches, sinus miseries, stress-linked ailments, depression, irritable bowel syndrome, ulcers and all the rest.

A new day is dawning in American medicine, and it can't get here soon enough.

But it won't happen magically and it won't happen for physicians who refuse to re-educate themselves about these new disease mechanisms.

In order to help the patient, we're going to have to understand *Desperation Medicine* . . . and we're going to have to know how to ask the patient the right questions, and then win the battle against these new forms of disease.

The Quest for the Holy Grail of Neurotoxin Effect

I guess you could say it was love at first sight.

After years of relentless research into the diagnosis and treatment of chronic, neurotoxin-mediated illness, I received a mighty boost to my morale on a recent summer afternoon in Pocomoke . . . at the moment when I first laid eyes on an awesome new machine known as the "Heidelberg Retinal Flowmeter," or HRF.

To say that the HRF represents a "giant step forward in the struggle to quantify the effects of toxins on the brain" is no exaggeration—because this elegantly engineered machine is capable of measuring such effects with crystal-clarity, while focusing on objects no larger than the typical human red blood cell.

Why is the HRF going to change the way a lot of medicine gets practiced in this country, and soon? Answer: this extraordinary "laser Doppler" device can collect enough data (in the space of exactly two seconds) to pinpoint the subtlest changes in blood flow through the capillaries of the retina, along with those found in the neural rim of the optic nerve and the nerve's deepest layer, the *lamina cribosa*.

Because it can accurately register minute changes in blood flow, the HRF allows physicians to measure the somatic evidence of injury from neurotoxins, and the effects of cytokines released by differential gene activation, after the genes have been turned on by those same neurotoxins. Such measurements are possible because the junction of the brain's nerves with the retina and its blood vessels (and also with certain key components of the optic nerve head) provides a transparent "window" onto the rapidly shifting changes in the perfusion of nerves caused by these low-molecular-weight toxins.

The HRF won't wind up in every family practitioner's office, mind you, nor will it be required there. For most practicing physicians, the Stereo Optical FACT kit will provide all of the tools necessary to make an initial diagnosis of neurotoxin-linked disease . . . and I predict that every physician in the land will soon know exactly what a patient means when he or she says: "I need a Contrast Sensitivity test!"

I'm sure I'll never forget the early-September day when the two body-sized trunks arrived from Heidelberg, accompanied by two other heavily boxed packages. I could hardly wait to open them. And I'm sure my excitement was evident to Dirk-Uwe Bartsch, Ph.D., a University of California at San Diego visiting professor of retinal diseases (and also the director of the Retinal Imaging Laboratory), who had been dispatched to my office by the manufacturer in order to school me on the use of this astonishing device.

Joseph Schwartz, M.D., a retinal specialist from Salisbury, Md., also arrived on schedule to help me through this long-awaited demonstration of how the HRF pinpoints the presence of neurotoxin-linked illness by measuring blood-flow through tiny capillaries.

After a quick guided tour of the machine, Dirk-Uwe showed us how to use the laser Doppler. It soon became apparent that the HRF could do much more than simply metering the flow along large retinal blood vessels. Shocked silent, we found ourselves actually measuring the movement of blood through the body's tiniest vessels . . . the location where the exchange of nutrients, oxygen and waste products actually takes place. In this micro-world of the picogram (10-to-the-minus-12 gm) and the zeptogram (10-to-the-minus-20 gm), it was possible to witness—up close and personal—the effect of movement of neurotoxin molecules and the release, locally, of TNF.

One key question loomed immediately: would blood drawn from a vein (the product of contributions from billions of capillaries) reflect the local release of cytokines by neurotoxin-primed adipocytes? No. On the other hand, did CS testing always pinpoint the definitive deficit of neurotoxins? No, it certainly did not! (Obviously, some patients carried neurotoxins . . . but not enough to trigger a "positive" outcome in the Contrast Sensitivity test. A positive CS test was a true positive, but a normal CS didn't rule out completely the possibility of a neurotoxic illness.)

I stood with my feet rooted to the floor on that remarkable afternoon, as the computer screen came alive and the images took light. Entranced, I gazed at an illuminated image of the optic nerve head, along with its rim and the spidery blood vessels emerging from the depths below. There seemed to be a billion capillaries . . . and each one blinked neon-bright with the movement of oxygen-bearing red blood cells.

Carl Sagan had gotten it right: the Milky Way *does* contain billions of stars, with a billion billion other stars looming in galaxies that stretch to the farthest horizon, world without end. . . .

And I was looking at them.

Quick . . . mark off a 10-pixel by 10-pixel area. Now click on the fast Fournier transform and you can analyze the flow, volume and velocity of individual cells in individual capillaries! Or you can zero in on the neuronal rim at the temporal side of the optic nerve. Go ahead . . . work the controls, fine-tune the focus . . . and celebrate the joy of looking at the final action-site of neurotoxins working on blood flow to a nerve.

As I told a local cardiologist: "Go ahead and fix blockages in large blood vessels (arteries). The neurotoxic action is in capillaries!"

The entire operation takes about one minute. Here are the "Velocity Reports," Controls, 360–450. And here are Cases, 210–260. Go ahead . . . run the same test again and again if you like, and you'll get *the same results!*

It doesn't matter if the illness has been caused by *Pfiesteria*, Sick Building Syndrome, Lyme or chronic soft tissue injury—because the results are always the same. And they demonstrate one crucial fact with compelling clarity: my theoretical model works! All that remains now is to complete the linkages and measurements and repeat the process enough times until the data is validated. Local release of TNF: how can I prove it? Local auto-regulation of blood flow: How can I control for that? And how about time of day, medications taken, cigarettes, fatigue, heart rate, caffeine ingestion and all the rest?

This was the first day of the search for the Holy Grail of neurotoxin research.

In the ancient days of primitive cultures, there would come a time when the tribesmen understood that the ineffective leadership of an old King had begun to convert their world into a wasteland. At that point, the tradition of the society mandated that he would be killed. Sacrificed on the altar of new knowledge and progress, the blood of the slaughtered King gave birth to a fresh beginning . . . to a refreshed and refurbished wonderland full of green grasses, bountiful crops and empowered citizens. In that simpler, myth-powered world, the Grail meant rejuvenation of the processes of light and life in human society.

So it is with the HRF. But its findings must be validated. The first, early results of holding the humble cup of the optic nerve —like the cup of the Grail—have fulfilled all of my dreams as a scientific researcher. Here is the bio-marker that will end the strife among opposing factions—while at last renewing the wasteland of medical science that had been paralyzed by acrimony, and establishing forever the reality of chronic, neurotoxin-mediated illness.

Within the next few months or so, I will be showing audiences the awesome benefit by demonstrating the HRF at Lyme meetings in Princeton, N.J. . . . at Florida DEP contamination sites near Leesburg . . . at ciguatera clinics in Puerto Rico . . . and at legal offices in Dallas where the attorneys specialize in cases involving chronic soft tissue injury. Here the legacy of the Grail will be fully tested. Are the old, widely accepted ideas about the limitations of medical science really true? Or can we push past them to a new, deeper understanding of the meaning of illness in our world? Can we answer the key medical question of our time: Are these toxin-linked illnesses part of a new, never-before-experienced disease threat to our nation?

If they are, then the weapon we will use most effectively against them will be the FACT backed up by HRF, which promises to make a 100-percent-accurate diagnosis of the condition, first time and every time.

It's accurate. It's utterly reliable. It's easy to operate . . . and like the Holy Grail, it's got four words written all over it:

Welcome to the future!

Let the Struggle Begin!

Like Dr. Faustus, that great classic hero who sold his soul to the devil in order to enjoy power over nature, the modern world hangs suspended over a yawning abyss. Will we come to our senses and rearrange our priorities in time to avert an evolutionary cataclysm?

For myself, I take great hope from the last lines of Goethe's 18th-Century version of the "Faust" myth, in which the threatened scientist cries out for help in his struggle against the demons who are carrying him off to Hell.

His anguished pleas do not fall on deaf ears.

At the very last instant—just before Faust's soul is to be flung into the abyss—a squadron of angels arrives to pluck him from the grip of the arch-fiend, Mephistopheles.

In one of the play's last lines, the Archangel Michael announces the rescue of Faust with a thundering proclamation: "Those who struggle ceaselessly toward the light—*these* we can save!"

Cholestyramine Recipes

- Put 4 oz. water, apple juice or cranberry juice in cup (glass or plastic is best)
- Add 1 scoop powder, stir vigorously
- Add more liquid to re-suspend remainder of powder in glass
- Wait 30 minutes before eating any food or taking any medication

- Hot coffee or tea at 140 degrees (use a meat thermometer)
- Add one scoop of powder
- Stir to dissolve
- Cool to drinking temperature (or pour over ice)
- Powder dissolves better this way

- 6–8 oz. low-fat milk
- 2 scoops ice cream (without fruit, nuts, chocolate chips, marshmallows or any other solid additives)
- Hershey's chocolate syrup to taste
- One scoop powder
- Blend in milk shake maker
  (with thanks to Rick and Ruth McGee)

Index

A

adhesin 267
adipocyte 59, 265, 267
Agency for Toxic Substances and Disease Registry (ATSDR) 145, 148, 151
Agent Orange 39, 244, 248
alligator xx, 24, 149, 167–170, 172, 176, 179–180, 185, 188, 190, 435, 437, 458, 464
amberjack 88, 91, 101, 114
American Society of Bariatric Physicians (ASBP) 111, 244
anabaena 182
Anderson Dr. Donald 90, 110
Aphanomyces 38–39, 135, 174
apoptosis 58, 254
Aspergillus 305
Aubain, Irene 369
Auerbach, Dr. Paul 247

B

Babesia 6, 60, 64, 207, 224, 239, 279–282, 296–297, 467–470, 472–473
Bacillus thurigensis 4, 460
Barkley, Sally 343, 355–359
barracuda 87, 99, 107, 114
Bartsch, Dr. Dirk-Uwe 270
Beavis, Dr. Kathleen 272

Bernstein, Dr. Joan 38
Bickling, Dr. Allan xxiii, 351
biomarker 83, 190–191, 315
bio-toxin 125, 317, 319–320, 359, 427
Blemlek, Linda 217
blue(-)green algae xx, 18, 26, 53, 63, 73, 147–148, 168, 172, 175, 177–178, 183, 185–187, 189, 199, 255–256, 260, 393, 435, 437, 455
blue mold 36, 73
Boesch, Dr. Donald 28, 37–38, 41–42
Borrelia 66–67, 207–208, 210, 212, 214, 221, 223, 233, 235, 253, 259, 387, 440, 470
brucellosis 118, 356
Buckheit, Kathleen 393, 452
Building-Related Illness 311
Burgdorfer, Dr. Willy 212, 471
burial 164, 304, 408, 456
Burkholder, Dr. JoAnn 21, 23–25, 74, 76, 391, 393, 424

C

campylobacter 92
carbamate 114, 117
Carmichael, Dr. Wayne 172, 393
Cartwright, Dr. Mark 67, 214

Cell from Hell 14, 16–17, 52, 135, 175, 186–187, 214

The Centers for Disease Control and Prevention (CDC) xix, 12, 29, 33, 71, 75, 85, 128, 143, 145–146, 150–153, 161, 207, 221, 228, 310–311, 345–346, 379–394, 423, 438, 440–446, 448–449, 451–452, 454, 470

Chaetominium 305

Charcot-Marie-Tooth Syndrome (CMT) 373, 375

Cheney, Dr. Paul 345, 347

Chesapeake Bay Program 37, 163, 422, 451

chlorothalonil 137

cholera 62, 115, 437

cholestyramine (CSM) xviii, 19, 29–30, 38, 41, 49, 53–54, 76, 82–83, 90, 101–105, 108, 110, 112, 123–125, 143–144, 147, 149–150, 170, 172, 176, 178, 184, 191–192, 198–200, 209, 215–217, 220, 223–227, 232, 245, 247–248, 250, 253, 258–266, 272, 274, 281–283, 285, 289–291, 302, 312, 319, 323, 335, 340, 344, 350–352, 358–359, 365–366, 368, 370–377, 382, 386, 390, 392, 397, 401–402, 411, 421, 423–426, 440, 452–453, 456–459, 463, 465–468, 472, 475

chronic fatigue syndrome xvii, 70, 85, 147, 213, 343, 345–346, 349–352, 359, 429, 463, 486

chronic toxin-mediated illness 20, 65, 146, 148, 197, 237

ciguatera xvi, 38, 87–91, 95–100, 102–110, 112, 115–116, 120, 147, 184, 210, 222, 252, 313, 394, 434, 462–463, 470, 475–476, 481, 486

ciguatoxin 88, 99–100, 104, 106, 115, 266

Ciliary neurotrophic factor 366

cladosporium 299, 305

clostridia 53

consensus statement 158, 188, 311, 435–436, 446

Contrast Sensitivity (CS) xviii, xxi, xxiv, 38, 41, 72, 75, 79–85, 90, 100–105, 108–109, 112, 120, 137, 139, 143–144, 146–153, 176, 179, 184, 191, 198, 200, 206–207, 209, 215, 222–224, 226–227, 232, 234, 247–248, 260, 267–269, 272–273, 282–283, 301–302, 312–315, 317, 319, 323–325, 331, 340, 349–350, 352, 358–359, 365–366, 370–372, 376–377, 387, 389–390, 392, 397–398, 401–402, 404, 409–411, 421, 423, 425, 438, 453, 463, 467–468, 470, 472, 476–477, 479

copper xii, 26, 28, 30, 34–36, 38, 41–42, 53, 76, 97, 131, 135, 138, 161, 169, 171–173, 175–176, 180, 183, 185–188, 416, 419–420, 422, 451

Copper-Pfiesteria 456

cyanide xxii, 134–136, 459
cyano-bacteria 73, 174, 176, 178,
    180–182
cyanophage 175
cylindrospermopsis xx, 42, 63,
    110, 168, 170, 174, 176–178,
    182, 307, 350, 393–394, 450,
    460, 462–463
cyst 5, 18, 208–210, 216
cytokine 58–60, 200–201

D

damage control 42, 142, 161–162,
    164, 436
Dashiell, Russell 368–369, 371
DDT 171–173, 464
Dead Zone, Gulf of Mexico 24,
    164
deleterious rhizosphere bacteria
    (DRB) 136, 163–164
Demas, Dr. George 42, 163,
    413–415, 417–419, 424–429,
    454
dengue fever 113
depression xvii, 65, 117, 147,
    152, 197–198, 201, 213, 216,
    246, 303–304, 306, 316,
    318–319, 343–344, 347–348,
    406, 461, 464, 477
Dietrich, Dr. Andrea 456
differential gene activation 18, 56,
    209, 478
dinoflagellate xxi, 5–6, 12, 15,
    20–21, 29–30, 34–36, 38, 41,
    52, 88–90, 95–96, 98–100, 138,
    147, 171, 186, 210, 255–256,

264, 271, 301, 373, 381, 402,
    419, 422, 424, 451, 453, 475
dissociation constant 108, 266
dithiocarbamates 26, 30, 34–35,
    41, 135, 138, 163
Donta, Dr. Sam 214
Dumler, Dr. J. Stephen 272

E

Economos, Jeannie 179
Ehrlichia 64, 207, 271, 384
Enbrel 272–273, 281
endocrine disrupters 180
endosymbiont 99, 106
endotoxin 214
enterohepatic recirculation 54,
    259
entomophaga 459–460
Environmental Protection Agency
    (EPA) xxi, 4, 37, 41–42, 72,
    75–76, 79, 112, 120, 122, 128,
    149, 151, 163, 186, 222, 393,
    404, 422, 451, 454, 457
exotoxin 215
extravascular circulation 250

F

Farmworker Association of Florida
    (FWAF) 179
fibromyalgia xxii, 66, 147,
    198–200, 213, 216, 344, 357,
    361–362, 367–368, 372, 406,
    462, 465, 475
filamentous algae 88, 95–97
flusilazole 137

Food and Drug Administration
(FDA) 19, 104, 144, 150, 259,
467, 473, 486
Foothill tick fever 239
Functional Acuity Contrast Test
(FACT) xxi, 75–77, 84–85,
101–105, 170, 178, 184,
190–191, 215–217, 223, 226,
267, 272, 281, 300–301, 323,
337, 339–340, 365–368, 372,
409, 434, 438, 449, 457, 463,
465–466, 478, 481
fungi 2, 11–12, 38, 53, 61–62,
110, 122–123, 129–132, 134,
136, 148, 150, 171, 183,
255–256, 299–300, 303, 305,
307, 310, 314–315, 320–321,
326, 329, 331, 333–334, 339,
381, 408, 475
fungicides 5, 26, 28, 34, 36, 39,
73, 121, 122, 127, 130–131,
133–134, 138–139, 172–173,
180, 186–187, 314, 329, 420,
451
fungus xx, 2, 36, 38–40, 58, 89,
122, 129–133, 135, 138, 143,
153, 172, 174, 299–300, 314,
318, 320–321, 335, 397,
459–460, 467
fusarium xx, 58, 135–137, 147,
187, 305
fusarium oxysporum 135–136,
147
Fuzzell, Frank 39, 121–128, 132,
135, 137, 139–140, 143–146,
148, 153, 162, 381, 389, 449,
458

G

Ginsburg, Dr. Arthur 75, 84
Glasgow, Dr. Howard 74, 393,
424
glitazone 59, 245, 254
Goerner, Skip 185
Griffin, Ann 169–170, 173–175,
177–181, 184
grouper 88, 91, 101, 109, 114
Gupta, Dr. Gian 161, 422

H

Hall, Dr. Sherwood 104–105, 108
heavy metal xii, 36, 82, 89, 94,
96–98, 163, 172, 416, 452
Heidelberg Retinal Tomogram
Flow Meter (HRF) 269–270,
463, 467, 478–479, 481
Heliobacter pylori 103, 164, 196
Hepatotoxins 177
Herxheimer Reaction (Jarisch-
Herxheimer, Herx) 214, 216,
226, 234–235, 250, 252–253,
254, 255, 261, 263, 267–268,
272–275, 281, 283–284, 367,
376–377, 410–411, 471
Hoggard, Dr. Mitch xxiv, 216, 237
homeostasis 56–57, 255, 257, 261
Hudnell Sign 223, 349, 401
Hudnell, Dr. Ken xxi, 37, 41,
70–73, 75–77, 79, 82, 109,
112, 120, 139, 149–151,
222–224, 340, 349, 367, 383,
391, 401, 415, 454, 457–458
hydrilla 189

hyena attack 161, 164, 303
hypoperfusion 85, 267–269, 472

I

Inman, Dr. Roger 161–162
insulin receptor 59, 244–245, 253–255, 260
Intensification Reaction 235, 247–248, 250, 253, 266, 272–275, 284, 457, 471
ionophore 31, 100, 250–251, 257–258, 262
irritable bowel syndrome xxii, 66, 103, 147, 306, 316, 477

J

Jasinski, David 306, 315–318, 320
Judy, Tom 84, 268–269, 282, 472

K

Koplan, Dr. Jeffrey 145, 383
Kuhn, Thomas 270, 353–355
Kujan, Russel xxiii, 253, 366

L

Lake Apopka xiii, 149, 167, 170, 172–174, 178, 436–437
Lake Griffin xx, 24, 42, 149, 167–170, 174, 176–178, 180–181, 184–186, 199, 437, 470
Leptospirosis 47, 118, 207
lightning-bolt pain 237
light sensitivity 65, 266, 278, 348, 382

Lone Star Tick 228–229, 386
Lyme xiv, xvi, xx, xxiii–xxv, 6, 60, 64, 66–68, 70, 82–83, 85, 100–101, 110–112, 116, 119, 123, 146, 184, 192, 198–199, 203–225, 227–228, 230, 233–238, 240–241, 243–245, 247–255, 260–265, 267, 271–272, 274, 279–284, 286, 290, 294–299, 313, 324, 349–350, 354, 356, 359, 376–377, 385–389, 394, 409–410, 429, 434, 439–442, 446–449, 457, 461–463, 465, 467–476, 480–481, 486
lymphocyte 59, 281

M

macrophage 59, 267
Maizel, Margaret 41
malaria 6, 113, 239, 468, 472
Malaria 60
manatee xx, 188–189, 464
margination 254
Martin, Bill 450
McDowell, Dr. Ted 162
memory loss xxii, 51, 66, 110, 123, 140, 149, 233–234, 352, 365
Merson, Steve 293–294
metalaxyl 36, 73, 133
metallic taste 65, 115, 286, 407
microcystin 147, 177, 182
microcystis 182, 256, 455–456
molecular dipole xxiii, 256, 259
monocyte 59, 200, 267

Moore, Marie 203, 217–220, 222, 224, 468–469, 474

muck farming 135, 169, 171, 172, 186, 314

Multiple Chemical Sensitivity (MCS) 310, 312–314, 463

mycotoxin 130–131, 147, 148, 244, 302–303, 314, 320–321, 323, 331, 335–336, 389, 397

N

National Institutes of Health (NIH) xix, 159, 212–213, 221, 345, 347, 440

natural selection xv, 39, 57, 171, 186

Nelms, Hunter 301–302

neurotoxin xi, xiii–xiv, xvii–xix, xxi–xxii, xxiv–xxv, 24, 31, 45, 64, 67–68, 70, 76–77, 79, 82–85, 88–90, 100–101, 103–104, 109, 111–112, 119, 137–138, 144, 148, 151–152, 170, 172, 176–179, 181, 184–185, 188, 193, 199–201, 203–204, 206–207, 209, 212, 214–217, 222–224, 234, 237, 239–240, 247, 250–252, 254–256, 258, 260–263, 268–270, 273–274, 280, 283, 285–286, 288, 293, 298, 301–302, 307, 310, 313, 321, 323–324, 331, 339–340, 344, 346, 348–353, 355, 357, 359, 362, 365–370, 373–374, 390, 393, 396, 399–400, 402, 405, 407, 423, 428–429, 434, 438,

449–451, 454, 458, 461–462, 464, 468, 471–476, 478–481

Neuse River 73

Newcastle Disease 435–436

Nguyen, Sonny 243, 245, 247–248

National Health and Environmental Effects Research Lab (NHEERL) xxi, 72, 112, 149, 393

Nichols, Bruce xi, xxiii, 4–5, 42, 418–419, 421, 423, 428

nitric oxide 56, 254

nodularin 255

Nostrom, Steven xxiii, 215

nuclear receptors 237, 255, 261, 265

nutrients xii, xx, 23–26, 28–29, 33–34, 36, 41, 56, 58–61, 97, 142, 162, 164, 311, 417, 457, 479

O

Obregon, Ishmael 127

Occam's Razor 70

Occupational Health and Safety Administration (OSHA) 305, 308, 321

ochratoxin 255

Ocklawaha 63, 169–170, 174–175, 178–179, 183

okadaic acid 255, 264

Oldach, Dr. David 422, 427

Olivieri, Dr. Arnaldo 106

Osler, Sir William 46, 204, 237, 433

P

PCR 56, 209, 250, 270–272, 384, 447

pelican 149, 169–170, 172–173, 179–181, 435–437

penicillium 299, 305

Peterson, Dr. Dan 345, 347

Pfiesteria xvi, xix–xx, xxiv–xxv, 5–6, 12, 15, 17–31, 33–38, 40–43, 46, 52–54, 58, 68, 70–72, 74–77, 79, 82–83, 88, 90, 96, 98, 100–101, 105, 107–110, 112, 123, 133, 137–140, 147, 149, 161, 164, 171, 175, 184, 186–187, 193, 196, 209–210, 214, 222–223, 237, 252, 260, 301, 307, 313–314, 349–350, 352, 380–382, 386, 389–394, 399, 402–403, 408–409, 412–414, 418–420, 422–429, 451–454, 456–457, 462, 465–467, 470, 473–477, 480

phosphatases 255, 260–261

pinta 207

pioglitazone 235, 248, 251, 254, 262, 265, 273–275, 281, 283, 285, 289–291, 313, 376, 440

piroplasms 296

Plum Island 113, 345

Pocomoke x, xi, xxiv, 1, 6, 9–10, 13, 16–17, 20–21, 35, 41, 50, 90, 155, 195, 203, 240, 245, 248, 249, 268, 282–283, 288, 293, 337–338, 341, 343, 361, 373, 376, 393, 395, 409, 420, 431, 453, 466, 478

Pocomoke River xi, xiii, xxiv, 5, 10, 12, 15–16, 23, 25, 36, 50–52, 400–401, 421–423, 452, 459

Poli, Dr. Mark 106, 108

porewater 38, 42, 76, 136, 138, 161, 416, 420, 422

Possible Estuarine-Associated Syndrome (PEAS) 12, 75, 453–454, 475

postural hypotension 349–352

PPAR-gamma 254–255, 273

predator-prey relationship 26, 99

pseudomonas 88, 99, 135–136, 147

Q

Q Fever 113–114, 118

quaternary ammonium 258, 336

R

Raines, Dr. Arthur xxiv, 237–238, 243

Ramsdell, Dr. John 77, 106, 108, 120, 391, 393, 427, 458

red snapper 88, 114–115

red tide 53

reflux 53, 103, 195, 198, 201, 306

relapsing fever 207

Ross, Dr. Perran 167

S

salmonella 92

Salmonidae 10

secretory diarrhea 10–11, 48–49, 51, 65, 140, 146, 206, 462

selective advantage 62, 147, 183, 294, 460

sick building syndrome (SBS) xvi, 82–83, 101, 110–111, 123, 184, 191, 199, 252, 301, 304–305, 307, 315, 319–320, 325, 389, 393–394, 429, 462–463, 470, 474, 475, 480

Smith, Pat xxiii, 216, 447

Smith, Rhonna 217, 225, 227, 458, 474

Smith, Theobald 239, 297

smokescreen 152, 161, 164, 213, 437

Sphyraena 87

Spielman, Dr. Andrew 294–296, 468–469

spirochete 66–67, 153, 207–212, 214, 221, 234, 255–256, 270–272, 296–297, 440, 448, 470–471

St. Johns River 170, 178, 181

St. Lucie River 29–30, 36, 373, 451

St. Martin's River 5, 6, 36

stachybotrys 299, 305, 314, 320, 331, 389, 397, 476

standing crop 1–3, 7, 186

Steere, Dr. Allan 212–215, 297, 387

Stephenson, Diane 203, 217, 228–229, 231–234, 249–250, 253, 272, 274, 283, 285, 370, 474

Stereo Optical Company xxi, 84, 268, 272

Strauss, Dr. Steven 347

Submerged Aquatic Vegetation (SAV) 162–163, 415, 417

Sullivan, Dr. Rob 155–156

syphilis 66, 192, 204, 207, 214

systems approach 34, 40–41, 212, 222, 314, 418, 465

T

Tarr, Norman 453–454

Thomas, Dr. Michael 402–403, 405

tick 60, 64, 66, 89, 110, 204, 206–207, 209–210, 212–213, 215, 218, 220–221, 225, 230, 232–233, 239–240, 264, 277, 295–298, 324, 421, 440–441, 447–448, 469–470

TNF 56, 58–60, 201, 253–255, 264–270, 272–273, 282–284, 313, 367, 468, 472, 479–480

Tosteson, Dr. Tom xxiii, 106–107, 266, 458

toxaphene 173, 435–436

toxin-mediated xvi, xxi–xxii, 29, 31, 62, 65, 83, 85, 109, 122–124, 153, 178–179, 184, 191–192, 201, 204, 263, 326, 340, 396, 408, 459

Trichoderma 305

tuberculosis (TB) 6, 208–210

Tuskegee Study 192

V

Venezia, Dr. Robert 392–393,
452–454

W

Wai, Dr. Chien 41
Webb, Paul 393, 452
West Nile virus 6, 113

Y

yaws 207
Yellow Rain 39, 244

Z

Zinser, Dr. Gerhard 269

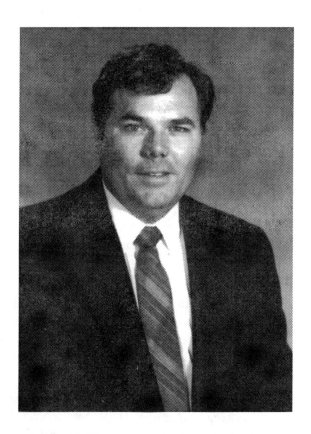

About the Author

Ritchie Shoemaker, named the "Maryland Family Practice Physician of the Year, 2000," has published numerous articles in medical journals and other publications on "chronic, neurotoxin-mediated illness," and his discoveries are now changing the way science thinks about disease. Trained as a molecular biologist at Duke University, Dr. Shoemaker used the experience he gained during 20 years of Family Practice to open the window on a frightening new disease threat now emerging from our chemically polluted environment.

Along the way, he fought numerous political battles with entrenched State and local public bureaucracies (along with the powerful CDC) who were intent on denying the existence of these new pollution-linked diseases.

Desperation Medicine reflects Dr. Shoemaker's broad, multi-dimensional approach to science. While exploring topics as varied as wetlands ecology, the genetic basis of cell functioning, philosophy from the Ancient Greeks to the Moderns, and the interactions of populations, the author raises disturbing new questions about the relationship between social ethics and disease.

As a determined patient advocate, this veteran family practice physician dared to attack one of the most troubling—and least understood—health issues of our time: how has our continuing pollution of the ecosphere altered the physiology of the disease pathogens everywhere around us?

After more than five years of intense scientific research, Dr. Shoemaker has developed a safe, accurate method for detecting the presence of pollution-linked, neurotoxin-based illnesses in patients . . . along with a powerfully effective treatment approach (based on a harmless, inexpensive and FDA-approved substance, *cholestyramine*) that promises to end the daily suffering of millions of "chronic" patients.

For those struggling with new, toxin-based illnesses such as Chronic Lyme Disease, Chronic Fatigue Syndrome, Ciguatera, *Pfiesteria*-Related Human Illness Syndrome and Chronic Soft Tissue Injury, *Desperation Medicine* offers a priceless opportunity: a chance to end the misery of chronic illness virtually overnight—while regaining the vitality and energy that will make you feel 20 years younger!

Crafted from Ritchie Shoemaker's wide-ranging interests and his willingness to challenge existing dogma, *Desperation Medicine* is based on a fundamental principle: "The key to understanding is casting out false knowledge!"

Ritchie Shoemaker, M.D., is the author of two previous books on science and health: *Pfiesteria: Crossing Dark Water*, and *Weight Loss and Maintenance: My Way Works*.